FEMININITY AND PSYCHOANALYSIS

For Freud, famously, the feminine was a dark continent, or a riddle without an answer. This understanding concerns man's relationship to the question of 'woman' but femininity is also a matter of sexuality and gender and therefore of identity and experience. Drawing together leading academics, including film and literary scholars, clinicians and artists from diverse backgrounds, *Femininity and Psychoanalysis: Cinema, Culture, Theory* speaks to the continued relevance of psychoanalytic understanding in a social and political landscape where ideas of gender and sexuality are undergoing profound changes.

This transdisciplinary collection crosses boundaries between clinical and psychological discourse and arts and humanities fields to approach the topic of femininity from a variety of psychoanalytic perspectives. From object relations, to Lacan, to queer theory, the essays here revisit and rethink the debates over what the feminine might be. The volume presents a major new work by leading feminist film scholar, Elizabeth Cowie, in which she presents a first intervention on the topic of film and the feminine for over 20 years, as well as a key essay by the prominent artist and psychoanalyst, Bracha Ettinger.

Written by an international selection of contributors, this collection is an indispensable tool for film and literary scholars engaged with psychoanalysts and anybody interested in different approaches to the question of the feminine.

Agnieszka Piotrowska is an award-winning film-maker and theorist, best known for her iconic documentary *Married to the Eiffel Tower*. She is the author of *Psychoanalysis and Ethics in Documentary Film*, *Black and White* and *The Nasty Woman and the Neo Femme Fatale in Contemporary Cinema*, editor of *Embodied Encounters* and co-editor of *Psychoanalysis and the Unrepresentable*.

Ben Tyrer is a film theorist and lecturer. He is the author of works on cinema, psychoanalysis and philosophy and is the co-editor of *Psychoanalysis and the Unrepresentable*.

'This new and highly readable collection of psychoanalytic essays, which is edited by Agnieszka Piotrowska and Ben Tyrer, provides a timely look at the meanings of femininity and women's desire as articulated in cinema through a range of stimulating and thought-provoking case studies and discussions. The book, which contains chapters from some notable authors in the field of feminist film scholarship and artistic and clinical practice (including Elizabeth Cowie, Bracha L. Ettinger, Vicky Lebeau and Caroline Bainbridge), deploys the ideas of Freud, Lacan, Klein, Riviere, Horney, Deutsch and Irigaray in order to unpack the complexities of the relationships between femininity, psychoanalysis and difference that will be of great interest to students and researchers who continue to tussle with the meanings of femininity in the contemporary cultural arena of cinema and beyond. The collection covers a lot of ground – revisiting older debates about the feminist politics of visual pleasure but adds a new layer of complexity to those earlier discussions by relating them to psychosocial and cultural concerns in contemporary contexts where the vexed relationship between intersectionality and psychoanalysis often comes to the fore. In so doing, the collection demonstrates its cultural and political relevance by paying attention to the unconscious dynamics of representation and to the raced and classed dimensions of cinematic experience and its relationship to wider processes of power and ideology.'

Candida Yates, Professor of Culture and Communication, Bournemouth University, UK

'This collective effort to think and rethink the psychoanalytic take on femininity could not come at a more appropriate time. *Femininity and Psychoanalysis: Cinema, Culture, Theory* pursues different facets of this question in a formidably interesting way, following a wide range of authors and critical approaches. A truly engaged and engaging volume.'

Alenka Zupančič, Professor of Philosophy and Psychoanalysis, Research Centre of the Slovenian Academy of Sciences and Arts, author of *What Is Sex?*

FEMININITY AND PSYCHOANALYSIS

Cinema, Culture, Theory

Edited by Agnieszka Piotrowska and Ben Tyrer

Routledge
Taylor & Francis Group
LONDON AND NEW YORK

First published 2019
by Routledge
2 Park Square, Milton Park, Abingdon, Oxon OX14 4RN

and by Routledge
52 Vanderbilt Avenue, New York, NY 10017

Routledge is an imprint of the Taylor & Francis Group, an informa business

British Library Cataloguing-in-Publication Data
A catalogue record for this book is available from the British Library

Library of Congress Cataloging-in-Publication Data
Names: Piotrowska, Agnieszka, editor. | Tyrer, Ben, editor.
Title: Femininity and psychoanalysis : cinema, culture, theory / [edited by] Agnieszka Piotrowska and Ben Tyrer.
Description: Abingdon, Oxon ; New York, NY : Routledge, 2019. | Includes index.
Identifiers: LCCN 2019004237 (print) | LCCN 2019006437 (ebook) | ISBN 9781315144054 (Master eBook) | ISBN 9781138500921 (hardback) | ISBN 9781138500938 (pbk.)
Subjects: LCSH: Femininity. | Femininity in motion pictures. | Femininity in literature.
Classification: LCC BF175.5.F45 (ebook) | LCC BF175.5.F45 F47 2019 (print) | DDC 155.3/33—dc23
LC record available at https://lccn.loc.gov/2019004237

ISBN: 978-1-138-50092-1 (hbk)
ISBN: 978-1-138-50093-8 (pbk)
ISBN: 978-1-315-14405-4 (ebk)

Typeset in Bembo
by Swales & Willis Ltd, Exeter, Devon, UK

For our mothers and for our sons.

CONTENTS

CONTRIBUTORS

Caroline Bainbridge is Professor of Culture and Psychoanalysis at Roehampton University. Her publications include *The Cinema of Lars von Trier* (Wallflower Press, 2007), *A Feminine Cinematics* (Palgrave Macmillan, 2008), *Television and Psychoanalysis: Media and the Inner World* (Palgrave Macmillan, 2013) and co-curated special editions of the journals *Psychoanalysis, Culture and Society* and *Free Associations*. Caroline is film editor for the *International Journal of Psychoanalysis*, and she co-edits Routledge's 'Psychoanalysis and Popular Culture' book series. She is a founding member of the BPC Scholar Steering Group and a Fellow of the Royal Society of Arts.

Sheila L. Cavanagh is a Professor at York University, former co-editor of the journal *Somatechnics* and outgoing chair of the Sexuality Studies Association (Canada). She edited a special double-issue on psychoanalysis in *Transgender Studies Quarterly* (2017) and co-edited *Skin, Culture and Psychoanalysis* (Palgrave Macmillan, 2013). Cavanagh wrote *Queering Bathrooms* (University of Toronto Press, 2010), a GLBT Indie Book Award finalist, and *Sexing the Teacher* (University of British Columbia Press, 2007), awarded honourable mention by the Canadian Women's Studies Association. Her scholarship appears in a range of psychoanalytic, gender and cultural studies journals.

Elizabeth Cowie is Professor Emeritus in Film Studies at the University of Kent, Canterbury. She was co-founder and co-editor in the 1970s of *m/f*, a journal of feminist theory, and author of *Representing the Woman: Cinema and Psychoanalysis* (Palgrave Macmillan, 1997). She has subsequently written on film noir, the horror of the horror film and on the cinematic dream-work. In *Recording Reality, Desiring the Real* (Minnesota University Press, 2011) she addressed documentary film as the serious, as spectacle and as an art of the real. Recent essays include 'Documentary Space, Place, and Landscape', in the online journal *Media Fields* (vol. 1, 2011); 'The Ventriloquism of Documentary First-Person Speech and the Self-Portrait Film', in *Embodied Encounters: New Approaches to Psychoanalysis and Cinema* (Routledge, 2014); 'The World Viewed: Documentary Observing and the Culture of Surveillance', in *A Companion to Contemporary Documentary Film* (Wiley-Blackwell, 2015); 'The Time of Gesture in Cinema and Its Ethics', in *Journal for Cultural Research* (vol. 19, no, 1, 2015); and 'The Difference in Figuring Women Now,' in *Moving Image Review & Art Journal* (vol. 4 nos 1 and 2, 2016, special issue on feminism and women's art).

Nava Dushi is an Associate Professor of Film and Media Studies at Lynn University. Her research traces the concept of the minor, its aesthetic manifestations and ethical consequences for culture and history. Her current work on a manuscript titled 'The Void in the Text: Minor Cinema and the Nation', proposes a theorisation of the untranslatable in minor national films, the singularity of their viewer mode of address and their potentiality to affect a creative encounter with the text.

Bracha L. Ettinger, PhD, is artist-painter and artist-theorist, philosopher and supervising psychoanalyst, Marcel Duchamp Chair and Professor of Art and Psychoanalysis at the EGS and Distinguished Professor of Philosophy at the GCAS. She is one of the world's leading thinkers in the realm of contemporary French philosophy, feminism and psychoanalysis. She participated recently with solo shows at the Kochi-Muziris Biennale (2018–2019) and the 14th Istanbul Biennial (2015). Other solo shows include UB Anderson Gallery, Buffalo (2018); Silesian Museum (Muzeum Śląskie), Katowice (2017); Museum of the City of St Petersburg (2013); Musee des Beaux-Arts d'Angers (2011); and Fundació Antoni Tàpies, Barcelona (2010). Her recent group exhibitions include *Colori*, GAM, Turin (2017); *Ontmoetingen*; MAS/KMSKA, Antwerpen (2017); and *The Human Condition*, Ekaterina Institute, Moscow (2017). Monographs dedicated to her art include *And My Heart Wound-Space* (Istanbul Biennial, Wild Pansy Press, 2015), *Art as Compassion* (ASA, 2011) and *Le Cabinet de Bracha* (Musée des Beaux-Arts d'Angers, 2011). She is author of numerous articles and books including *The Matrixial Borderspace* (University of Minnesota Press, 2006). A *Reader* of her selected essays in two volumes is currently in print with Palgrave-Macmillan (ed. G. Pollock).

Pia Hylén is a poet, painter and psychoanalyst, who moves on the edge of femininity in desire, creativity and analysis. She was educated at the University of California, Berkeley, the University of Copenhagen and the École de la Cause Freudienne in Paris. She lives and works in Portugal, participates in seminars from Iceland to Tel Aviv, writes and paints and has her practice in Lisbon. Her first book of poetry was presented at the opening night of 'La Semaine de la Poèsie' at her stand in Place St Sulpice in Paris 2010.

Joseph Jenner is close to completing his PhD in Film Studies at King's College London. He is drawing together his research interests in posthumanism, spectatorship and the science-fiction genre to posit a posthuman model of spectatorship that engages with contemporary political questions about gender, race and the human. Joseph has recently had an article published with the journal *Science Fiction Film and Television* entitled 'Gendering the Anthropocene: Female Astronauts, Failed Motherhood and the Overview Effect'. He works as a teaching assistant at King's College London and lecturer and tutor at MetFilm School.

Vicky Lebeau is Professor of English at University of Sussex and a trainee member of the British Psychoanalytic Council. She is currently completing a book on psychoanalysis and class.

Wendy Leeks went to university as a mature student, after a short career in journalism. She studied art history because she knew next to nothing about it. She received a first-class degree from Leeds University and developed her interest in psychoanalytic (specifically Lacanian) and feminist perspectives in her PhD on the nineteenth-century painter Ingres and his female nudes, with a focus on lesbian spectatorship of those images. She has subsequently published on these issues in relation to Ingres and other areas of visual culture. Since retirement form academic management in 2014, she has pursued a project of queer interpretation and investigation within the psychoanalytic realm.

Allister Mactaggart is a Lecturer in Media at Chesterfield College. He has published widely on various artistic endeavours of David Lynch, including the monograph *The Film Paintings of David Lynch: Challenging Film Theory* (Intellect, 2010), as well as articles and book chapters on topics in fine art, film, television and popular music. His work sets out to analyse the dialectical relationship between the psyche and the social as it manifests itself in culture, society and politics.

Agnieszka Piotrowska, PhD, is an award winning film-maker and a theorist. She is best known for her award-winning cult documentary *Married to the Eiffel Tower* (2009) screened globally in 60 countries. Piotrowska has written extensively on psychoanalysis and cinema and is the author of the monographs *Psychoanalysis and Ethics in Documentary Film* (2014), *Black and White: Cinema, Politics and the Arts in Zimbabwe* (2017) and *The Nasty Woman and Neo Femme Fatale in Contemporary Cinema* (2019), all published with Routledge. She made an acclaimed feature film in Zimbabwe entitled *Escape* (2017) in partnership with Zimbabwean artists. She is a Reader in Film Practice and Theory at the University of Bedfordshire, UK and the Visiting Professor in Film at Gdansk University, Poland.

A. R. Price is a psychoanalyst and the translator of Lacan's Seminars IV, X, XIX and XXIII.

Davina Quinlivan is a Senior Lecturer in Film at Kingston University. She is the author of *The Place of Breath in Cinema* (Edinburgh University Press, 2014) and *Filming the Body in Crisis* (Palgrave Macmillan, 2015). Her current research includes a monograph on the cinema of Joanna Hogg (Edinburgh University Press, forthcoming) and a project that considers Barbara Hepworth's art as cinematic practice and philosophical, feminist aesthetic.

Igor Rodin is a PhD candidate at the Hebrew University of Jerusalem. His research is situated at the intersection of ecosophy, Lacanian/post-Lacanian psychoanalytic theory and film theory. His PhD thesis entitled 'The Econtology of Cinema: Subjectivity, Text and Reading: From Matter to *Sinthomaton*', deals with the ontology of the two-dimensional image via the work of theoreticians such as Jacques Lacan, Gilles Deleuze, Félix Guattari, Bracha L. Ettinger, Timothy Morton and Reza Negarestani. Rodin is the translator of Bracha L. Ettinger's texts that were published in the Russian psychoanalytic journal *Lacanalia*.

Ben Tyrer is the author of *Out of the Past: Lacan and Film Noir* (Palgrave Macmillan, 2016) and co-editor of *Psychoanalysis and the Unrepresentable: From Culture to the Clinic* (Routledge, 2016). He is co-coordinator of the Psychoanalysis in Our Time international research network and a member of the editorial board of the *Film-Philosophy* journal.

ACKNOWLEDGEMENTS

This collection emerges out of two symposia organised by the Psychoanalysis in Our Time research network – an international initiative coordinated by the editors, Agnieszka Piotrowska and Ben Tyrer. We would like to thank the Nordic Council of Ministers and the British Association of Film, Television and Screen Studies for their support of this initiative over the last five years. The two wonderfully productive events, directly inspirational for this volume were: 'Psychoanalysis and Femininity', which took place at the National Maritime Museum in Gdansk, Poland, 8–10 April 2016; and 'Psychoanalysis and the Symptom', which took place in Sopot, Poland, 7–9 April 2017. In this volume we are bringing together some of the presenters at these symposia as well as the writings of a number of other renowned international thinkers. We are also grateful for the feedback of the colleagues at the Film-Philosophy conferences where we had opportunities to present some of the work included in the collection.

An earlier version of Chapter 5 was initially published in English by Bracha Ettinger in two parts in the now defunct journal, *The Almanac of Psychoanalysis*. Ettinger retained all rights to the texts, and they are compiled, revised and updated here with the author's direction and permission. We are also very grateful to Ettinger for supplying the fantastic cover image for this volume, 'Eurydice – Medusa – Pieta n.3' (2015–2018), as well as a selection of her sketches, paintings and notebook pages that are reproduced in this book with permission. We would like to express our thanks to the Freud Museum for their kind permission to include two photographs from their collection – of Anna and Sigmund Freud in Chapter 10 – and to Bryony Davies in particular for her help in securing these permissions. We are also very grateful for Carol Morley's permission to use an image from her 2014 film, *The Falling*, and to Matthew Barrett at Sayle Screen Ltd for his assistance with this.

INTRODUCTION

Agnieszka Piotrowska and Ben Tyrer

We are proud to present this volume on *Femininity and Psychoanalysis*. It is an unruly collection, covering a vast area of thought. It is controversial no doubt because of the contributors' choice of topics and the inevitably difficult decisions we had to make as editors in terms of whose voices we include in this volume, what is going to be discussed and put forward and what to leave for another occasion – simply at times for reasons of space. The book continues from the volume that Agnieszka edited in 2015 (*Embodied Encounters*) and *Psychoanalysis and the Unrepresentable* (2017), which we both edited, as we have done with this volume. It is interesting to observe how some debates continue and develop: one of them is the discussion about the importance of (or not) of sexual difference and its representations in culture and the clinic.

First of all, it is important to stress that the book's title and its whole ethos is indeed concerned with femininity more broadly and *not* feminism per se. However it pains us, as we are both rather clearly feminists, it is perfectly possible to be very feminine and not be a feminist. The book is about what femininity is from a psychoanalytical point of view – or what it might be. The reason why this is worth saying here is that the responses from reviewers and colleagues appear to conflate the two: we believe that feminism and the feminine connect of course and rather obviously, but are indeed different concepts. Nonetheless, as the book is psychoanalytically inspired, and we pay attention to unconscious slips and bungled actions, it is worth pondering briefly why there is the confusion: feminism deals with an unequivocal demand for equality of the sexes, femininity focuses on the essence of womanhood. The history of psychoanalysis is in part a history of a debate over what a woman, or the woman, might be. Is she equal to the man and in what way? This is of course putting the issue simply not to say simplistically. However, this is indeed still the core of the matter. The notable psychoanalyst and feminist thinker Jacqueline Rose put it slightly differently: "The history of psychoanalysis can in many ways be seen entirely in terms of engagement with this question of feminine sexuality" (Mitchell and Rose 1983: 28). Sigmund Freud, the esteemed father of psychoanalysis to whom we are all indebted, was also a deeply conservative patriarch as well as a man of great insight and a genius. Some of his comments about womanhood we still shudder over and now, in the era of the #MeToo movement some of Freud's comments would have to be declared as near offensive: his insistence on "penis envy" (already disputed by Karen Horney, as discussed by A. R. Price in Chapter 12 of this volume), his negation of a possibility of same-sex encounters, his open declarations that women are incapable of changing after the age of 30 and his deeply ambivalent attitude towards the figure of a female hysteric who used her body in order to express her deep dissatisfaction with the patriarchal world – all of these make us feel uncomfortable today.

And yet psychoanalysis is still the only theoretical, and indeed clinical, paradigm that acknowledges the Other in us and that therefore allows for the bizarreness and idiosyncrasies of everyday life to be examined without searching for a rational explanation: psychoanalysis teaches us that there is no such thing. Because the unconscious is founded in response to the untranslated messages of the Other, it operates as a site of continued incoherence within the subject, yet also as a site of truth. This truth being that *truth* is contradictory and *incoherence* is the subject's way of being true to contradiction. At times this "incoherence", when not "worked through", will explode as a bodily irregularity, a physical symptom, which has its source in a mental struggle – and it is worth remembering here that Freud's whole system was built on a woman suffering in this way. His whole discovery of the unconscious was thanks to the symptom of the female hysteric who he examined, with Breuer, so thoroughly in their groundbreaking *Studies on Hysteria* (1895).[1]

The issue of the symptom, and sinthome, and female agency vis-à-vis femininity is, one way or another, the subject of most contributions of this volume, although there is only one chapter (Chapter 2, by Davina Quinlivan) dealing head on with the figure of the hysteric. It is perhaps ironic that despite the critical role of the hysteric in Freud's oeuvre, he found femininity, womanhood, such a scary and unknowable proposition. Many famous female psychoanalysts early on tried to reclaim the hysteric and these include Karen Horney, Melanie Klein, Joan Riviere and Sabina Spielrein to name but a few.

In her re-telling of the case of one of the hysterics, namely Anna O., the more contemporary notable psychoanalyst Colette Soler (2006) recalls the bizarre tale of Breuer falling into transferential love with Anna O. without recognising the process, and completely losing his professional cool when he learnt that his patient not only relapsed dramatically after his departure, but moreover had a hysterical phantasmatic experience of giving birth. Perhaps the gaze of the hysteric did temporarily leave Breuer castrated and petrified as in the Medusa myth (which incidentally is another unfortunate example of Freud identifying a feminine castrating potential: see Piotrowska 2019: 18). Soler draws our attention to the real Anna O. who re-emerges as a fully engaged member of society doing important social work in exotic places under her real name (Soler 2006: 4–6). It is not clear (despite the claims of Freud et al.) whether the extraordinary encounter with the petrified Dr Breuer did contribute to her cure; it might well have done, although the curious abandoning of her in the middle of the treatment appears a cruel if understandable move. It is perhaps itself symptomatic that Freud does not record the inherent issues in the treatment of Anna O. – her torment and Breuer's confusion temporarily written out of the mainstream history of the practice. But the shades of the archetypal panic over the strength of the woman's sexual desire, so well known from Gothic novels, are indeed visible in this case study as in many others. Perhaps an experience of love, be it brief and indeed phantasmatic, was enough for this particular person to find her place in the Symbolic. Perhaps all she needed was to talk to somebody who appeared to listen – for a while. Perhaps the shock of being abandoned was enough to make her go into the world and do work devoted indeed to women in trouble in different continents (ibid.: 6). Nonetheless, one thing is clear: her strength and resolve appear to have overcome her passionate dependency on the man who may have helped her too. These tendencies stand firm between her death drive and her creativity. They do in the end flow Antigone-like from her own desire and she succeeds in the external world, in the Symbolic – alone but victorious, and full of agency.

In our volume the figure of the hysteric hovers over many chapters but many of the contributors engage instead with Lacanian reformulations of the symptom and of the notion of the body (the Real) versus the Imaginary and the Symbolic. Lacan struggled throughout his life with the task of taking femininity out of the tale of sexual difference, out of the Oedipal tale, out of the biological definitions only – allowing for, in Seminar XX in particular, a possibility of the feminine within a biological man. Lacan, the great heir of Freud, created a system that in its openness is both generative of new ideas but also therefore forever open to interpretations and perhaps misinterpretations, which this book embraces enthusiastically, presenting a variety of new visionary presentations of his thought, alongside many others.

We are especially privileged to include Elizabeth Cowie's magisterial chapter, "The certainties of difference and their difficulty: desire and the symptom" (Chapter 1), on femininity and the symptom, but also on creativity in the sinthome. The chapter marks a significant reformulation of her original texts (such as "Woman as Sign" first published in 1978 in the groundbreaking feminist journal, *m/f*, which she founded with Parveen Adams and Rosalind Coward).[2] In her chapter, Cowie focuses on feminine desire, jouissance and the relationship to love and art, which offers both an opportunity to revisit Dreyer's last film, *Gertrud* (1964), first discussed in *Representing the Woman: Cinema and Psychoanalysis* (1996), as well as a new discussion of Jane Campion's *The Piano* (1993). Adele, of course, is a hysteric of sorts, and her symptom is closely related to her sinthome, her music. Cowie touches upon the connection between sexual desire and the relationship between mother and daughter. We are delighted that Elizabeth Cowie's contribution to this volume marks the first time in over 20 years that she has written on the subject of Woman in a project that rethinks some of her foundational early ideas.

Every chapter in this volume discusses feminine agency, female desire and/or its position in the world vis-à-vis issues of identity. Davina Quinlivan's contribution, "Her skin against the rocks, the rocks against the sky: revisiting Weir's *Picnic at Hanging Rock* (1975) after Morley's *The Falling* (2014) and Freud's fable of female hysteria" (Chapter 2), revisits both the foundational figure of the hysteric in psychoanalysis and strange sensations of Peter Weir's *Picnic at Hanging Rock* in order to examine Carol Morley's tale of mass faintings at an English girls school in terms of collectivity and transgression that takes us beyond the patriarchal origins of psychoanalysis and towards a narrative of female self-possession.

The contributions of Caroline Bainbridge and Vicky Lebeau each discuss the ways in which racial difference and the postcolonial insist on moving the conversation on femininity outside the strict bounds of sexual difference. In Chapter 3, "Growing up girl in the 'hood: vulnerability, violence and the girl-gang state of mind in *Bande de Filles/Girlhood*", Bainbridge reflects on her own position as well as that of director Céline Sciamma as white women exploring the lives of African-French teenage girls of the *banlieues* in the latter's 2014 drama, *Girlhood*, while Bainbridge also draws on Donald Meltzer's "girl-gang state of mind" and Luce Irigaray's *parler femme* as a means of understanding the world of the film's protagonist, Marieme. In Chapter 4, "Revisiting Joan Riviere", Lebeau provides a detailed re-evaluation of the foundational work on "Womanliness and Masquerade" by Riviere, exploring the racialised fantasies that cut through the analysand's psychic life as much as they do the analyst's own interpretations. Lebeau argues for the importance of understanding the social in relation to the psyche so as not to blind psychoanalysis to the vital perspectives on race and desire in, for example, the work of Frantz Fanon.

The artist and psychoanalyst Bracha L. Ettinger's chapter, "Supplementary jouissance and feminine sexual rapport" (Chapter 5), presents a revised version of her groundbreaking 1995 essay on femininity in which she set out her original model of sexual difference after Lacan. Taking inspiration from her own clinical encounters and artistic practice, as well as the work of Deleuze and Guattari and Merleau-Ponty, Ettinger theorises a new perspective on the feminine *beyond the phallus*, taking instead the metaphor of the womb to posit a "matrixial" femininity grounded in co-emergence and what she calls "borderlinking": a spectrum of trans-individual experiences that cannot be accounted for by the divisional, phallic logic that she sees in Lacan. Updating work first published in Hebrew in a limited run of ten copies, and then translated into English in two parts for the now defunct *Almanac of Psychoanalysis* in 1998 and 2000, this chapter gathers both sections, "Supplementary Jouissance" and "Feminine Sexual Rapport", together for the first time in English: making the work – with Ettinger's new corrections and clarifications – available to a far wider readership than previously possible. The chapter also includes Ettinger's own translations into English from both Lacan's seminars and *écrits*, and from Jacques-Alain Miller's own courses, many of which remain unpublished even now.

Applying Ettinger's theories of sexual difference to the cinema, Chapter 6 by Nava Dushi and Igor Rodin, "Self-recreation through the uncanny encounter: reading the feminine close-up in cinema", proposes a re-thinking of the technique of the close-up in cinema. Rather than the "phallic" mode of photographing the subject that privileges the topology of the *face* (and resisting the weight of film theoretical tradition from Balázs to Mulvey), Dushi and Rodin propose an understanding of film based on Ettinger's "matrixial gaze" and an aesthetics of contingency, uncertainty and traumaticity.

Working in a more avowedly Lacanian register, while also drawing on Kristeva, Arendt and Marxist cultural theory, Allister Mactaggart's chapter, "*River*'s edge: the ebb and flow of feminine ex-sistence" (Chapter 7), offers a distinctive view on love and loss through a look at the popular television series, *River* (BBC, 2015). Starting from a coincidence of psychoanalysis and detection, Mactaggart argues that the eponymous River's passage through mourning takes him into an encounter with femininity and an understanding of love.

Ben Tyrer's chapter, "*Under Her Skin*: on Woman without body and body without Woman" (Chapter 8), examines the recent science fiction films of Scarlett Johansson in relation to her "sex symbol" star image in order to chart the differing accounts of sexual difference that Lacan gives in his work from the 1950s to the 1970s. Focusing on *Her* (2013) and *Under the Skin* (2013), Tyrer argues that a "phallic" model of sexual difference can only position woman as object, while a properly feminine logic can be discerned through an understanding of the ontology of sexual difference as put forward in Seminar XX and Alenka Zupančič's *What Is Sex?* (2017).

Agnieszka Piotrowska's chapter co-written with Joseph Jenner, "Desire, commitment and the transformative power of touch: the posthuman femme fatale in *Under the Skin*" (Chapter 9), is in a dialogue with Tyrer's chapter, offering a different take on *Under the Skin* and some disagreements over its significance as their chapter focuses on the proposition of how to imagine the creation of posthuman female subjectivity. Combining Piotrowska's research on touch with Jenner's on posthumanism, the chapter aims to chart the journey of the alien woman from posthuman femme fatale to an Antigone-like subject of desire, focusing on the transformative encounter between Johansson's character and the man with neurofibromatosis played by Adam Pearson.

We have two chapters that deal directly with and challenge the notion of the binary of sex(uality): Chapter 10 by Wendy Leeks about Anna Freud and Marilyn Monroe, and Chapter 11 by Sheila Cavanagh on Oedipus and Tiresias. Leeks' contribution, "AnnaMarilyn: queer tales of femininity", examines biography and psychoanalysis in relation to the life stories of two famous women, Anna Freud and Marilyn Monroe. Exploring the unexpected coincidences and points of contact in the lives of these two women, Leeks notes their differing symbolic status – as sexuality embodied (Monroe) and sexuality denied (Freud) – and considers the queer potentials of their histories, beginning with the question "Was Anna Freud a lesbian?" and moving on to consider the speculation around

Monroe's bisexual/lesbian "tendencies". In "Tiresias: Bracha L. Ettinger and the transgression with-in-to the feminine", Cavanagh makes a radical proposition to abandon the Oedipal metaphor of sexual difference altogether, and – drawing on the theories of Ettinger – instead proposes a transgender fluidity as the way of thinking about the world through her discussion of the figure of Tiresias in *Oedipus Rex*. We also include the contribution of Pia Hylén, a psychoanalyst and artist, whose poetry and drawing gives expression to feminine desires, experiences and "vulnerabilities" in Chapter 14, "VuLNeRaBILITies".

Psychoanalyst A. R. Price's notes on Lacan's controversial *L'étourdit* in Chapter 12, "A specimen of a commentary on Lacan's '*L'étourdit*'", throw some light on Lacan's views on the decades of disputation between acclaimed psychoanalysts such as Karen Horney, Helene Deutsch, as well as Ernst Jones regarding on the one hand the "impossibility" of the sexual relationship, and on the other the fear of feminine castration. Bringing the eye of an experienced clinician as well as translator (Price has translated Lacan's Seminars IV, X, XIX and XXIII – on object relations, anxiety, sexual difference and the sinthome – into English for publication in recent years) to Lacan's famously difficult, even *untranslatable*, essay *L'étourdit* (an impossible pun somewhere between *dizziness* and *bewilderment*), Price has chosen to break down the original French text line-by-line, sometimes even word-by-word, rather than offering a more general description of the piece or a straightforward translation. The effect is to transform Lacan's essay on sexual difference into a series of vertical moments, where the literal, poetic, theoretical and clinical implications of each signifier are explored in depth: close analysis as textual psychoanalysis, we might say. The result is a chapter that is sometimes no less challenging than Lacan's original, but one that rewards careful attention for its insights into a major essay of Lacanian psychoanalysis, which has thus far not received sufficient attention in the Anglophone literature.

Piotrowska's short story (or creative non-fiction) on a moment of #MeToo in Communist Poland (Chapter 13) corresponds interestingly with Price's chapter. In a way this story is also indeed about the vagina and castration anxiety (or misunderstood menstruation), which is what the Jones–Horney–Lacan debate is focused on in Price's chapter. For Antonia to apologise would have been to submit to castration, while the other character Joanna does just that. Price focuses in his notes on the deutero-phallic phase of development, which is, arguably, the topic of Lacan's text. In this context there is a deeper significance of the "running around" game for the boys in finding their own identity and coping with (castration) anxiety.

It is also interesting to consider how the failure of the Communist ideal of gender-equality is yet another proof of the value of psychoanalysis, especially in the area of female sexuality and asymmetrical gender and power relations.

We hope that this collection opens a space in which these ideas and phenomena can be debated once more and look forward to the time when all the binaries, and particulary that of sexual difference, can finally be rethought.

Notes

1 For further discussion of the unconscious as a site of incoherence see Frosh, S. (2012) Psychoanalysis and Relational Ethics After the Turn. In S. Frosh and S. Roseneil (eds.) *Social Research After the Cultural Turn*. London: Palgrave, pp. 56–72.

2 As Cowie notes, "I published several key essays in *m/f*, in particular, 'Woman as Sign', 'The Popular Film as Progressive Text: A Discussion of Coma', and 'Fantasia'. These have appeared in a number of anthologies, most recently in 2000 and 2009, as well as appearing in revised form in my book, *Representing the Woman: Psychoanalysis and Feminism* (1997)". See: http://reframe.sussex.ac.uk/repsychoanalysis/about/elizabeth-cowie.

Bibliography

Mitchell, J. and Rose, J. (eds.) (1983) *Feminine Sexuality: Jacques Lacan and the école freudienne*. London: Macmillan Press.

Piotrowska, A. (2019) *The Nasty Woman and the Neo Femme Fatale in Contemporary Cinema*. London: Routledge.

Soler, C. (2006) *What Lacan Said About Women*. New York: The Other Press.

1

THE CERTAINTIES OF DIFFERENCE AND THEIR DIFFICULTY

Desire and the symptom

Elizabeth Cowie

For Freud, woman's desire was an enigma; writing to the French psychoanalyst Marie Bonaparte he famously declared that, "the great question that has never been answered, and which I have not yet been able to answer, despite my thirty years of research into the feminine soul, is 'What does a woman want?'" (cited by Jones 1953: 421).[1] Lacan, taking up Freud's question in *Encore*, poses it in relation to woman's enjoyment, her *jouissance* that he argues is other than phallic *jouissance*, which she also enjoys. Asking women about this other *jouissance*, "to try to tell us", he declares: "We've never been able to get anything out of them. So we call this jouissance by whatever name we can come up with" (Lacan 1999: 75). What is addressed in this chapter is this questioning by both Freud and Lacan of woman as other and thus the enigma of her desire. Asking women questions, however, cannot advance knowledge of the unconscious of feminine desire, just as the child cannot fathom the m/Other's desire. For the question "What does a woman want?" is also the question "What does she want of me, that is, what am I for her?" Thus, Lacan suggests, the problem expressed in the question is the problem of the Other, "woman being, in this case, equivalent to truth" (ibid.: 127). For Lacan, however, the central truth that he insisted upon throughout his later work is that "*Il n'y a pas de rapport sexuel*", "there is no sexual relationship"; instead there is the possibility of love (2006: 147).[2] In *The Sinthome*, Seminar XXIII, the consequences for the subject that the sexual relation does not exist are explored in relation to the psychoanalytic concept of the symptom (Lacan 2016: 68). It is here that Lacan introduces his new syllogism of the "sinthome" in his discussion of the writings of James Joyce, and through which he addresses the limitations of "going through the fantasy" as an ending of analysis. Instead Lacan formulates the symptom-as-sinthome as a knotting of the Real, Imaginary and Symbolic. In this Seminar Lacan not only develops his conceptualisation of the Real but also addresses how art – the artifices of art – might be engaged through the symptom in relation to Joyce's writing, while at the same time Lacan complicates the role of the phallus and the Name-of-the-Father. As a result, Lacanian analyst Geneviève Morel suggests that Lacan's theory of the symptom "allows us to think the relations between the sexes and the generations without necessarily referring to the Name-of-the-Father nor to the phallus, as transcendent norms of a symbolic order" (Morel 2005: xvi). While Paul Verhaeghe and Frédéric Declercq write, "the Lacanian conclusion of the treatment (. . .) is a particular process that is situated entirely in the line of femininity" (2002: 76).[3]

This chapter seeks to trace the complications for his account of sexual difference that Morel and Verhaeghe suggest that Lacan introduces here, and relate them to the story of femininity. For "femininity" is a "story", a construction, that all those who become placed as "feminine" find themselves within, and part of that story is the assumed interchangeability or equivalence of woman and femininity in the writing of both Freud and Lacan. It is a story, however, that remains incomplete, creating a gap that is the Real of knowledge. Lacan repeatedly returns to the question of femininity and the woman but he does so not to close the gaps, instead a certain "gapping", or incommensurability, appears as constitutive. Freud himself suggested that "if you want to know more about femininity, enquire from your own experiences of life or turn to the poets" (1933/1964: 135). I will be turning not to poets but to two film directors, Carl Theodor Dreyer and Jane Campion, to examine ways in which woman's desire finds articulation in cinema's stories, drawing on Lacan's re-thinking of the symptom in relation to femininity. I am drawing here on the discussions that I was part of in the 1970s and 1980s on feminine sexuality in the turn to psychoanalysis and Lacan's re-reading of Freud, which were central for my book, *Representing the Woman: Cinema and Psychoanalysis* (1997). In my analysis of the representation of women in film I drew upon a psychoanalytic understanding of fantasy in its role in desire, identification and sexuality for male and female characters. I argued that for both men and women their sexual identification is neither singular nor a choice, rather it arises as a concatenation, a palimpsest, realised in the context of the contingency of the Other who responds to our demand for love. For one enacts the emplacements – both unconscious and conscious – of one's psychical history in relation to one's parental figures and one's encounter with the demands and desires – enjoined or prohibited – that they convey, consciously or unconsciously. This chapter returns to the question of desire and sexual difference in film's representations through Lacan's concept of the sinthome.

Freud had acknowledged that there is an "uninterpretable navel" to dreams and the unconscious,[4] while Lacan called for a training in antiphilosophy for analysts,[5] and in *Encore* he declared that "The Discordance between knowledge and being is my subject" (1999: 120), but nevertheless acknowledges that "We are still (*encore*) caught up in the insufficiency of knowledge" (ibid.). It is the "insufficiency of knowledge" in relation to sexuality and to the categories of sexual difference that this chapter explores, for we might see in Lacan's re-thinking of Freud's ideas – with his graphs, mathemes and concepts – an attempt to wrestle with the uninterpretability Freud writes of, and the insufficiency of knowledge he laments. Charles Shepherdson has suggested that,

> These attempts at a logical formalization of Freud are not merely descriptive, however, but are used as a means of discovery. It is almost as if Lacan believes that the conceptual impasses which his logical formulations produce are themselves capable of revealing something about the real.
>
> *(2003: 141)*

Taking up again the question of our psychical relation to sexual difference, to "sexuation" as Lacan poses it, and the different relation of men and women to jouissance – as Lacan continued to do in his late Seminars – I suggest that femininity is as much an enigma for women as for men, inasmuch as "being feminine" is something other than anatomical difference, or biology in the sense of hormones. Indeed Lacan himself comments, in *The Psychoses*, in relation to Freud's case study, "What is Dora saying through her neurosis? (. . .) Her question is this – *What is it to be a woman?*" (1993: 175). Femininity is what is added to the biological difference of "being a woman" in a performance, through gestures of movement and speech, in forms of response and through appearance: a masquerade.[6] This is no less true for men, of course, and that it is equally an enigma – and a problem – is attested by the regular appearance of claims that masculinity is in crisis. At the same time the categories "woman" and "man" are not singular but involve further categories, not only in terms of age – for "girls" are not-yet-fully "women" – but also categories that are social, that is, *relational*: women as mothers, sisters, daughters, wives and workers. Being a mother or father to a son, or daughter, or being daughter or a son to a mother or father are each different kinds of being a woman, or a man, and each centres a relationship. Indeed, for Lacan what is central is that our subjectivity arises in relation to an Other and others through discourse: that is, in a social relation, which is the focus of his discussion of the "Four Discourses" in Seminar XVII. For language is trans-individual and speech, discourse, always implies – anticipates – another subject as addressee, and interlocutor.

How then, as Juliet Mitchell asked in a recent interview, "does the construction of sexual difference become so embedded that we experience it as who we are?" (2015: 115). Her book *Psychoanalysis and Feminism* (1974) presented Freud in a new and vital way for feminists in 1974, while in the collection of essays that she co-edited with Jacqueline Rose, she writes that for Lacan,

> the analysand's unconscious reveals a fragmented subject of shifting and uncertain sexual identity. To be human is to be subjected to a law which decentres and divides: sexuality is created in a division, the subject is split; but an ideological world conceals this from the conscious subject who is supposed to feel whole and certain of a sexual identity.
>
> *(Mitchell and Rose 1982: 26)*

The account of femininity in both Freud and Lacan is of a construction, not as an essence or as simply biological. This also means that for Lacan there is no feminine outside language because, as Jacqueline Rose notes, first "the unconscious severs the subject from any unmediated relation to the body as such (. . .) and secondly because the 'feminine' is constituted in a division in language" (ibid.: 55).

At stake is how we think the "ideological" – the social organisation of difference that is usually addressed in terms of gender assignment – in relation to the unconscious formations that arise in relation to the constitutive splitting of the subject in its relation to lack, prohibition and desire.[7] What arises is both an attributed sexed identity, and a psychological relation to difference and to sexuality. It is this that Jean Laplanche's discussion, in his essay, "Gender, Sex, and the Sexual" emphasises, and that I want to draw upon here. He argues that gender – the social and linguistic identification of a difference of sex – precedes sexuality, but, he says, "Yes, gender precedes sex. But far from organizing it, it is organized by it" (2007: 215). Gender is the social assignment of difference, and Laplanche emphasises the primacy of the other, the social, in the messages of gender assignment both at an official level – the level of Foucault's discursive ordering – in the registering of the birth of a child who is always thereby sexed and, more importantly, by its carers. The baby's being for others is not only as a boy or girl, but also as a son or daughter. But these messages assigning gender, Laplanche argues, are "also carriers of many 'noises', all those brought by the adults who are close to the child: parents, grandparents, brother and sisters. Their fantasies, their unconscious and preconscious expectations" (ibid.). Here Laplanche draws on a key element of his work in describing these messages from the other – mother or carer – as seductive but also enigmatic, as "preconscious-conscious" in which "the parental unconscious is like the 'noise' – in the sense of communications theory – that comes to disturb and *compromise* the preconscious-conscious message" (ibid.). It is a gendered child that the parent addresses, but "their unconscious wishes also come to infiltrate gender assignment". And, Laplanche suggests, it is "above all what is *le sexual* in the parents that *makes noise* in the assignment" of gender and that "in the presence of the child, the adults ultimately come to reactivate their *infantile sexuality* above all" (ibid.).[8] For the child, he says, "Gender is acquired, assigned, but enigmatic up to about fifteen months. Sex comes along to fix, to translate gender in the course of the second year (. . .) The *castration complex* is its center". Laplanche also argues, however, that "The certainty of the castration complex is maintained on the basis of ideology and on the basis of illusion, namely, in the early genital phase" (ibid.: 216, emphasis in original).[9]

Mustapha Safouan, a member of the Lacanian school, points out that:

> Not only does *the essence of the Oedipus complex not lie in the rivalry* for which it is the precondition, it is even that very rivalry that obscures its essence. The Oedipal complex is in the end no more than *one cultural form* among others, those others being equally possible providing they perform the same function of *promoting the function of castration* in the psyche.
>
> *(1990: 281, emphasis in original)*

It is as *signifier* that the phallus comes to play its role as an ideal "precisely, of that whose insufficiency is discovered for the boy and its nonexistence for the girl, at an early age, in an attribute of the father" (ibid.: 280). Lacan (re)defines the phallus (which is not the penis) as the structural function of whatever "*x*" the child hypothesises the paternal figure possesses making him the focus of the maternal figure's desire, that is, the possession enabling the father to domesticate and control the mother's otherwise unpredictable desire. If the Name-of-the-Father, as the O/other of the mother, "forbids" by standing in the way of the child's wish for unlimited access to the mother, it is because until this intervention the mother is for the child not a woman, but the m/Other. This intervention is the "answer" to the problem of the m/Other's desire, and the constitutive lack in the subject. As Safouan also notes,

> Only the play of the signifier [the Imaginary] can explain this introduction of a phallus that is in some sense absolute, along with what follows from that introduction, that is, the subordination of access to genitality to a movement that the subject feels as an exclusion from that very phallus.
>
> *(Ibid.: 280)*

It is, he suggests, a special case of the "induction of the imaginary by the symbolic that can be illustrated even in the formation of the 'scientific mind'" (ibid.). This move, namely the experience of an "insufficiency", or an absence as "castration", in relation to the "*x*" that is the phallus, does not thereby ensure the child identifies according to his or her biological sex, and thus accords with his or her "gender", or that she or he desires the other of her biological sex/gender, that is, as their object-choice. Moreover the carnality of mutual sexual acts that open on to enjoyment, to jouissance, also open the subject to the abyss of lack that is at the same time apprehended. It is through the masquerade, for the woman, or parade for the man, that each player in the sexual act sustains themselves in having or being the phallus for the other.[10]

While for Freud there was no mystery about the boy's desire – he wants the mother, but must turn away from her or risk the father's wrath, which is imagined as a threat of castration – the enigma of castration for the girl continues to haunt discussions of sexual difference, which Lacan's discussion in *Encore* does not resolve. Developing Freud's account of the Oedipal complex, Lacan states,

> there is no chance for a man to have *jouissance* of a woman's body, otherwise stated, for him to make love, without castration (*a moins de castration)*, in other words, without something that says no to the phallic function (. . .) But what he approaches is the cause of his desire that I have designated as object *a*. That is the act of love.
>
> *(1999: 72–73)*

The woman, however, does not have this *jouissance* in the same way because she is not subject to this "no to the phallic function", instead – as noted earlier – Lacan posits that she has her own *jouissance* of the body "beyond the phallus" (ibid.: 74) but about which she knows nothing (ibid.: 75), nevertheless she also has phallic jouissance (ibid.: 78).

In *Encore* Lacan, drawing on set theory, presents two groups of "propositional formulas" through which he specifies two different relations to the prohibition that is instituted by the phallic function, symbolic castration and two different modes of jouissance. Both groups of formulas contain an assertion that all are subject to the phallic function, and a negation of that assertion. The formula on the left side describes the relation that defines the masculine – though that may not be all or only men – whereby all those *x*'s choosing the left side are submitted to the phallic function, but "with the proviso that this function is limited" (ibid.: 79). Its limitation is the existence of one *x* that is not submitted to the phallic function, "the father function", and it is this exception that guarantees the universal law of symbolic existence. In this "exception" Lacan keeps faith with Freud's idea of the primal father who enjoys without limit, who is not submitted to the phallic function but who was removed by the band of sons who were thereby freed to enjoy but conditionally, subject to a prohibition, namely symbolic castration. The man who places himself on the left side, "is unable to attain his sexual partner, who is the Other, except inasmuch as his partner is the cause of his desire" which is "nothing other than fantasy" (ibid.: 80). Hence Lacan's assertion, "*Il n'y a pas de rapport sexuel*", there is no sexual relation, no coming together in mutual enjoyment as a complementarity of what is given and what is taken, in what one is or one has for the Other.

Addressing the right side of the graph, the side of femininity – though this may not involve all or only women – Lacan's formulae designate that there is not one *x* that is not submitted to the phallic function, but also includes the negation that not every *x* is submitted to the phallic function. Where for those on the side of the masculine there is a universal, thus a set of "all men", on the side of the feminine "women" is not a singular or universal group because woman lacks a limit. Thus Lacan writes of Woman crossed through, barred, and he places her as having a relation to the big Other, the Symbolic, "the locus in which everything that can be articulated on the basis of the signifier comes to be inscribed" (ibid.: 81). The big Other is barred, however, so the Woman barred has a relation to the signifier of the Other, which, however, is also barred S(A-barred) (Autre, Other). The feminine relation to jouissance is doubled, both a phallic jouissance and, as noted earlier, a jouissance beyond the phallus that Lacan defines as a jouissance of the Other, A. Yet now Lacan equivocates, using the conditional tense for this other jouissance: "Were there another jouissance than phallic jouissance, it shouldn't be/could never fail to be that one" (ibid.: 59). Here Lacan is playing on the logic of the Stoics when he states that "It is false that there is another one, but that doesn't stop what follows from being true, namely, that it shouldn't be/could never fail to be that one" (ibid.: 60). That women say nothing about an/other jouissance neither confirms nor denies its non-existence, yet Lacan finds its confirmation in the women mystics: in the writings of Hadewijch d'Anvers, for example, or

Bernini's statue of Saint Teresa in Rome, seeing which one "would immediately understand that she is coming (. . .) What is she getting off on? It is clear that the essential testimony of the mystics consists in saying they experience it, but know nothing about it" (ibid.: 76). This jouissance may also be experienced by those who are male, "because one is not obliged, when one is male" to situate himself on the side of "all", but "can also situate oneself on the side of the not-all, as mystics" (ibid.).[11] This other jouissance that "shouldn't be/could never fail to be that one" is an "extra (*en plus*)" jouissance rather than another (ibid.: 77). And it is the one that Lacan will invoke as the jouissance of the symptom in the declaration that woman is a symptom "for those encumbered with the phallus" (1982: 168), and later as the jouissance of the sinthome.

What Lacan is also addressing in *Encore* is philosophy itself, and the question of knowledge and truth that is intrinsic to "the four discourses – on which the social link is based" (1999: 78).[12] In Lecture VIII of *Encore*, "Knowledge and truth", Lacan also investigates the question of knowledge and of reason as a procedure that thereby produces what is not speakable, knowable, in the imaginary or in the symbolic, which is the Real that is connected to the body. He writes, "The Real can only be inscribed on the basis of an impasse of formalisation" (ibid.: 93), and it is the Real that arises because "the sexual relation doesn't stop not being written. *Because of this, the apparent necessity of the phallic function turns out to be mere contingency*" (ibid.: 94; my emphasis).

It is the Real that haunts *Encore* as that which is incompletely accounted for in the formulae of sexuation and that Lacan will continue to address in Seminar XXII *RSI*, and Seminar XXIII, *The Sinthome*. Where for the man the *objet a* cause-of-desire is Woman barred, on the side of femininity, no *objet a* is indicated for her; instead Lacan writes that for Woman barred, "something other than object *a* is at stake in what comes to make up for (*supplier*) the sexual relationship that does not exist" (1999: 63), which in the formulae is the barred Other, that is, the m/Other. The *objet a* is not an object of desire but the object-cause of desire, and it is so because it stands in for not *something* lost, but for "lostness", the "goneness" of the absent object, and not the object as such. The *objet a* in the Real is the impossible Real of the lack in the mother/Other. In Seminar XII Lacan says that *objet a* is not simply a hollow or "initial zero of the reality of the subject being incarnated in pure lack", it is a "residue (. . .) which through its simple presence, modifies, inclines, inflects the whole possible economy of a libidinal relationship to the object, of any choice whatsoever which is qualified as objectal" (1965: 138). While, in *Encore*, Lacan says that "Woman serves a function in the sexual relation only *qua* mother" (1999: 35), but also that the woman has a jouissance arising from being "not-whole" [not-all], but for which she "finds the cork" to stop up jouissance "in the *a* constituted by her child" (ibid.). But is woman's function *qua* mother a function for herself in the sexual relation, or for the man, or both? Lorenzo Chiesa – exploring Lacan's Seminars "as they revolve around a logical and critically onto-theo-logical investigation of the basic axiom 'There is no sexual relationship'" (2016: xi) – suggests that in

Lacan's assertion that the woman is in the sexual relation *qua* mother, he seems to understand this "primarily in the sense of '*from the man's perspective*'" (ibid.: 13). This implying, therefore, that men – as adults post-Oedipally – relate to woman-as-mother, which Chiesa points out "conceals another, more troubling statement: as soon as, *from woman's perspective*, woman starts to serve a function in the sexual relationship *only* as mother, sexual difference, and the symbolic order with it, are at risk" (ibid.). For woman is doubled, in being "mother" for another, and in being a daughter to a mother, as well as – for some women – nurturing her child as its mother. While, as Laplanche emphasised, the child experiences her mother in relation to this doubling and to the complex messages it involves, which for a daughter then also becomes part of her experience as a woman and, if or when, she becomes a mother.

Lacan returns to the question of the woman's desire in Seminar XXII, *R.S.I.* (1975), when he says, "What she busies herself with are other *objet a*, being children" (1982: 167). He then declares that "The phallus is not phallic *jouissance*", and that "for whoever is encumbered with the phallus, what is a woman? A woman is a symptom". This arises because:

> there is no jouissance of the Other as such, no guarantee to be met with in the body of the Other to ensure that the enjoying other exists. A manifest instance of the hole, or rather of something whose only support is the *objet a* – but always in a mix-up or confusion.
>
> *(Ibid.: 168)*

Nevertheless, he continues,

> In point of fact a woman is no more an *objet a* than is a man – as I said earlier, she has her own, which she busies herself with, and this has nothing to do with the object by which she sustains herself in any desire whatsoever. To make of this A-Woman a symptom, is to say that phallic jouissance is equally her affair, contrary to what is said. *The woman has to undergo no more or less castration than the man. As for what is involved in her function as symptom, she is at exactly the same point as her man.*
>
> *(Ibid., my emphasis)*[13]

Lacan does not explore what this means for the woman, instead commenting that "We have yet to articulate what corresponds in her case to that real ex-istence I spoke of earlier as the phallus" (ibid.). Chiesa, however, suggests that Lacan is

> using the term *jouissance* in two different ways: feminine *jouissance*, the *jouissance* of the not-all as such, is corked or contained by means of a child *qua* the object *a*, which, as a supplementation to the negatively additional character of feminine *jouissance*, produces itself a form of *phallic jouissance*.
>
> *(2016: 14)*

As a result, Chiesa argues,

> This undecidable – concerning fundamentally whether woman is or is not phallic – will then be more generally the undecidability of the phallic function *tout court*: there is no sexual relationship, *but* there are sexed liasons, *but* there ultimately are sexed relations only because woman opens onto the absence of the sexual relationship.
>
> *(Ibid.: 171)*

There is, indeed, a haunting undecidability in Seminar XX, heralded in its title, *Encore*, used by Lacan to refer to his audience as – still, or again, *encore* – coming to hear him, but also referring to what there is "still" to know about wanting to know and not know – of woman's sexuality, her "femininity". Thus Jacques-Alain Miller's inclusion for the English translation of the subtitle "On Feminine Sexuality, the Limits of Love and Knowledge" restates the hesitation as "limits", which are intrinsic to the very idea of both love and knowledge. It is still, *encore*, or again, in the following seminar, XXII, *R.S.I*, where Lacan develops his thinking about the Real, that is the hole, the fundamental lack that is a lack-in-being, while introducing the formulation, "A woman is a symptom for man". It is the symptom and its relation to the Real, Symbolic and Imaginary that are the focus of Seminar XXIII where Lacan uses the word sinthome – adopting the old French spelling of the word symptom – to identify a particular way in which the subject engages with her symptom, and its role for the subject's Real, Imaginary and Symbolic relations.[14]

In Seminar XII Lacan had placed the symptom as central to the Real, defining this third term in relation to the Symbolic and the Imaginary:

> it is in the symptom that we identify what is produced in the field of the Real. If the Real manifests itself in analysis and not only in analysis, if the notion of the symptom was introduced, well before Freud by Marx, so as to make it the sign of something which is what is not working out in the Real, if in other words, we are capable of operating on the symptom, it is insofar as the symptom is the effect of the Symbolic in the Real.
>
> *(1965: 20)*

For Lacan the symptom is not a coded message addressed to another, rather "if symptoms can be read, it is because they themselves are already inscribed in a writing process. As particular unconscious formations, symptoms are not significations" (2005: 371). The symptom is inscribed in a writing process and that is a Real "enjoying", a jouissance, "they are what gives Symbolic form to the Real of the the drive" (Verhaeghe and Declercq 2002: 2). Where Freud had viewed the symptom as "like the grain of sand around which an oyster forms its pearl" (1905/1953: 83), Lacan proposes the "grain of sand" as the Real of jouissance around which the symptom, as a Symbolic construction, forms. This may emerge in the body, as in the conversion symptoms of paralysis, blindness, etc. in war neurosis that Freud addressed,[15] or as the bodily felt, as a terror, anxiety, etc. The symptom, as Žižek notes, is a particular pathological signifying formation in the unconscious that enjoys, resisting interpretation, "a stain which cannot be included into the circuit of discourse, of social bond/network", which is the Symbolic, "but which is at the same time a positive condition of it" (1991a: 207).

Returning to the question of the symptom in Seminar XXIII, Lacan uses the term *sinthome* in order to mark a difference in the psychical formation of the symptom in that the sinthome, unlike the symptom, involves a creative process that upholds the consistency of reality for a subject, "knotting" the Real, the Imaginary and the Symbolic. This spelling gave Lacan much scope for wordplay through which he explores the multiple associations, the creative connections, of this mode of the symptom: synthetic-artificial man, synthesis between symptom and fantasy, Saint Thomas, etc. While Lacan developed and explored this new concept in Seminar XXIII in relation to the work of James Joyce, his concern was not only an analysis of Joyce and his writing, but the practice of psychoanalysis and of how to conceive in a new way the possibility of the end of analysis for the analysand. Namely, not only by "going through her fundamental fantasy", gaining distance from the fantasy framework of her reality, but now also by "identifying" with her sinthome. Fantasy for Lacan is central for the subject in managing lack in the Other, and its constitutive alienation, such that, "The subject situates himself as determined by the phantasy (. . .) whether in the dream or in any of the more or less well-developed forms of day-dreaming" (1979: 185).[16] The subject's "fundamental fantasy", Chiesa writes, "should be regarded as a 'compromise formation' par excellence: indeed, it is both the consequence of and a reaction (a defence) against the fact that the symbolic Other of the signifiers is a structurally lacking order". Thus, "It both relates the barred subject to the Real lack in the Symbolic, that of the real object *a*, and at the same time, 'veils' this lack in the unconscious through the imaginary dimension of the object *a*." Thereby it is "the locus in which the subject emerges as a consequence of the knotting together of the three orders of the Symbolic, the Imaginary, and the Real" (2016: 142). The goal of psychoanalysis thus became "*la traversée du fantasme*", the traversing, the going through, of the fundamental fantasy by which the subject is able to assume a new relation to the Other, to desire, as a relation of lack. The question Lacan then poses is:

> What, then, does he who has passed through the experience (. . .) who has traversed the radical phantasy (. . .) become? How can a subject who has traversed the radical phantasy experience the drive? This is the beyond of analysis, and has never been approached.
>
> *(1979: 273)*[17]

In *Seminar XXIII* it is now the symptom-as-sinthome that achieves the knotting of Real, Imaginary and Symbolic, in a re-thinking of the Real that effects a displacement of the Symbolic: instituted and upheld by the Name-of-the-Father, the phallic signifier. Instead, with the concept of the sinthome, Lacan articulates a mode of a subjectivity not formed by the desire of the other, the Name-of-the-Father or the Imaginary. Lacan develops this through a series of permutations of the tying of the Borromean knot, which thereby produce "holes". It is a *creative process* of naming in working with the holes and knots that are the Real. Central here is Lacan's thinking of the Real: "the Real must be sought on the other side, on the side of the absolute zero", it is "tied to nothing" (2016: 102, 104). Chiesa suggests that this zero, or nothing, "equates to the always-already lost mythical jouissance of the real Real". What is required is the *semblant*, the "fake" jouissance of *objet a*, "in order to "make One" – to cork the hole in the symbolic structure", thus retrospectively creating "the illusion of an absolute *jouissance* (or suffering) which has been lost" (2005: 163). Lacan now proposes a jouissance of the symptom/sinthome in the Real distinct from "so-called phallic jouissance" that is "located here at the conjunction between the symbolic and the real" (2016: 43). Lacan writes this as JA-barred, "jouissance of the barred Other" for "there is no jouissance of the Other because there is no Other of the Other" (ibid.). The jouissance that "would be if it were", and that was the not-all of feminine – other – jouissance of *Encore*, can no longer be JA (which does not exist); instead, replaced by JA-barred, it is the jouissance of the sinthome, for in identifying with his sinthome the man too, like the woman, is "not all". Thus Geneviève Morel argues that, "the 'not-all' is not exclusively reserved for women, in the sense that everyone's sinthome, rooted in the mother tongue, is also 'not-all' for him" (2006: 69).[18] And the subject is individualised/individuated (Chiesa's term), rather than being the "one" of the symptom that is always addressed to an other (2005: 169).

Thus, rather than the interpretation of the symptom, or the going through of the fantasy, there is in this mode of ending analysis, an identification with the symptom-as-sinthome. Lacan declares that, "It is insofar as the unconscious is knotted to the sinthome, which is singular to each individual, that we may say that Joyce (. . .) identifies with the individual (. . .) embodying the symptom in himself" (2016: 147). In Seminar XXIV Lacan speaks of "Knowing how to deal with your symptom, that is the end of analysis", and that this knowing, "Might it be or might it not be to identify oneself – while taking some insurance, a kind of distance – to identify oneself to one's symptom? I put it forward that the symptom could be (. . .) it can be the sexual partner" (1976/1977).[19]

Roberto Harari, in his complex and subtle reading of Seminar XXIII in *How James Joyce Made His Name: A Reading of the Final Lacan* (1995), emphasises that in contrast to the subject of the symptom, who is a barred or divided subject, "One who says 'I cannot live like this' (. . .) Conversely, one is sure that 'one cannot live without' the sinthome" (1995: 358–359). The goal then of psychoanalysis for Lacan is to bring about the creative process involved in the sinthome for the subject, which Joyce achieved through his writing. Verhaeghe and Declercq declare that this creative process of identification with the sinthome is, "situated entirely in the line of femininity", due to the woman's "special relationship to the *objet a* and the jouissance", she is "'naturally' invited to create something of herself, in the very process of becoming a woman" (2002: 76). But this process of becoming "one", of an individuation, cannot be referred back to the sexual differences of the Imaginary/Symbolic that are instituted by castration. Rather it might be that "becoming a woman" itself is a process of identifying with her sinthome, for, as Lacan states, "The Oedipus complex is, as such, a symptom". "Everything is sustained in so far as the Name-of-the-Father is also the Father of the Name, which doesn't make the symptom any the less necessary" (2016: 13). Moreover, "The Name-of-the-Father can just as well be bypassed (. . .) on the condition that one makes use of it" (ibid.: 116). The Name-of-the-Father intervenes to knot the Symbolic and the Real, interposing itself between the child and the desire of the m/Other and its ravages, and it is a role that is not necessarily required to be undertaken by the child's biological father, or even by a man. Rather, it is the function that is central, namely as figuring the social laws and conventions that are also recognised by the mother. Further, Lacan writes that:

> this fourth element (. . .) in the knot of the symbolic, the imaginary and the real. There is, however, another term for this (. . .) what is involved in the Name-of-the-Father, at the very degree to which Joyce bears it out, with what it would be most suitable to call *the sinthome*.
>
> *(Ibid.: 147)*

We suffer our symptom, and it was Freud's work with his patients' symptoms that led him to propose the unconscious of psychoanalysis. But if there is no sexual difference in the unconscious, rather there is the symptom, there can be no "feminine way" that is not also a symptom-as-sinthome. What also emerges is the possibility of a sexual relation, but only,

> To the extent that there is a sinthome, there is no sexual equivalence, that is to say, there is a relation (. . .) Where there is relation, it is to the extent that there is sinthome, that is to say, to the extent that the other sex is supported by the sinthome.
>
> *(Ibid.: 84)*

The "other sex" here for Lacan is woman for the man, however I suggest that this is more simply the "other of my (sexual) desire" if, as Lacan said, one may line up on one side or the other in the formulae of sexuation. Indeed this is what Lacan suggests in Seminar XXIV where he says that this other "can be the sexual partner" (1976/1977: 3). In Seminar XXIII, however, Lacan declares "If a woman is a sinthome for any man, it's quite clear that another name needs to be found for what is involved in man for a woman, since the sinthome is characterized precisely by non-equivalence" (2016: 84). Harari argues, however, that a different view emerges in his talks from the *Journées de l'École freudiènne de Paris* (9 July 1978), for Lacan now suggests that "So much so that I consider you all out there, insofar as you are, you have every Jack as *sinthome* his Jill. There is a he-sinthome and a she-sinthome (. . .) that's all that's left of the so-called sexual relation" (Lacan, quoted in Harari 1995: 209). Harari adds that what is left

> is for every man to take his woman and vice versa, always as *sinthome*. Thus the sexual relation, or all that's left of it, is an *intersinthomal* relation. This is the "repaired" remains of the "remaining" bound sexual relation in accordance with whatever one's *sinthome* incarnates.
>
> *(Ibid.)*

This is why femininity and masculinity are performances, masquerades, a taking on of a role that also divides the subject in herself.

In his reading of Seminar XXIII, Roberto Harari writes: "What, then, did Joyce carry out by means of his writing, according to Lacan? Nothing less than the *mise en scène* of this quadruple knot" (1995: 62). In his discussion of Joyce's writing, Lacan comments as well on the difficulty of his language, its deformations:

> Joyce writes English with these peculiar refinements that mean that he disarticulates the tongue, the English tongue (. . .) Don't imagine that this only begins with *Finnegans Wake*. Long before, notably in *Ulysses*, he had a way of chopping up sentences that inclined that way. It is truly a process that is exerted in the direction of finding another use for the language in which he writes, a use that is far from ordinary. This is part and parcel of his *savoir-faire* [his know-how].
>
> *(2016: 59)*

And later Lacan speaks of Joyce's

> speech that comes to be written while being broken apart, pulled to pieces – to the point that he ends up dissolving language itself (. . .) imposing on language itself a sort of fracturing, a sort of decomposition, which makes it so that there is no longer any phonatory identity.
>
> *(Ibid.: 79)*

But also that,

> Joyce didn't know that he was fashioning the sinthome, I mean that he was simulating it. He was oblivious to it and it is by dint of this fact that he is a pure artificer, a man of *savoir-faire*, which is what is likewise known as an artist.
>
> *(Ibid.: 99)*

Lacan then asks, "Why is Joyce so unreadable? We must indeed endeavour to imagine why this is so. It might be because he doesn't stir any sympathy in us." To answer this Lacan returns to the question of the link and asks, "Why shouldn't it happen that a knot should fail to be Borromean, that it should be botched?" (ibid.: 131).

This arises if the third ring, the Imaginary, passes between the ring R, the Real, and ring S, the Symbolic. "It slides, and the imaginary relationship has no locus" (ibid.). Lacan then introduces the possibility of a correction to "this mistake, this fault, this lapsus", which is achieved by

> the *Ego* as rectifying the wanting relationship, namely what, in the case of Joyce, does not tie the imaginary in a Borromean fashion to the link between the real and the unconscious. Through this artifice of writing, I would say that the Borromean knot is restored.
>
> *(Ibid.)*

In the very fabrication of his writing, Joyce is restoring the knot through tying together the Real, the Imaginary, and the Symbolic, which is sinthome (ibid.: 44).

Harari posits the "subversive implications of the *sinthome*" (1995: 358), and argues that for analysts, it is not a matter of creating Joycean doubles, but rather of bringing "about in the analysand an inventiveness (. . .) to realise a change of discourse to allow access to a new perception of what is implied by letters and invention, thus to new signifiers" (ibid.: 359). It is this that can arise, as well, in the creative process without analysis, as Joyce did. For Lacan, Harari argues, Joyce marks a rupture in the very conception of art and literature so that "the reader can only feel elided, brushed aside" (ibid.: 231). Indeed, Lacan declares, "The symptom in Joyce (. . .) stands no chance whatsoever of hooking anything of your unconscious" (2016: 145). And Harari writes that "Joyce is forbidding, dumbfounding, in that he prevents imaginary identification. In the face of this, interpretations emerge that are inductive or induced, induced by this *sinthomatic* writing that 'forbids' our access to its supposed clear sense" (1995: 231).[20] We are nevertheless *engaged* by the sinthomatic in Joyce's writing, "addressed", which as such involves a certain form of identification as addressee, as one who "hears" Joyce, but a hearing that will be "awry", as Žižek suggests of the anamorphosis in Holbein's painting of the Ambassadors (1991b: 90–91), following Lacan's discussion of it in *The Four Fundamental Concepts of Psycho-Analysis* (1979: 88–89). In the painting we only see the smear of paint as a skull when we move position, a parallax where two different positions of view produce meanings that are incompatible, and no synthesis or mediation is possible. Similarly, the holding of meaning made possible by the Imaginary and Symbolic is penetrated and made uncertain by the Real of Joyce's project in his writing, in an undoing of "proper" sense. Joyce's wordplay or word deformation/defamation opens us to the problem of sense and sense-making; producing a gap in meaning that is the Real in Lacan's sense.

The sinthome and cinematic enjoyment

Lacan asks, in Seminar XXIII, "In what way is artifice expressly able to target what presents itself in the first instance as a symptom? In what way can art – the artisanal – foil, as it were, what imposes as a symptom?" (2016: 14). And,

> How can an art target in an expressly divinatory way the substantialization of the sinthome in its consistence, but also in its ex-sistence and in its hole? (. . .) How is it that someone has been able to target through his art the rendering of this fourth term [that is] essential to the Borromean knot.
>
> *(Ibid.: 28)*[21]

It is this question that I address in the next section. For Lacan it is the letter and writing that are central, as signifiers, and he rarely discussed films or the photograph, instead he developed his theory through considerations of painting and literature.[22] The art that I am concerned with in this chapter is the cinematic: film, moving pictures and the ways in which the Real – as that which disturbs Imaginary unity and Symbolic forms by reposing lack – might be engaged in film and thereby enabling a questioning of our imagined and Imaginary constructions of self and other – of ideology – that are themselves social constructions. My question here is: can film – as image and sound – not only confront us by a Real, a gap in meaning and in meaning-creation, but also knot the Real, the Imaginary and the Symbolic such that, as well as producing "induced" interpretations, we are also engaged by the sinthomatic that imposes in relation to a certain non-sense? I will explore this question by considering the sinthome in film in three interrelated ways: in relation to a particular filmic character and the emergence in the film's narrative, its storyworld, of what might be understood as her sinthome. In relation to how a film as an artefact, a figural work, might figure as sinthome for the author/director, such as Lacan examines in the work of James Joyce. And in relation to the way in which we as embodied viewers and listeners might be engaged by film in relation to it as sinthome, in a creative response. The two films that I want to consider as sinthomatic, *The Piano* (Jane Campion, 1993) and *Gertrud* (Carl Theodor Dreyer, 1964), each centre the problem of desire and the sexual between men and women but, unlike in Joyce, their focus is a woman character. And both films conclude with a poem that both jars the sense – and the satisfaction – of their endings, and renders the fourth term, the sinthome.

The Piano is a Gothic romance set in the lush and exotic sub-tropical forests of nineteenth-century New Zealand. It centres on Ada McGrath who, at the film's opening, has arrived to marry Alisdair Stewart, the New Zealand colonist with whom her father has arranged her marriage, for she is an unwed mother of a young daughter. *The Piano* is also a story of masculine desire: on the one hand of Stewart, for whom Ada is a wife he has obtained through an arrangement much as he will later obtain land from Baines. To him she is a possession, but also an object of desire, yet who he wishes to be desired by, but doesn't know how to address his demand for love, and approach her. On the other hand, and in contrast, Baines will desire Ada because she *is* a subject of desire, and he wishes her to desire him as she desires her piano. The film's powerful effect on audiences is testified in many writings on it, as Barbara Klinger notes, "taking up sustained residence in their imaginations and emotions" (2006: 19).

It is in the entanglement of desire and piano that Ada moves from symptom to identifying with her sinthome, going through her fundamental fantasy to identify with her sinthome. The voice that the audience hears in the film's opening narration is, we are told, "not my speaking voice, but my mind's voice", for Ada has not spoken a word since she was 6 years old and no one, including herself, knows why. She says that she does not think of herself as silent because of her piano, and through its sounds she expresses herself, but her music is not a language and instead she employs sign language, for which her daughter – Flora – serves as the interpreter. When Ada tells Flora about her father she explains through gestures that she didn't need to speak, for "I could lay thoughts out in his mind like they were a sheet", but they didn't marry because he became frightened, "and stopped listening". It is Ada's muteness that, I suggest, is her symptom, and that she enjoys through her piano as her "voice" – as the way she makes sounds. Her muteness, as her symptom, is, as Žižek notes, not part of the circuit of discourse, and thus of the social bond/network (1991a: 207). Her intense attachment to her piano is both a plot element, and, as her enjoying/jouissance, it is entangled with her sexuality and desire. Lacan, in Seminar XXIII, writes of analysis as teaching the analysand, "to perform a splice between his sinthome and the parasitic Real of jouissance" that is *jous-sens*, enjoyment-in-sense (2016: 58). Thus Žižek argues that "Symptom as *sinthome* is a certain signifying formation penetrated with enjoyment" (emphasis in original), and it is "the only positive support of our being, the only point that gives consistency to the subject" (1991b: 207). It is in the "splicing" that the sinthome is joined to jouissance.

Ferried from the ship on to shore after her long journey, Ada and Flora are forced to stay all night, finding shelter under the canopy of Ada's boned hoop petticoat, until Stewart arrives with Maori porters for their luggage. But her piano is left on the beach, as a burden whose transport Stewart sees no justification for. Missing it, Ada persuades Baines to take her and Flora to it; as she plays he becomes fascinated by her vivid enjoyment, while Flora dances cartwheels and constructs a shell sea horse on the sand. Baines wants the piano-as-Ada, and offers Stewart a piece of land he has wanted, but cannot afford, instead Baines says he will exchange it for Ada'a piano, but he'd then need to have piano lessons. Stewart is eager to make the deal and offers Ada as a teacher. Baines' fascination is now desire, for he then bargains with Ada, offering her a piano key in exchange for each piece of clothing she disrobes, and allowing him to touch her, so that she can "earn" her piano back. He becomes disgusted, however, at his effective prostitution of Ada, saying, "I want you to care for me, but you can't", and gives her back her piano, and thus her body (in one scene, Baines, naked, caresses and embraces the piano), a gesture that reverses his earlier exploitation of her in a recognition of Ada as a subject of desire. It is now that she comes to desire him, sexually, as she had not her husband, and she goes to him. Flora, spying on them, sees them together and tells Stewart – who she now calls papa – of their relation. He then observes them making love, and next day Stewart intercepts Ada after her visit to Baines and attempts to rape her but is interrupted by Flora calling "Mama! Mama! They're playing your piano". Stewart then boards Ada and Flora up in their house, imprisoning them. Learning that Baines is leaving the area, Ada seeks to send Baines a declaration of her love – a piano key – via her daughter but Flora, fearing for the loss of their home, takes it instead to Stewart, who in a rage of jealousy cuts off Ada's index finger, thereby depriving her of her ability to play her piano, the symbol/symptom/sinthome of her jouissance, and of her desire for Baines. That night, as Ada sleeps restlessly, he tells her of his anger, that he meant to love her, but had "clipped your wings". Then, while singing a lullaby, he sees she is very hot and gently removes the bedclothes and caresses her – as she had done to him earlier one night after her incarceration. Now, however, he is sexually aroused and starts to remove his clothes to penetrate her but is stopped when he sees her looking at him, and he murmurs "What?" as if she had spoken.

Stewart now takes his gun and goes to Baines, but instead of killing him, asks "Has Ada ever spoken to you . . . in words?" When Baines says no, Stuart tells him he heard her, "here . . . in my head", and though he did not see her lips move, she said, "I am afraid of my will, of what it might do, it is so strange and strong . . . I have to go, let me go. Let Baines take me away, let him try to save me". He tells Baines to go, take her away, for Stewart just wants it all to be a "bad dream". Ada and Flora leave with Baines, together with her piano that is carefully loaded on to the small boat alongside them. Once at sea she asks Baines to throw her piano overboard but, in error, a rope around it catches her foot and she is dragged into the water with it. She struggles free, choosing life (without the piano) over death by drowning. In the epilogue we see her learning to speak again as we see her playing another, different piano, enabled by her new shiny metal index finger, heard tapping on the piano keys. She says that she imagines her piano in its grave in the sea, and herself suspended above it, which "lulls me to sleep" and that "It is a weird lullaby, and so it is; it is mine". She then recites the first three lines of Thomas Hood's poem "Silence", which also opened the film: "There is a silence where hath been no sound. There is a silence where no sound may be – in the cold grave, under the deep deep sea". This now-remembered scene in which she declares "not that" to death, and to her piano, is the *mise en scène* of her "choice", to live and to speak, it is her identification with her symptom-sinthome.[23] In its remembering it is the scene of an epiphany for Ada. An epiphany takes something existing and makes something new of it. Lacan writes in relation to Joyce, "It's there for the reading in Joyce that epiphany is what makes it so that, by virtue of the fault, the unconscious and the real are tied together" (2016: 134). The "fault" here is the "error" of the rope entwining her foot that arises from Ada's declaration "not that" in relation to her piano. "The 'but not that'", which Lacan declared, "is what I am introducing in this year's seminar on the sinthome" (ibid.: 6). Such a "not that" Harari argues, "is a "reaction", and the "beginning of an escape from the subjection to the neurotic symptom – regarding which the sinthome, in its singularity, would entail a break from these subjective positions" (1995: 32).

As spectators of this sinthomatic scene/seen do we not feel a disappointment with the strangeness of this abrupt happy ending, and thus a break in our identification with Ada and her story of resistance? This we must, for it is Ada's sinthome, which has "no chance whatever of hooking anything of your unconscious"

(Lacan 2016: 145). Yet audiences *are* "hooked" by the film, in an embodied response of both delight and puzzlement. Delight in a Gothic heroine who defies patriarchy and makes her escape.[24] What disturbs, however, is a "strangeness", a gapping of meaning, which Campion has introduced – indeed that is present in all her films.[25] We experience this "gapping" not only in relation to the sudden happy ending, but at the very beginning, with the impossibility of Ada's "mind's voice" speaking to us, which the film opens with. There are also the abrupt cuts to scenes not directly contributing to the film's plot, for example, the performance by the white settlers of the story of Bluebeard and his wives – a story of male power and violence over women – to which the Maori spectators react as if the murders are really happening. Or the cut to Flora hugging trees, copying her Maori playmates, with its sexual implications, for which Stuart forcibly reprimands her for what he calls her "dirtying" of the tree trunks, and then makes her scrub them "clean".[26]

Most signally, this strangeness pervades the final shots. Ada's symptom – her muteness – was supported by her piano, but in choosing to live she abandoned it and the piano lost, drowned, becomes her muteness lost. In her identification with the poem that is "a weird lullaby", her muteness/the piano drowned is consigned to its grave under the sea. Her shiny new metal finger is then the signifier of her identification with her sinthome – her "piano lost" – and it figures both a jouissance that is phallic and a "castration", a limitation on enjoyment; and it does so not only visually but also in its sound, the jarring noise as it hits the key. Here is the *mise en scène* of the quadruple knot of Real, Imaginary, Symbolic and sinthome that Harari noted, a creative process of invention. As sinthome, Ada's prosthetic finger signifies the tying of the Real with the Imaginary and Symbolic, closing the gap, the aporia, which, for example, the gaze as *objet a* opens us to, namely of an irreducible Real. At the same time the Real is figured in the violence that the metal prosthetic finger references, namely Stewart's violent attack on her enjoyment of her symptom/her piano playing when he hacked it off in anger at her adultery with Baines. Not only does the film narrate a feminine desire, and sinthome, but it also re-poses the difficulties – as well as different possibilities – of masculine desire, and love.

In *Gertrud*, too, feminine desire and its difficulties are central, and in this film as well a poem figures the sinthomic. *Gertrud* was Carl Theodor Dreyer's last film, and that he felt was one of his most important works, what is also centered is a woman's desire for love, which remains unfulfilled, and that is explored in relation to masculine desire through its three male characters' relation to Gertrud.[27] The film's plot, its central enigma in Roland Barthes' sense[28] – both for the other characters and for the spectator – is the love that its protagonist, Gertrud, seeks from each of the men, and it is in the filmic narration of her quest that the symptom/sinthome appears. Dreyer has said that "I'm interested in generally a single person in the film – *Joan of Arc* (1928), *Day of Wrath* (1944), and generally women" (1966: 62), and these are often a female character who stands opposed to masculine hypocrisy, to the oppressive structures of church, state and patriarchal convention, even at the cost of her life. Gertrud is another such character, but whose steadfast commitment does not lead to her death. While Dreyer's films are not autobiographical, the emergence of what I shall argue is the "rendering of the fourth term, the sinthome" (Lacan 2016: 28) can be understood as also a figuring for Dreyer himself.[29]

The film is based on the play *Gertrud* by the Swedish writer, Hjalmar Söderberg, set in the early twentieth century, about his unhappy affair with the opera singer Maria von Platen, in which he stages the question that baffled Freud: *What does woman want?* Dreyer, however, has reversed the narrative perspective of Soderberg's play from that of the men and their loss of Gertrud, to that of Gertrud and her gospel of love, and in doing so poses the problem of the question itself, namely, as Lacan identifies it, that there is no sexual relation. Dryer retains the three main characters from the play,[30] as well as using scenes and dialogue, but he places the spectator very differently: narratively, by centering Gertrud, and by changing the play's story arc in the epilogue he added. And he changes the play filmically, by his highly formal and stylised filming and *mise en scène.* It is through Dreyer's deployment of both narrative form and film form that the sinthomic appears.

Gertrud is a former singer, now married to an ambitious politician, Gustav Kanning, but this marriage has become (or always was) without love on her part, though not without sexual passion. Gertrud instead finds love with a young composer, Erland Jansson. He is revealed, however, to be unworthy of her by Gabriel Lidman, her former lover and a celebrated poet returned home to receive the honours of his country and, perhaps, to persuade Gertrud to return to him. Gertrud had left Lidman when she discovered that he saw her love for him as a distraction from his work and hence as secondary to his more serious project as a poet. At the end of the play she leaves all three men, each of whom has failed to meet her ideal of love, but in the film she goes to Paris with her friend Axel Nygren – a character not in the play – to study dreams and psychoanalysis.

In the film each man Gertrud has loved fails her by showing that she is not sufficient to his desire; Kanning says, "But Gertrud, dear, love can't fill a man's life. It would be ridiculous, for a man"; while Lidman had earlier written alongside his sketch of her profiled face, "woman's love and man's work – enemies from the start"; and for Erland she is "too proud", in refusing to share him with other women. Gertrud, for these men, is the *objet a*, cause of their desire and their symptom, which is not love. Thus Gertrud also fails each of them, her jouissance being elsewhere in her demand for love, which appears in her response to Erland's music, seen when he plays for her and she sings the words of his "Serenade": "The darkness has formed a pearl, The night has borne a dream. Hidden, it will grow inside me, Blindingly white and tender". This scene is the prelude to their love-making, while the song references Freud's account of the formation of the symptom as like that of a pearl (1905/1953: 83). Gertrud had, she says, pursued Erland, and she "doesn't understand" her love for him.

While in the play Gertrud's pursuit of love leads her to loneliness, in the film this is reversed; Gertrud identifies as a woman of free will, consciously choosing to forsake these men's love, and thereby she follows Lacan's demand that one should not give up on one's desire, "given that desire is understood here (. . .) as the metonymy of our being" (1992: 321). Moreover what Gertrud declares to each of her three lovers is not simply "not you", but more importantly, it is an affirmation of "love" and thus a declaration of "not that": not that kind of love each offered her, namely of woman-as-symptom. Here arises, as in *The Piano*, the "but not that" which Lacan introduced (2016: 16), and Harari argued was the "beginning of an escape from the subjection to the neurotic symptom" (1995: 32). The love that Gertrud sought was on the one hand a love that each man was not capable of because, as symptom, she was "not all" for them in their lives; on the other hand their lives were "not all" without her. For Gertrud, there is an "all of love" in loving that she demands, and it is here that we can see her symptom-as-sinthome in the repetition of her demand, while in leaving each of the men she acts out the impossibility of being for them their symptom.

Dreyer, however, added an entirely new sequence in the film as an epilogue, in which we see Gertrud – now very elderly – meet for the last time with her old friend Axel Nygren. Dreyer, while he justified the scene as drawing on comments Söderberg had later made (cited by Rosenbaum 1995: 111), he writes that his central concern in introducing the epilogue was to ensure sympathy for Gertrud at the film's closure, rather than ending with her running away to Paris, "and the public had the satisfaction to see this woman didn't break down and she didn't regret. She had chosen solitude and she accepted it" (Dreyer 1966: 36). Dreyer replaces loneliness with solitude, removing the sense of absolute tragedy in Söderberg, and by giving her a life after her lovers – namely her work in Paris – Dreyer makes Gertrud a woman of her own choices and not a woman who sacrifices herself to a fatalistic ideal of a reciprocated love.

The sympathy, or even identification, that the film could invoke might include being moved by and admiring her commitment to love, perhaps even being envious of the integrity of her commitment, and of the way in which it sustains her. That is, we might envy her sinthome, to which nevertheless we cannot connect! We may of course identify with the place of addressee of Gertrud's love – as one who fails her, as Gabriel did when he ridiculed her love; or perhaps identify as the one who could return her love and thus who does know, in reviewer Kirk Bond's words: "really what love is" (1966: 68). Tom Milne describes *Gertrud* as a film "about a rather tiresome woman mid-way between an Ibsen bluestocking and a Strindberg shrew whose behaviour seems almost like an advertisement for women's rights" (1971: 168).[31] Nevertheless, he sees beneath "its naturalistic surface, its near-Ibsen conflicts, that it is Dreyer's most mysterious and personal, most supernatural film, glowing with a more secret magic than any previous work" and "the whole film echoes like counterpoint for two voices – 'I love you' and 'Come with me' – which never quite coincide" (ibid.: 170–171). Rejecting the story and what he calls its "almost dogged literalness" of treatment, another meaning is obtained whereby Milne comes to find a position, a place of address, of the impossibility of the two discourses: of the masculine and the feminine.

Love for Lacan, is similarly not straightforward for, in his seminar on anxiety, he declares that,

> What we give in love is essentially what we haven't got and when this not having comes back at us there is most certainly regression and at the same time a revelation of the way in which we have left him wanting, so as to represent this lack.
>
> *(2014: 141)*

Instead, in *Encore*, Lacan points to love as the illusion that the sexual relation "stops not being written", and thus "doesn't stop being written" (1999: 144). It is this illusion that *Gertrud* addresses.

In the epilogue, many years later Axel visits Gertrud on the occasion of her birthday, bringing her a copy of his new book, and she returns to him the letters he had sent her for, with their "warm and good words spoken from your heart", she does not want strangers to read them, and he then burns them in the fire – a corresponding act of closure. He asks her if she has ever written poetry, and in reply Gertrud reads to Axel her short poem written at the age of 16, that she calls her "gospel of love":

> Just look at me. Am I beautiful?
> No.
> But I have loved.
> Just look at me. Am I young?
> No.
> But I have loved.
> Just look at me. Do I live?
> No.
> But I have loved.

And with quiet satisfaction she tells Axel that she has asked the words "*Amor Omnia*" – love is everything – to be on her gravestone. It is here that Gertrud's identification with her symptom-sinthome appears, namely in the identification realised in Gertrud's avowal in her poem, "Just look at me. Am I beautiful? No. But I have loved", whereby she asserts her being and her agency without reference to the other of her loving, and thus independently of either the other's reciprocation or its absence. The anticipatory grammar of the poem written as a young girl, in which being beautiful is denied while having loved is claimed, implies a future time that is identified with, in which "being beautiful" – object of desire/symptom for men – is denied. Instead she affirms herself as "having loved", in an identification that secures her consistency as an individual, her individuation. Her identification with the sinthome is a naming of her Real, individualising the lack in the Symbolic as other than the Name-of-The-Father, and thereby assuming the real lack in the Other (Chiesa 2005: 188).

Gertrud was for Dreyer a highly personal project, demonstrated both by his very different scripting of Gertrud's story, and in his film form that, pared down and simple but at the same time foregrounded, is like Joyce's wordplay. The filmic strategies in *Gertrud* continually distance the spectator to produce a sense of separation, while also experienced as portending. The very long takes result in a sense of elongation or extension to scenes unrelieved by shot changes or point-of-view "insights"; and the similarity of scenes organised around dialogue exchanges – with characters moving between chairs, sofas, chair arms, benches, etc. as they talk to each other but rarely gaze at one another or are shown exchanging looks – produces an awareness of form as such.[32] It is through his film form that Dreyer enables the film's "secret magic" that Milne writes of, and that Jean-Luc Godard saw as "equal, in madness and beauty, to the last works of Beethoven" (cited in Rosenbaum 1995: 114).[33] As such it is a mode of "gapping", a perceived incompleteness of visual meaning. In the epilogue, however, Dreyer relents on this highly formal style, and now shows Gertrud and Axel exchanging looks as they reminisce about their past together, introducing an intimacy absent earlier. The scene in which she takes her poem from her desk, then joins Axel at the sofa and reads it to him is a single shot some five minutes long. They are initially framed in medium-close two-shot, with the fire, burning brightly, seen in the background between them, and they look directly at each other as they talk. Gertrud, answering Axel, affirms that she regrets nothing, and declares, "I suffered much and often made mistakes, but I have loved". The shot ends as they each rise from the sofa and walk to the door, as Gertrud describes how she has imagined Axel in the future visiting her grave and picking the anemones growing on it, and she tells him "Take it as a word of love that was thought, but never spoken". But she says this in closure, for she now asks him to go, "otherwise we'll end up by running off to Paris", and the shot ends as they say goodbye and she stands at the door he has exited, in medium shot, watching him leave. It is only now that there is a POV sequence, filmed in four reverse field shots, first of Axel in long shot walking away, then turning to wave goodbye, second of Gertrud as she waves back to Axel seen from her vantage point, but now in the medium shot thus we do not see her from Axel's position. The third and fourth shots repeat the first two, as Axel picks up his hat and coat then looks back and again waves to Gertrud, then the film cuts to Gertrud as in shot three, who also waves then slowly shuts the door. The sound of church bells ringing and music that were heard at the beginning of the epilogue are now heard again as the film ends.

Dreyer's shot composition and absence of POV and shot/reverse-shot editing earlier in the film can be understood figuring Gertrud as "caught" by the gaze/desire of these men who cannot love her as she desires. Indeed it is this that is directly alluded to in the painting Dreyer positioned behind Gertrud at the reception for Lidman, of a naked woman pursued by hounds, which startles and distresses her, as well as the mirror Gabriel gave her so that she might see how beautiful she is. But in filming Gertrud and Axel's leave-taking through these POV shots Dreyer is visually presenting an epiphany, of Gertrud now "free" of the gaze. Dreyer suspends narrative, storytelling, in this sequence while the closed door beyond which is Gertrud is both a closure and a holding, the woman, perhaps mother, gone but there, free in herself.[34] What is framed by the cinematic is the knotting of the Real, Imaginary and Symbolic that is the sinthome, for "through his art", as Lacan suggests, Dreyer is producing a "rendering of this fourth term" (2016: 28). The sinthome is a naming of the Real, and it is given a material existence, a consistence, in the film form through these four reverse field shots, but, because only two of the shots – namely Gertrud's – are true POV shots, it also introduces the camera's gaze that is external to Gertrud as a subject. It is an otherness, a strangeness – ex-sisting, that nevertheless insists and thus a hole, a gap in the repeated shots/views that nevertheless re-mark lack for the subject for the spectator and perhaps for Dreyer, as his sinthome. As such, this highly conventional shot sequence is a visual, that is cinematic, equivalent of Gertrud's poem, in its knotting of the Real, the Symbolic and the Imaginary.

In this discussion what I have sought to show through my exploration of each film in relation to what Lacan identifies in his term "sinthome" and his concept of the "not that", is the subject's individuation without the phallic signifier. I see this arising not as a "feminine way", but rather as other or as indifferent to the sexual difference that, I argued earlier, is posited by the Symbolic order for, as Lacan asserts: "The subject's sexual position (. . .) is tied to the symbolic apparatus" (1993: 171). Our identification as sexed beings is an identification as sexual, and as sexually different in the unconscious and in the subject as a conscious felt, but the two may not be the same. The unconscious is the discourse of the Other and thus belongs to the Symbolic order, for as Lacan argues in Seminar XXIV, "It is the Other with a capital O that is at stake in the unconscious. I do not see how one could give a sense to the unconscious, except by situating it in this Other, the bearer of signifiers" (1976–1977: 3).[35] This Other, which is also the m/Other, introduces the Real of lack in that it desires. The naming and names of sexual difference both institute and attempt to assuage this lack but whose failure the symptom attests to. For Lacan, the concept of the sinthome as knotting the Real, Symbolic and the Imaginary is a naming of one's Real, one's lacking, which is, it seems, indifferent to sexual difference. In conclusion, therefore, I speculate that what we name as our sexual difference is itself a sinthome.

Notes

1 Cited by Ernest Jones in his biography *Sigmund Freud: Life and Work* (1953: 421). Bonaparte's answer, if any, is not recorded by Jones. Freud writes, in "The Question of Lay Analysis", "We know less about the sexual life of little girls than of boys. But we need not feel ashamed of this distinction; after all, the sexual life of adult women is a 'dark continent' for psychology" (1926/1959: 212). The implicit reference to the African continent has been much commented upon for its problematic implication of the unknowability of those placed as other. Equally problematic is the suggestion in the metaphor that "the feminine", like Africa, is a singular territory and that it is only men for whom feminine desire is a riddle.

2 The phrase is used in following Seminars, especially in *Encore* in relation to the sexual relation not being "able to write the sexual relationship" (Lacan 1999: 35).

3 The conclusion of the treatment is "the identification with the Real of the symptom, the choice of jouissance, and the creation of a neosubject" (Verhaeghe and Declercq 2002: 76), which I explore later in this chapter. Bracha Lichtenberg Ettinger has similarly identified the radical implications of Lacan's concept of the sinthome for the sexual relation and for femininity in developing her concept of the "matrixial". She writes: "We need to give the *sinthome* a matrixial twist in order to discover what a 'woman' can become in-difference for a woman" (2006: 191).

4 "There is often a passage in even the most thoroughly interpreted dream which has to be left obscure; this is because we become aware during the work of interpretation that at that point there is a tangle of dream-thoughts which cannot be unraveled and which moreover adds nothing to our knowledge of the content of the dream. This is the dream's navel, the spot where it reaches down into the unknown" (Freud 1900/1953: 525).

5 Cited by Justin Clemens in *Psychoanalysis is an Antiphilosophy* (2013: 4); Lacan, *Autres Écrits* (2001: 314).

6 Joan Riviere used the term in her article "Womanliness as Masquerade", where she concluded that there is no difference "between genuine womanliness and the 'masquerade' (. . .) whether radical or superficial they are the same thing" (1926: 306). I explored the role of the masquerade in *Representing the Woman: Cinema and Psychoanalysis* (1997: 239–245).

7 Mitchell in her earlier work had rejected the term gender because its use too often simply replaced biological determinism with social determinism, leaving out the unconscious. But she comments that in her recent work she has drawn on the term to address the ways in which "'gender' is different from 'sexual difference'. I use 'gender' for lateral relations, and 'sexual difference' for vertical relations. Vertical relations implicate identifications with parents, and lead on to descent via reproduction (. . .) Within a psychoanalytic framework I would say that sexual difference is 'achieved' after the castration complex", whereas she argues "gender emerges earlier as a distinction between bisexual children into girls and boys" (2015: 126).

8 Laplanche's term in French for "sexual" is in the broader sense that is given in the term sexuality in English, whereas the usual term "*le sexuel*" in French retains its connection to *sexue*, which designates anatomical difference. Thus he argues "For Freud, *le 'sexual'* is thus external, if not actually prior, to sexual difference, indeed to gender difference: it is oral, anal or paragenital [polymorphous perverse]" (2007: 203).

9 The contingency of upright stance in humans that obscures the female genital organs that in other animals are "perfectly perceptible, visible" (Laplanche 2007: 216). Thus, Laplanche asks, "Isn't *this contingency an extraordinary destiny?* The upright stance makes the feminine organs inaccessible to perception. Now, this contingency has been elevated by many civilisations, and no doubt our own, to the rank of the major, universal signifier of presence/absence" (ibid.: 217). In questioning the inevitability of the castration complex Laplanche points out "After all, in analyses, memories linked to the castration complex are often found in attenuated form. Attenuated: that is, themselves compromised by what they want to repress (. . .) '*le sexual*'" (ibid.: 218). This repressing thereby creates it.

10 Lacan, drawing on Riviere's discussion, writes, "Paradoxical as this formulation may seem, I would say that it is in order to be the phallus – that is, the signifier of the Other's desire – that a woman rejects as essential part of femininity, namely, all its attributes, in the masquerade. It is for what she is not that she expects to be desired as well as loved" (2005: 583). And that, because the woman performs femininity, it "has the curious consequence of making virile display in human beings seem feminine" (ibid.: 584).

11 The English translation gives the formulation of male side, then refers to "not-whole" for those placing themselves on the formulation of the right side, but "not-all" is a preferable translation as used by Lorenzo Chiesa (2016: 3, and throughout).

12 Joan Copjec has shown that the formulae of sexuation and their exceptions should also be understood through Kant's classical logic of antinomies of pure reason in which he argued that mathematical antinomies demonstrated the limits of reason. "His point",

Copjec argues, "is that our reason is limited because *the procedures of our knowledge have no term; what limits reason is a lack of reason*" (1994: 223, emphasis in original). Her argument here is that "All pretentions of masculinity are, then sheer imposture; just as every display of femininity is sheer masquerade. Through his desubstantialisation of sex, Lacan has allowed us to perceive the fraudulence at the heart of every claim to positive sexual identity" (ibid.: 234).

13 I have used Cormac Gallagher's translation here, which is slightly different, including "contrary to what is said ..." at the beginning of the sentence "The woman has to ...", producing a slightly different meaning, which is the one I am drawing upon.

14 I am drawing here on comments by Adrian Price, the translator of *The Sinthome* in English, in his keynote paper given at the symposium "Psychoanalysis and the Symptom", Sopot, Poland, 7–9 April 2017.

15 On this see Freud's "Introduction to *Psycho-Analysis and the War Neuroses*" (1919/1955).

16 Adrian Johnston explains that the matheme of fantasy ($ ◊ a), the diamond-shaped "lozenge" (poinçon) ◊ can be read as a condensation of four symbols in logic: "conjunction"; "disjunction" [or]); "greater than"; and, "less than". The subject's desires are scripted and orchestrated by an unconscious fundamental fantasy in which the desiring subject ($) is positioned in relation to its corresponding object-cause of desire, each of the four aspects thus being possible variants of this positioning of $ vis-à-vis *objet a*. "Singular subjects flesh out conjunction, disjunction, being 'greater than', and being 'less than' in their own styles, namely, as their unique fantasies of merger or symbiosis (conjunction), scorn or refusal (disjunction), mastery or domination ('greater than'), slavery or submission ('less than'), and any number of other possible particularizations of these four basic categories of rapport". https://plato.stanford.edu/entries/lacan (accessed 19 February 2018).

17 Lacan devoted the year of his Seminar XIV *The Logic of Phantasy* (1966–1967), to unravelling the theoretical implications of the inscription of fantasy in the unconscious signifying structure. He argued that fantasy would perform the essential function of "knotting" the psychical registers of the Symbolic, the Imaginary and the Real – and thus of constituting what Freud called "psychic reality".

18 Morel is addressing here the central role Lacan gives the "mother"-carer, "The child who learns to speak remains marked for the rest of his or her life both the words and the jouissance of the mother (or her substitute). This leads to a subjectivation to her demand, desire, and jouissance, 'the law of the mother', from which one should separate him – or herself". This law, she says, "inherits the properties of the feminine 'not-all': it is an unlimited law", unlike the law of the father. Both Morel and Lacan, as Laplanche too, qualify the term "mother" as the central carer, not the biological personal who gave birth to the child. We might question, therefore, the role of the descriptor "feminine" in the "not-all" of jouissance (Morel 2006: 69). Morel develops her discussion of the sinthome in relation to two fascinating case studies.

19 As Adrian Price has noted, Lacan does not consistently use the term sinthome in relation to the identification with the symptom (see above).

20 Harari writes this as, "The *sinthome* in Joyce is a *sinthome* that has nothing to do with you" (1995: 230).

21 The sinthome ex-sists, eccentric or outside the symbolic order, while the sinthome's knotting of the symbolic, imaginary and real, always at the same time inscribes a "hole", a gap or gapping, which Lacan demonstrates through his different tying of the Borromean knots in Seminar XXIII, for holes thereby appear in the space delineated by the threads of the knotting, just as the knitting of wool in holes are created between the links of wool. Žižek writes that ex-sistence is Lacan's expression for "the impossible-real kernel resisting symbolization" (1991b: 136).

22 In Seminar XXIII, however, Lacan does, having just seen Oshima's *The Realm of the Senses* (1976), which he says he was "taken aback by (...) because of its female eroticism", by which he means what is involved for the woman in castrating the man after his death by erotic strangulation, but that "We all know that it's a fantasy" (2016: 107).

23 Barbara Klinger notes of the piano lost that returns in the film's final image that "the viewer is not sure how to interpret its surprise return and the accompanying depiction of Ada's other possible fate (. . .) Indeed the mysteries of the interpretive and affective dimensions of this image have become a mainstay of my viewing of *The Piano*" (2006: 24).

24 Vivian Sobchack writes that, "Campion's film moved me deeply, stirring my bodily senses and my sense of my body. The film not only 'filled me up' and often 'suffocated' me with feelings that resonated in and constricted my chest and stomach, but it also 'sensitized' the very surfaces of my skin (. . .) a body that was achingly aware of itself as a sensuous, sensitized, sensible material capacity" (2004: 61–62). See also: Sue Gillett, "Lips and Fingers: Jane Campion's *The Piano*" (1995: 286), and her *Views from Beyond the Mirror: The Films of Jane Campion* (2004).

25 Klinger writes of the "inscrutable visual and the inevitable associative processes at work" in the *The Piano*, and refers to Barthes' formulation of a "third meaning" that resonates with an excess signification (2006: 21; Barthes 1977: 52–68). This is the sense in which I use the term "gapping", now in a psychoanalytical context.

26 As many writers have noted, Campion's use of sexual relations in Maori culture as open and freer plays to Western ideas of the sexuality of the racial other while nevertheless foregrounding the problematic role of the white colonialists. This too introduces a gapping, an uncomfortableness, for feminist audiences. For example, Dyson, "The Return of the Repressed?" and Leonie Pihama's "Ebony and Ivory: Construction of the Maori in *The Piano*", in Harriet Margolis', *Jane Campion's "The Piano"* (2000: 114–134). And Laleen Jayamanne, *Toward Cinema and Its Double: Cross-Cultural Mimesis* (2001: 48).

27 My discussion here develops my earlier analysis of *Gertrud* (1997: 248–260).

28 In *S/Z* Barthes terms the "hermeneutic code" the series of enigmas that are posed by the narrative, of questions whose answers are suspended, until a final disclosure (1975: 18–19).

29 This concern may be understood in relation to Dreyer's personal history, for he was an illegitimate child whose birth mother was reviled by his adoptive parents, and who had died painfully as the result of an unsuccessful abortion attempt of another unwanted pregnancy outside marriage. Growing up lonely and taciturn, as he writes later in a brief autobiographical sketch, "he reveres and idealizes the image of his real mother (. . .) regarding her as a victim rather than a villainess", writes Jonathan Rosenbaum in his essay "*Gertrud* as Non-Narrative" (2017: 4), online.

30 Jonathan Rosenbaum notes that in the play all the characters are somewhat unpleasant, "especially Gabriel, who is more of a wastrel, and Gertrud whose cruel streak and chatter make her distinctly less heroic" (1995: 111).

31 It is in reviews of the film that the ambivalence to which the demand for love gives rise is apparent. Kirk Bond writes of it as a soap opera "in which the woman cannot or will not understand the man has interests of his own that are necessary in the scheme of things. She must have the man's total devotion (. . .) here is the rather gratuitous suffering of a 'woman's story'". Yet he also acknowledges that "Dreyer is saying (. . .) that man must once more know really what love is" (1966: 68, 69).

32 Jacques Rivette, commented that: "If Dreyer's film (. . .) doesn't function formally as a dream, it nevertheless (. . .) prescribes an 'oneiric' vocabulary: at once the telling of a dream and a session of analysis, an analysis in which the roles are ceaselessly changing; subjected to the flow, the regular tide of the long takes, the mesmeric passes of the incessant camera movements, the even monotone of the voices, the steadiness of the eyes – always turned aside, often parallel, towards us: a little above us – the strained immobility of the bodies, huddled in armchairs, on sofas behind which the other silently stands, fixed in ritual attitudes which make them no more than corridors for speech to pass through, gliding through a semi-obscurity arbitrarily punctuated with luminous zones into which the somnambulists emerge of their own accord" (Rivette 1969, cited by Rosenbaum 1995: 111).

33 Rosenbaum comments that "one wonders whether [Godard] might have been partly thinking of the question and answer written by Beethoven as an epigraph to the finale of the last quartet (the corresponding musical passage figures centrally in *2 Ou 3 Choses que je sais d'elle*): "Muss es sein? Es muss sein!" (Must it be? It must be!)" (1995: 114–115).

34 Rosenbaum, in his very fine discussion of the film, addresses the strangeness of this ending in a way that suggests the sinthome when he writes that this "static image" refers back to Dreyer's mother, and is a "nonnarrative realm", which he describes as "a state that both precedes and follows any need to acknowledge his father, any necessity to tell a story, placing narrative within parentheses" (1995: 116).

35 The reference is to the unofficial translation by Cormac Gallagher, www.lacaninireland.com/web/wp-content/uploads/2010/06/insu-Seminar-XXIV-Final-Sessions-1-12-1976-1977.pdf.

Bibliography

Adams, P. and Cowie, E. (1990) *The Woman in Question*. Cambridge, MA: MIT Press.

Barthes, R. (1975) *S/Z*. London: Jonathan Cape.

Barthes, R. (1977) *Image, Music, Text*. New York: Hill & Wang.

Chiesa, L. (2005) Lacan *Le-sinthome. (Re)-Turn: A Journal of Lacanian Studies*, Spring, 157–170.

Chiesa, L. (2016) *The Not-Two: Logic and God in Lacan*. Cambridge, MA: MIT Press.

Clemens, J. (2013) *Psychoanalysis is an Antiphilosophy*. Edinburgh: Edinburgh University Press.

Copjec, J. (1994) *Read My Desire*. Cambridge, MA: MIT Press.

Cowie, E. (1997) *Representing the Woman: Cinema and Psychoanalysis*. London: Macmillan Press.

Bond, K. (1966) The Basic Demand of Life for Love. *Film Comment*, 4, 67–69.

Dreyer, C. T. (1966) My Way of Working Is in Relation to the Future: A Conversation with Carl Dreyer. *Film Comment*, 4, 62–67.

Dreyer, C. T. (1991) *In Double Reflection*. New York: Da Capo Press.

Ettinger, B. L. (2006) *The Matrixial Borderspace*. Minneapolis, MN: University of Minnesota Press.

Jonathan, J. (2017) *Gertrud* as Non-Narrative: The Desire for the Image. Available at: www.jonathanrosenbaum.net/2017/08/gertrud-as-nonnarrative-the-desire-for-the-image.

Fink, B. (1996) *The Lacanian Subject: Between Language and Jouissance*. Princeton, NJ: Princeton University Press.

Freud, S. (1900/1953) The Interpretation of Dreams. In J. Strachey (ed.) *The Standard Edition of the Complete Psychological Works of Sigmund Freud*, Vol. V. London: Hogarth Press.

Freud, S. (1905/1953) Fragment of an Analysis of a Case of Hysteria. In J. Strachey (ed.) *The Standard Edition of the Complete Psychological Works of Sigmund Freud*, Vol. VII. London: Hogarth Press.

Freud, S. (1919/1955) Introduction to *Psycho-Analysis and the War Neuroses*. In J. Strachey (ed.) *The Standard Edition of the Complete Psychological Works of Sigmund Freud*, Vol. XII. London: Hogarth Press.

Freud, S. (1926/1959) The Question of Lay Analysis. In J. Strachey (ed.) *The Standard Edition of the Complete Psychological Works of Sigmund Freud*, Vol. XX. London: Hogarth Press.

Freud, S. (1933/1964). On Femininity. In J. Strachey (ed.) *The Standard Edition of the Complete Psychological Works of Sigmund Freud*, Vol. XXII. London: Hogarth Press.

Gillett, S. (1995) Lips and Fingers: Jane Campion's *The Piano*. *Screen*, 36(3), 277–287.

Gillett, S. (2004) *Views from Beyond the Mirror: The Films of Jane Campion*. St Kilda: Australian Teachers of Media.

Harari, R. (1995) *How James Joyce Made His Name: A Reading of the Final Lacan*. New York: The Other Press.

Jayamanne, L. (2001) *Toward Everyday Cinema and Its Double: Cross-Cultural Mimesis*. Bloomington, IN: Indiana University Press.

Jones, E. (1953) *Sigmund Freud: Life and Work*, Vol. 2. London: Hogarth Press.

Klinger, B. (2006) The Art Film, Affect and the Female Viewer: *The Piano* Revisited. *Screen*, 47(1), 19–41.

Lacan, J. (1965) *Seminar XII, Crucial Problems for Psychoanalysis*. Trans. C. Gallagher. Available at: www.lacaninireland.com.

Lacan, J. (1976–1977) *Seminar XXIV, L'insu que sait . . . . Final Sessions 1–12* Trans. C. Gallagher. Available at: www.lacaninireland.com.

Lacan, J. (1979) *The Four Fundamental Concepts of Psycho-Analysis*. Trans. A. Sheridan. London: Penguin Books.

Lacan, J. (1982). *Seminar XXII, RSI* (1974/1975), extract from the Seminar of 21 January 1975. In J. Mitchell and J. Rose (eds.) *Feminine Sexuality: Jacques Lacan and the école freudienne*. New York: Norton. Complete translation by C. Gallagher, Cormac. Available at: www.lacaninireland.com.

Lacan, J. (1992) *The Ethics of Psychoanalysis*. Trans. Dennis Porter. London: Routledge.

Lacan, J. (1993) *The Psychoses*. Trans. R. Grigg. London. Routledge.

Lacan, J. (1999) *Encore: The Seminar of Jacques Lacan Book XX: On Femininity, the Limits of Love and Knowledge, 1972–3*. Trans. B. Fink. New York: Norton.

Lacan, J. (2001). *Autres Écrits*. Paris: Éditions du Seuil.

Lacan, J. (2005) *Écrits*. Trans. B. Fink. New York: Norton.

Lacan, J. (2006) *Le séminaire. Livre XVIII. D'un discours qui ne serait pas du semblant*. Paris: Editions du Seuil.

Lacan, J. (2014) *Anxiety: The Seminar of Jacques Lacan, Book X*. Trans. A. R. Price. Cambridge: Polity Press.

Lacan, J. (2016) *The Sinthome: The Seminar of Jacques Lacan, Book XXIII*. Trans. A. R. Price. Cambridge: Polity Press.

Laplanche, J. (2007) Gender, Sex, and the Sexual. *Studies in Gender and Sexuality*, 8(2), 201–209.

Margolis, H. (ed.) (2000) *Jane Campion's "The Piano"*. Cambridge: Cambridge University Press.

Milne, T. (1971) *The Cinema of Carl Dreyer*. London: Tantivy.

Mitchell, J. (1974) *Psychoanalysis and Feminism*. London: Allen Lane.

Mitchell, J. (2015) Interview with Juliet Mitchell – *Psychoanalysis and Feminism*: Then and Now, with Wendy Hollway and Julie Walsh. *Psychoanalysis & Society*, 2(2), 12–130.

Mitchell, J. and Rose, J. (1982) *Feminine Sexuality: Jacques Lacan and the école freudienne*. New York: Norton.

Morel, G. (2005) Sexe, genre et identité: du symptôme au sinthome. *Cités*, 21, 61–78. Translated and available online at: http://.cairn-int.infor/article-E_CITE_021_0061.

Morel, G. (2006) The Sexual Sinthome. *Umbr(a): Incurable*, 1, 65–83.

Riviere, J. (1926) Womanliness as Masquerade. *International Journal of Psycho-Analysis*, X. Reprinted in V. Burgin, J. Donald and C. Kaplan (eds.) *Formations of Fantasy*. London: Routledge.

Rosenbaum, J. (1995). *Placing Movies: The Practice of Film Criticism*. Los Angeles, CA: University of California Press.

Safouan, M. (1990) Men and Women: A Psychoanalytic Point of View. In P. Adams and E. Cowie (eds.) *The Woman in Question*. Cambridge, MA: MIT Press.

Shepherdson, C. (2003) Lacan and Philosophy. In J.-M. Rabaté (ed.) *The Cambridge Companion to Lacan*. Cambridge: Cambridge University Press.

Sobchack, V. (2004). *Carnal Thoughts: Embodiment and Moving Image Culture*. Berkley, CA: University of California Press.

Verhaeghe, P. and Declercq, F. (2002) Lacan's Goal of Analysis: *Le Sinthome* or the Feminine Way. In L. Thurston (ed.) *Essays on the Final Lacan: Re-Inventing the Symptom*. New York: The Other Press.

Žižek, S. (1991a) The Truth Arises from Misrecognition. In E. Ragland-Sullivan and M. Bracjher (eds.) *Lacan and the Subject of Language*. New York: Routledge.

Žižek, S. (1991b) *Looking Awry: An Introduction to Jacques Lacan through Popular Culture*. Cambridge, MA: MIT Press.

2

HER SKIN AGAINST THE ROCKS, THE ROCKS AGAINST THE SKY

Revisiting Weir's *Picnic at Hanging Rock* (1975) after Morley's *The Falling* (2014) and Freud's fable of female hysteria[1]

Davina Quinlivan

Picnic at Hanging Rock is Peter Weir's stunning 1975 adaption of Joan Lindsay's 1967 classic novel that follows the mysterious disappearance of a group of schoolgirls after a Valentine's Day picnic in the Australian Outback. Weir's film is lush, evocative and elliptical, as oneiric and shimmering as the sun-bleached day itself in which the girls vanish from existence: girls lie curled on rocks, their dresses folded around them while they sleep, voices scatter into the wind. More recently, the film-maker Carol Morley has directed a similarly sensuous tale, *The Falling* (2014), in which a group of British girls experience a wave of hysterical exhaustion, fainting, falling into a deep slumber during a dizzying spell of eerie contagion. While both films focus on a particular period in the lives of a group of schoolgirls, moments set against the backdrop of balmy summer heat, I am interested in their individual reflections on female hysteria and its embodiment through the diegetic bodies on-screen as well as formal attributes such as sound, composition and colour. Freud is well known for his studies in hysteria and the epidemic of this condition that was most prevalent during the nineteenth century; my choice of films reflect their contemporary response to hysteria and, specifically, challenge conceptions of hysteria as a forgotten phenomenon of the past.

Most significantly, Morley is fascinated by the symbolism and imagery of fainting, which, in her film, comes to represent a manifestation of denied or displaced sexuality, inspired by 'the explanation traditionally offered for hysterical outbreaks – particularly in late 17th-century Salem' (2015a). Salem's 'hysteria' is especially called to mind during one of *The Falling*'s most memorable sequences in which we view the central protagonist, Lydia, carried by other girls, her back against their hands, her body lifted by their fingers, uncannily evoking the potent imagery of witchcraft, sleep and the sensuous, female body, so powerfully associated with Weir's masterpiece. This chapter will consider the concordances and rich visual and sonic correspondences between Morley's film and *Picnic at Hanging Rock*, tracing

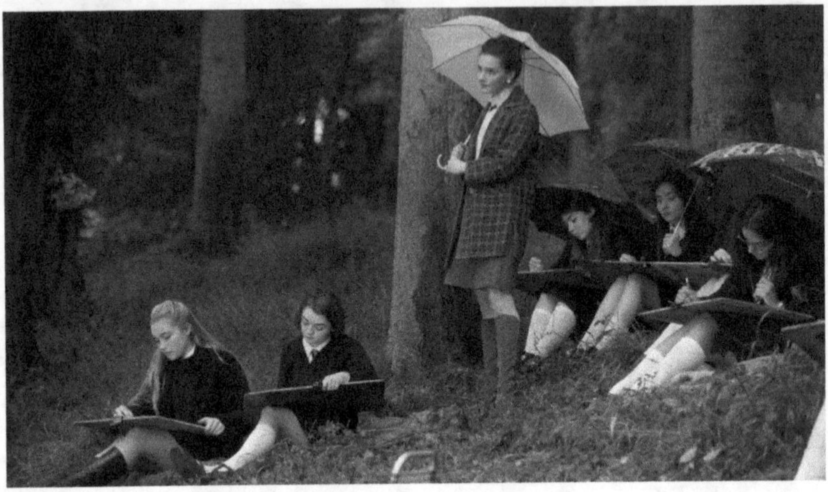

FIGURE 2.1 *The Falling.*

Source: Courtesy of CAMP/Independent Film Co.

a cinematic genealogy of girlhood, of the mystical and mythic and the questions surrounding embodied experience and sensuality that both films invite. This will, then, lead me to a closer examination of each film's imaging of female hysteria and the French feminist thought of Héléne Cixous, especially, whose critique of Freud's original conception of this notion emphasises not the 'faulty' (Cixous and Derrida 2001: 34) behaviour of girls, but the fecundity of female sexuality and self-pleasure, each film's concentrated gestures confounding the logic of the Freudian, female hysteric. In bringing both *The Falling* and *Picnic at Hanging Rock* together through my examination of the female hysteric, I hope to flesh out further the affirmative potential of the female hysteric in film and thus reclaim this position from a feminist perspective, building on the work of feminist critics such as Caroline Bainbridge and Lucy Bolton.

Psychoanalysis, feminism, hysteria

Historically linked with femininity for hundreds of years, hysteria's involuntary, uncontrollable, somatic symptoms were coming to be understood in the emerging critical feminist discourse not as a medical condition but a cultural one, an embodied index of forms of repression (Devereux 2014: 19). While the focus of this chapter is concerned with Morley and Weir's films, it is useful to consider another pertinent representation of hysteria that asserts its cultural position in contemporary film: David Cronenberg's *A Dangerous Method* (2012). According to Cronenberg's exploration of the love triangle that existed between Sigmund Freud, Carl Jung and Sabina Spielrein, female hysteria is a disturbing condition that binds both body and soul; *A Dangerous Method* opens with images of Spielrein (played by Keira Knightley) being transported to the Swiss clinic in which most of the film is set. While Knightley's body remains intact, her psychic pain is conveyed through a series of contortions and jerks, her jaw juts forward and her hands grapple against the sides of her carriage, smacking down on its windows. The female hysteric is laid bare for all to see. While Cronenberg's film ultimately foregrounds Spielrein's subjectivity and her journey towards recovery, Knightley's performance in those very first few troubling moments of the film are emblematic of cinema's obsession with the image of the female hysteric. Knightley's portrayal of Spielrein follows a long line of cinematic 'hysterics' indelibly linked with the history of cinema itself. Certainly, the female hysteric has long provided potent subject matter for popular Hollywood cinema, from the melodrama genre of classical Hollywood cinema (*Now, Voyager* [Irving Rapper, 1942]; *Sunset Boulevard* [Billy Wilder, 1950], *Whatever Happened to Baby Jane* [Robert Aldrich, 1962]) to the psycho-sexual thrillers of the late 1980s and beyond (from *Fatal Attraction* [Adrian Lyne, 1987], to *Gone Girl* [David Fincher, 2014]). The female hysteric is invariably a cypher for feminine lack, dysfunction and, as epitomised by Hitchcock's oeuvre, the object of misogyny (*Vertigo* [Alfred Hitchcock, 1958], *The Birds* [Hitchcock, 1963]). While patriarchal cinema tends to perpetuate Freud's 'myth' of female hysteria with representations of paranoid and narcissistic women, art cinema tends to offer up more nuanced, visceral explorations of the female psyche and sexual repression such as Michael Haneke's *The Piano Teacher* (2001) or Andrea Arnold's *Red Road* (2006). Weir and Morley are both auteurs whose evocative treatment of the subject of female hysteria is represented not only through the narrative but through the very fabric of their images. For example, Weir's depiction of his Australian locations take on an eerie, oneiric presence as if embodying the psychic ruptures felt by the girls within the narrative, haunting and strange. Morley films a canopy of branches and grassy textures as if they are emblems of her protagonist's interiority, malevolent as well as lush and beautiful. Furthermore, the specificity of *adolescent* female hysteria in Morley and Weir's films, coupled with their aesthetic innovations, uniquely questions the embodied implications of hysteria and the bodily registers of female subjectivity such as sensation, sensuous experience and sexuality.

It has been the project of first-, second- and third-wave feminist psychoanalytic thought to evaluate and critique Freud's views on female hysteria: that is, either directly through rethinking its usefulness and applicability as a way of articulating female experience, or as a contested site, re-examined within the bounds of post-Freudian analysis. For example, French feminist thinkers such as Luce Irigaray (1985), Julia Kristeva (1989) and Hélène Cixous (1976) are well known for their appropriation of Freudian thought, privileging much more generative and enlightening reflections on the female psyche, of which issues such as depression, melancholia and desire come to stand for a nexus of emotional and physical conditions complexly reshaping the contours of the (Freudian) feminine. Second-wave feminism, in particular, saw the development of a new discourse in which, as

Elaine Showalter puts it, 'hysteria was reclaimed in the name of feminism' (quoted in Devereux 2014: 19). Indeed, Morley and Weir's films can be seen to operate on this level, as examples of second-wave feminism that appropriate archaic notions of hysteria and assert female subjectivity, not as enigma (as Freud argues), but as mobile and fluid.

In the words of Juliet Mitchell (2000), cases of neuroses gave Freud clues to normal mental formations: dreams were everybody's every day, or every night, psychoses, and sexual perversions or inversions were both widespread and could constitute a choice. In 1905, Freud wrote in his 'shocking' case study of a young hysterical girl, 'Fragment of an Analysis of a Case of Hysteria', otherwise known as 'Dora':

> [N]ow in this case history sexual questions will be discussed with all possible frankness, the organs and functions of sexual life will be called by their proper names, and the pure minded reader can convince himself from my description that I have not to hesitate to converse upon such language even with a young woman.
>
> *(Mitchell 2000: 11)*

Dora had a nervous cough, she lost her voice and experienced migraines and thus she was depressed in a way that Freud called hysterical unsociability. Famously, Dora walked out on Freud, finally finding her own voice without his help, behaviour he merely shrugged off as a form of vengeance. For feminists, Dora remains a powerful caesura in Freud's chain of logic, which privileged the Oedipus complex and thus underestimated the power and complexity of female sexuality and desire, especially desire between female subjects. Indeed, as Mitchell reminds us, for Freud, 'the homosexual female, would merely present a crucial ambivalent mother attachment and paranoia owing to the pre-oedipal period of narcissism and nothing more' (ibid.: 55). *The Falling* and *Picnic at Hanging Rock*, precisely avoid such Freudian analyses of female homosexuality; their narratives are erotic and do depict tenderness and affection between young women, but the classification of sexuality itself (as either heterosexual, homosexual or bisexual) remains ambiguous and, more importantly, irrelevant.

Importantly, for Marcia Landy, Hollywood melodrama often employs the 'psychopathology of hysteria' in which 'there is always material which cannot be expressed in discourse or in the actions of the characters furthering the designs of the plot, a conversion can take place into the body of the text' (1991: 272). While Weir's and Morley's films do not subscribe to any of the conventions of the melodrama genre, both *Picnic at Hanging Rock* and *The Falling* adopt varying aesthetic modes and formal configurations in order to articulate, in Landy's words, a hysterical 'psychopathology' (ibid.). Indeed, the trope of Dora's 'hysterical' silence, her withdrawal from linguistic meaning, is echoed through each film's sound design, from the subtle, crackling heat and murmuring ambience of Weir's landscapes to Morley's employment of Tracey Thorne's vocal textures to inspire a sense of longing, retreat and disharmony. In this sense, sound and the displacement of the female voice serves to counter Freud's unconscious misogyny and foreground silence and non-verbal utterances as emancipatory acts. While the sound of the female scream, as well as, more generally, the female voice as 'other' characterises the representation of the hysteric in films such as *The Birds*, the silences and non-verbal utterances in both Weir and Morley's films such as the sound of breathing and sighing conjure the vanished voice and body of Freud's Dora, a vanishing point whose subjectivity remains precious and vital to feminist criticism and psychoanalysis. Before sound can be further discussed in relation to female hysteria in *The Falling* and *Picnic at Hanging Rock*, it is important to consider how hysteria is more broadly implicated in the visuality of each film.

Rethinking Hanging Rock

Weir's film opens with a painterly, beautifully rendered image of Hanging Rock itself, the last place in which the girls will be seen before they mysteriously vanish from existence. A faint turquoise sky looms over clusters of dense foliage, bare, wiry branches and tendrils of soft leaves and clouds interlace above the tip of the mossy rock. This image is overlaid with the film's title in an overtly decorative font, its curling flourishes picked out in white, contrasting the dark canopy of trees in the foreground. The significance of this landscape in the opening image is, for a number of critics, geographical and evocative of a national context. Indeed, for a critic such as *Sight and Sound*'s James Bell (2012), Weir's film represents a broader, post-colonial critique of Australia:

> [T]hough not in the Outback, the rock, which rises ominously out of pastoral countryside, is a signifier of the older, pre-colonised Australia, and a reminder of how tenuously the Victorian attitudes of the school sit with the rugged realities of the country.

Similarly, for Chris Cabin, writing for *Slant* (2014), the film's symbolic representation of its location is most significant: 'It's the characters' ceaseless need to fully understand, outsmart, and undermine nature's sway that drives them into fervour and, often enough, leads them to shuffle off this mortal coil'. While such criticism is right for acknowledging the tensions between order and chaos, the wild heartlands of Australia and the repressed ideals of colonial identity, it is the film's articulation of female hysteria and its very specific, intricate connection with imagination, desire and collective experience that haunts me most of all, indelibly inscribing a different sense of girlhood within cinematic history. Indeed, at first glance, the title images that open Weir's film portray a romantic landscape twinned, acutely, with normative notions of femininity, as evoked through its very use of a romantic font style and pictorial imagery. The titles overtly elicit notions of softness, whiteness, purity and decorative perfection, yet the longer I dwell on this sublime image, its calm and stasis pricks at the viewers' skin, it unnerves and unsettles. Such moments of queasy anxiety will be prescient of Weir's unravelling of both landscape and girlhood, of femininity and the stultifying, suffocating ideals of beauty that the girls are forced to reckon with as repressed subjects of Western patriarchal culture as well as, more specifically, the colonial violence associated with Australian's history.

Ostensibly, the film begins at Appleyard College, a girls' boarding school, in 1900. Even before they set out for their picnic, tensions ensue: one of the girls, Sara, is banned from the expedition and is forced to read a classical poem that she rebelliously switches for one of her own; while one of the central protagonists, Miranda, is described by a schoolmistress as a Botticelli angel, hinting not only at her angelic beauty, but the fable of her existence as an idealised construct of female identity, condescendingly referring to the unreality of her being. Famously, the girls are dressed in white Victorian lace, adorned with white gloves and sunhats. Much of the film's potent imagery calls attention to the sensuality of these girls: streaks of hair falling over heavily starched tunics and unfurling from prim, high collars, then, later, barefoot on the rocks, pale, milky bodies basking in the sun. These images of abandon and delight play out as key, evocative, sequences that come to represent the film's depiction of female hysteria most acutely associated with the girls' exploration of Hanging Rock, while the film's latter sequences of collective fury and revolt (shouting and defying their school mistresses) represent the girls remaining at the school and their response to the absence of the others.

Nearly 40 years later, Morley's *The Falling* stages a return to similar themes of female hysteria, female collectivity and madness. Set in the late 1960s, Morley's narrative is loosely based on a real case of mass hysteria in Blackburn in which dozens of girls suddenly fell prey to a bout of collective fainting. In an article for the BFI, Morley (2015b) herself acknowledges the debt she owes to *Picnic at Hanging Rock*, as well as films such as *The Virgin Suicides* (Sofia Coppola, 1999), *Don't Look Now* (Nicholas Roeg, 1973), *Heavenly Creatures* (Peter Jackson, 1994) and *The Devils* (Ken Russell, 1971); these choices alone offer up a distinct sense of the film's alchemy, its eroticism and dark subject matter, and its transgressive evocation of femininity. Most revealing of all, in a beautiful collage of photographs featured in the article, Morley writes in blue ink beside an image taken from *Picnic at Hanging Rock*: 'mystery, crushes, sound to evoke strangers' (ibid.). Further, on the key influence of Weir's aesthetic and thematic style, Morley writes:

> [Weir's] schoolgirls seemed poetic and enigmatic, like they had stepped out from a painting. I wanted to be in their gang. The supernatural quality of the natural world is something I was aiming to achieve in *The Falling* and so *Picnic* was most certainly a film that kept floating about in my mind as I researched and wrote the script.
>
> (*Ibid.*)

With her cinematographer, Claire Denis' frequent collaborator, Agnes Godard, Morley's film evokes the eerie pleasures of *Picnic at Hanging Rock* and its uncanny universe in which the conservative, patriarchal ideals of external, ordered beauty and the protocols of school life are steadily undone through the ambivalent, collective power of female adolescents.

While Weir's film-making style makes use of colour, scale and sound within the diegesis, adopting an austere, classical form of film-making, Morley's is rather more experimental, naturalistic and richly textured through its score by Tracey Thorne and its brittle, dizzying camerawork and washed out colour palette that has more in common with 1960s new wave British cinema, apt given the film's period setting. Such painterly attributes betray a specific heritage for Peter Bradshaw, invoking the female hysteric in a culturally specific context: 'It comes from the heart of a certain kind of Englishness: as murky, wet and luxurious as the water in which Millais drowned Ophelia' (Bradshaw 2014). Certainly, *The Falling* expands and elaborates Weir's sensual climates, its airy miasma of intense female kinship, passion and psychic disturbance, transposed to English soil, but Bradshaw's comments tend to draw too easily parallels between Morley's film and dominant cultural perceptions of female mental illness through *Hamlet*'s Ophelia, the love object whose overwrought emotional state leads to suicide. In contrast, both Morley's and Weir's films transgress such objectifying imagery through their refusal to pathologise female behaviour (characters in *The Falling* are seen to make attempts at pathologising female behaviour, but the film does not).[2]

Set deep within the British countryside at a strict girls school in 1969, the film represents an intense, affectionate and intimate friendship that develops between 16-year-olds, Lydia and Abbie. We know little about these girls except Lydia's dsyfunctional home life and Abbie's keenly developing experimentation with boys; what we do know of them is gleaned almost entirely from Morley's depiction of their entanglement, their fascination with each other and the strange feelings of kinship, doubt and desire that their interactions forge (there are resonances with another British girl-centred narrative set in the Yorkshire wilds, *My Summer of Love* [Pawel Pawlikowski, 2004] and the dark, delirious teenage friendship it represents, as well as of course *Heavenly Creatures* [Peter Jackson, 1994]). When Abbie dies in a bout of fainting shortly after she discovers she is carrying a child, Lydia and the rest of the school begin to faint, 'falling' as the film's title reminds us, as if under a spell, like Snow White, or collectively in some sort of trance, communing with the dead Abbie. During a key sequence, Lydia is seen standing among her classmates, closing her eyes as she falls slowly backwards, trusting the weight of her body to the other girls as she arches her back and stretches her arms out, Christ-like, in a ritual that both commemorates and reenacts Abbie's death; her willfulness to understand and ritualise Abbie's last moments is embodied through fainting as both an intimate act of love and imaginative play that undermines the strict moral and social codes of behaviour at the school. Horizontal, with a wave of hands beneath her like watery reeds and rushes, she reclaims, perhaps, Ophelia's final pose, not as passive female object, but dominant emancipator, freeing herself and her schoolmates from the inertia of repressed emotion, rising from a thicket of tangled fingers and hands.

While *Picnic at Hanging Rock* opens up questions about mental illness without necessarily providing answers, addressing the fragile psychic states of its traumatised young girls, especially through the suicide of Sara at the film's close, Morley's film confronts this subject head-on; from a young male character's derisive taunt, 'you're all mad bitches', to the school mistress' frustrated denial that demands her school not be treated like a mental institution, the girls are at once labelled as unwell, mentally unstable and hysterical, weak and powerless. However, as Lydia's grief is made clear, Morley's film offers up an increasingly different way in which to view female hysteria, pointing at the emancipatory powers of collective thought, embodied subjectivity and erotic fixation. Here, as with *Picnic at Hanging Rock*, the girls' displaced or denied sexuality, as Morley puts it, charges the film with a static pressure that is felt both within the diegesis and on the body of the film itself. In order to understand, more closely, the evocation of female hysteria and its affirmational qualities in both films, it is useful to draw attention to the thought of Hélène Cixous and her response to Freud.

For Cixous and Catherine Clement, in their 1975 book, *la jeune nee*, there is much political potential in the concept of hysteria. As Toril Moi writes, both Cixous and Clement agree that Dora's hysteria developed as 'a form of protest, a silent revolt against male power' (2001: 330). Certainly, Cixous also uses language in a way that reclaims the power of silence and the silence of the body, especially. Most compellingly, in her 1975 play *Portrait of Dora*, Cixous explores the possibility of feminine theatre by rewriting Freud's case study, underscoring the theatricality of psychoanalytical discourse as the talking cure, using voice, gestures, staging, ritual and myth in order to scrutinise the relationship between the semiotics of symptoms as the acting out of the hysteric body and the Symbolic Order. As Erella Brown persuasively writes in her article 'The Lake of Seduction: Body, Acting and Voice in Helene Cixous Portrait de Dora',

> Cixous, who takes hysteria as a key to both feminine sexuality and performance, stages Freud's failure with Dora as a dysfunctional dramatic operation by depicting his insistence on reading his paternal Oedipal model into Dora's hysteria as ineffective in regard to the real performative throbbing of the hysteric stage.
>
> *(1996: 626)*

Brown's thought is especially significant because she highlights the role of gesture and enunciation, the hysteric as performer par excellence.

Cixous' thought seems highly relevant to the role of performance, theatricality, ritual and the emphasis placed on embodiment and the hysteric's body in both *The Falling* and *Picnic*. Here, hysteria is not simply narratively, or thematically explored, but felt through the fabric of each film, their mise-en-scène, static as well as mobile camerawork, Thorn's soundtrack and performances; above all, the sensuality of the body and the highly tactile imagery each film conjures. When Cixous refers to the ways in which her play allows Dora to carry out 'the indispensable ruptures and transformations in her history, giving her liberation by bringing her into the text' (quoted in ibid.), she might just as well as be describing the female protagonists of *Picnic at Hanging Rock* who undergo such radical transformations or Lydia's actions in *The Falling* in which she is seen to play up to conceived notions of the female hysteric, as performer and 'liar'.

With these thoughts in mind, there are certain moments in both films that emerge as revelatory, corresponding closely with Cixous' reflection on hysteria and its dramatic arts, its inherent theatricality and a form of feminine theatre that, by extension, applies here, to a feminine cinematics. Indeed, for theorists such as Emma Wilson, Bolton, Bainbridge, Sarah Forgacs and Liz Watkins, French feminism presents multiple, exemplary models of thought through which to develop fruitful explorations of women on-screen, from Jane Campion to Lynne Ramsay. Such feminist cinematics are not predicated on the representation of Freudian lack and/or absence, but rather the specificity of 'women, the feminine and cinema' (Bainbridge 2008: 1), to echo Bainbridge's sentiment in her book *A Feminine Cinematics*. I want to consider how *The Falling* and *Picnic at Hanging Rock* offer up a kind of film-making in the feminine that opens up viewers to the ruptures and contradictions in female identity and patriarchy's assertion of these traits as feminine lack or failure within society, as Freud would contend.

There are two sequences I wish to explore here: the first in which the girls in *Picnic at Hanging Rock* bask in the sun at Hanging Rock and Lydia's fainting. In Weir's film, we see the girls assembled like living sculptures such as those the British feminist sculptor Barbara Hepworth might have cultivated, curled up and eyes closed so that the light passes through the small 'o' shape carved out of their curving midriffs, breathing gently as the image frames them collectively, like an ancient ruin. The girls are neither asleep nor fully awake, meditative and subtly empowered. This image contrasts dramatically with the pictorial glimpses of femininity the film has offered up until this point, emphasising their outward appearances, their linguistic and behavioural conformity. Similarly, the silences contained within the sequences at the rock become evocative of the girls' inner lives, their relinquishing of external reality and their drive towards self-discovery. Such silences and breaths on the soundtrack directly rupture and transform our notion of hysteria and of patriarchal cinema, evoking what Wilson might call an 'inner cinema', which she richly explores in her article 'Identification and Melancholia: An Inner Cinema of Hélène Cixous' (2000). This sequence uncannily evokes Dora's 'silent revolt' (Moi 2001), appropriating Dora's loss of language and shifting its meaning through the film's aural soundtrack.

For Irigaray, air corresponds with a particularly feminine form of being in which the sounds and rhythms of breath, as well as silence, are part of an embodied communion with oneself, 'returning to oneself' breath after breath, preserving one's subjectivity: 'woman communicates through air, through blood, through milk and even through voice and love before and beyond any perceptible thing' (2004: xiii). It is worth noting that the hysteric in patriarchal society loses her breath, she is stifled, hyperventilating, struggling to breathe or give voice to her words, as Knightley's portrayal of Spielrein suggests, but Weir's girls are different, they are *heard* differently, as emancipated women in control of their bodies and minds.

The Falling also bears comparison with Cixous' 'Portrait of Dora' through its more concentrated form of self-reflexivity, its visceral formalism and compelling account of Lydia as emancipatory presence, the ritual maker and master performer. In one particular scene, Lydia incites a riot with her response to medication: 'Kill the system, it's killing you!!!' she screams, rounding up the other girls. Most importantly, while Lydia mimics Abbie's symptoms through fainting, she also mimics her mannerisms. Provoking her peers as well as the school's authorities, Lydia is seen with a hand raised to touch the skin under her eye, a game where she puts her finger in her friends' mouth, calling to mind the use of mimicry in Cixous' play. Here, Lydia masquerades as Abbie, resurrecting her while simultaneously poking fun at those who do not understand her grief. In close-up, an intimacy is fostered between viewers and Lydia, as we hear her voice mimic Abbie's, her face and gestures slowly, subtly resembling the friend she grieves for.

Further, on a formal level, Morley's film adopts, in one of its most memorable sequences, a dissolve technique that overlays Abbie's face, notably, her lips and cheeks, with a canopy of trees and abstract, stretched shapes suggestive of sunlight and watery reflections, wryly casting her as a modern Ophelia, prescient of Lydia's suicide attempt at a lake. This beautiful image might best be seen to restate the impossibility of representation and the inevitable twinning of female loveliness with its patriarchal equivalent: nature. Importantly, it is the precise overlaying of female sensuality (her lips, her skin) with elemental imagery that marks it out as a visual disturbance within the mise-en-scène, a romantic ideal that is appropriated by Morley (Sofia Coppola does this in *The Virgin Suicides* to similar effect).

At the end of Morley's film, Lydia is saved from drowning by her mother Eileen, an agoraphobic, usually too afraid to venture outdoors. Thinking her dead, Eileen cradles Lydia's body, deeply regretting her lack of care for her daughter up until that point. Lydia awakens and finally expresses her grief over the loss of Abbie. Both women experience compassion for each other anew, opening themselves up to recovery and some sense of futurity. The girls in *Picnic* are never found, except the body of Mrs Appleyard, a governess. Writing themselves out of the narrative, they are a vanishing point within patriarchal cinema, as Dora is a vanishing point in Freud's case study. In conclusion, both Weir's and Morley's work are highly suggestive of the political potential of hysteria but, more importantly, they articulate a de-familiarising zone, an uncanny, silent space in which an inner life of female desire and horror can be played out, consciously responding to, and challenging, dominant cinema's fascination with Ophelia-esque tortured adolescents or Lolita-esque nymphets. In sum, I have argued that the depiction of female hysteria in Morley and Weir's films is ultimately generative, positive rather than simply representational of Freud's thought. However, female hysteria has not always been portrayed in such affirmative ways and, often, it is the galvanising narrative point within Hollywood cinema's ever popular thriller or horror genre in which women are victims of their own paranoid-depressive states (see *Gone Girl*, for example). If Freud's Dora, in her many cinematic guises, is forever beholden to a patriarchal economy, then, the question is how to redefine her trajectory and re-read her story as a vital narrative of female self-possession.

Notes

1 I am extremely grateful to the editors for their invitation to contribute to this volume; this chapter started its life as a conference presentation at Royal Holloway University, 2016, as part of the international conference 'Childhood, World Cinema and Nationhood'.
2 Lucille Hadzihalilovic's *Innocence* (2004) is also notable here for its boarding school-bound inversion of Freudian femininity, a film I have discussed elsewhere at length. See Quinlivan (2009).

Bibliography

Bainbridge, Caroline (2008), *A Feminine Cinematics: Luce Irigaray, Women and Film*, Basingstoke: Palgrave.

Bell, James (2012), 'DVD Review: *Walkabout + Picnic at Hanging Rock*', *Sight and Sound* online, http://old.bfi.org.uk/sightandsound/review/5596. Accessed December 2016.

Bradshaw, Peter (2014), '*The Falling*', *Guardian*, www.theguardian.com/film/2014/oct/10/the-falling-review-london-film-festival-carol-morley. Accessed September 2016.

Brown, Erella (1996), 'The Lake of Seduction: Body, Acting, and Voice in Helene Cixous' Portrait de Dora', *Modern Drama*, 39(4), 626–649.

Cabin, Chris (2014), '*Picnic at Hanging Rock*', *Slant*, www.slantmagazine.com/dvd/review/picnic-at-hanging-rock. Accessed June 2017.

Cixous, Hélène (1976), 'The Laugh of the Medusa', *Signs* (trans. Keith Cohen and Paula Cohen, 1(4), 875–893.

Cixous, Hélène and Jacques Derrida (2001), *Veils* (trans. Geoffrey Bennington), Stanford, CA: Stanford University Press.

Devereux, Cecily (2014), 'Hysteria, Feminism and Gender Revisited', *English Studies in Canada*, 40(1), 19–45.

Irigaray, Luce (1985), *Speculum of the Other Woman* (trans. Gillian C. Gill), New York: Ithaca University Press.

Irigaray, Luce (2004), *Luce Irigaray: Key Writings*, London and New York: Continuum.

Kristeva, Julia (1989), *Black Sun: Depression and Melancholia* (trans. Leon S Roudiez), New York: Columbia University Press.

Landy, Marcia (1991), *Imitations of Life: A Reader on Film and Television and Melodrama*, Detroit: Wayne State University Press.

Mitchell, Juliet (2000), *Psychoanalysis and Feminism: A Radical Reassessment of Freudian Psychoanalysis*, London and New York: Penguin.

Moi, Toril (2001), *What Is a Woman? and Other Essays*, Oxford: Oxford University Press.

Morley, Carol (2015a), 'Carol Morley: Mass Hysteria Is a Powerful Group Activity', *Guardian*, www.theguardian.com/film/2015/mar/29/carol-morley-the-falling-mass-hysteria-is-a-powerful-group-activity. Accessed 10 July 2016.

Morley, Carol (2015b), 'Carol Morley: These Are the Films That Inspired *The Falling*', BFI Online, www.bfi.org.uk/news-opinion/news-bfi/features/carol-morley-films-inspired-falling. Accessed 20 December 2016.

Quinlivan, D. (2009), 'The Kineasthesia of Sound in *Innocence*', *Studies in French Cinema*, 9(3), 215–224.

Wilson, E. (2000), 'Identification and Melancholia: An Inner Cinema of Hélène Cixous', *Paragraph*, 23(3), 258–269.

3

GROWING UP GIRL IN THE 'HOOD

Vulnerability, violence and the girl-gang state of mind in *Bande de Filles/Girlhood* [1]

Caroline Bainbridge

Introduction

This chapter explores the dynamics of vulnerability, violence and relatedness at work in the psychological development of Marieme/Vic (Karidja Touré), the protagonist of Céline Sciamma's *Bande de Filles/Girlhood* (France, 2014). Drawing initially on psychoanalytic notions of "the girl-gang state of mind" articulated in the work of Donald Meltzer (1973), and on Luce Irigaray's concept of *parler femme* (speaking [as] woman) (1977/1985), it argues that dimensions of "unspeakable" feminine experience are brought to life on the cinema screen for viewers as "gestures of girlhood". In order to consider the thematic significance of discourses of "race" that surround the film, this chapter also turns to Black feminist theory to reflect on what it means to view it (and to write about it) from a position inscribed in white privilege. The methodological implications for intersectional scholarship are addressed in the next section and provide an important frame of reference for the discussion that follows.

Girlhood is a coming of age film that focuses on the experiences of its protagonist, Marieme, who lives in a *banlieue* on the outskirts of Paris. The film was written and directed by Céline Sciamma, a white woman with a track record of festival success for her earlier films, *Water Lilies* (France, 2007) and *Tomboy* (France, 2011). *Girlhood* has enjoyed widespread critical acclaim, but there has also been important commentary on Sciamma's decision to focus the story on a young Black woman, and on the film's sometimes troubling tendency toward "cultural appropriation"[2] and the associated legacy of white liberal guilt (Blay 2015; Chew-Bose 2015; Tewolde-Berhan 2015). Media coverage has highlighted the casting decisions made by Sciamma, who selected non-professional actors for lead roles having scouted them in public places. Sciamma and the four key female actors in the film reportedly lived together for three weeks while shooting the film to deepen their collaboration (Anonymous 2015a). As Agnieszka Piotrowska's reflexive account of historical inter-cultural collaborations and her film practice in Zimbabwe indicates, seeking to conscientiously overturn the legacies of colonial power and history through encounter, entanglement, and collaborative creativity constitutes a "'minor' political gesture" (2017: 166), albeit the case that ethical questions nevertheless persist: it is a start. A feminist perspective on Sciamma's motivations must keep this intentionality in mind, despite the obvious limitations.

The formative experiences of girlhood as depicted in Sciamma's film are written on and through the body, paying particular attention to raced and classed facets of experience. I argue that the film's evocation of the highs and lows of adolescent experience – and its phased fantasies of binding, splitting and competition – offer a compelling commentary on the close imbrication of lived experience, cultural politics, identity and growth. Overall, I make the case that the film offers a timely opportunity for exploring the emotional work entailed in growing up for girls seeking survival in complex sociocultural and political environments, where the inflections of intersectional experience are often contradictory. However, I also suggest that a psycho-cultural approach to questions of cinematic representation enables new ways of thinking about reflexive feminist practice, provoking consideration of the ethical and methodological responsibilities linked to scholarship that maps the contemporary cultural terrain of intersectional femininity.

Ethical considerations

In her work on *Precious* (Lee Daniels, USA, 2010), Katariina Kyröla notes with sensitivity the difficulties involved for white scholars who are interested in discussing the cultural politics of "race" and ethnicity:

> How we see ourselves (and others) as ethical subjects relates intimately to not only how we feel about things, but to how we feel we *should* feel about things, and to how we express, articulate and intellectually process those feelings.
>
> *(2017: 2, original emphasis)*[3]

Highlighting the crucial significance of bell hooks' work on "learned helplessness" (2003: 26), Kyröla cautions against "a white liberal attitude towards racism which, despite acknowledging racist structures and one's own privilege enabled by them, helps keep whiteness and white (bad) feeling in the center" (2017: 2). This resonates with Reni Eddo-Lodge's observation

> that, at first, talking about race is uncomfortable, because too many white people are angry and in denial . . . [A]fter white people begin to get it, it's even more uncomfortable for them to think about how their whiteness has silently aided them in life.
>
> *(2017: loc. 2432)*

It thus becomes urgent for white scholars to reflect on how best to "own" their part in the oppressive regime of structural racism, and to consider how it might be possible to contribute to undoing its insidious dynamics – strategic, reflexive, conscientious interventions can contribute towards this project.

One means of beginning to do such work involves reflexive scholarly practice that is grounded in and informed by Black scholarship and its various commentaries on the ontological and epistemological failures and silences of unthinkingly white theory. In aiming to explore unspeakable dimensions of identity and experience as represented in mainstream cinema culture, this chapter therefore attempts to understand how meaning is made and interpreted through the mechanisms of film. To do this, it takes an object relations psychoanalytic approach to the psychological and emotional processes at work, but this is underpinned with feminist intentionality. To this end, I reflect on how previous methodological practices I have used to explore the cinematic treatment of femininity (Bainbridge 2008) can be deepened and made more politically conscious by foregrounding Black feminist scholarship on theory, identity and politics. My aim here is to write more reflexively about the racialized, sexualized and gendered dimensions of power and ideology, while at the same time attempting to resist the pull into a "well-meaning but guilty-feeling white liberal" mentality (Eddo-Lodge 2017: loc. 1601).

This seems all the more crucial given the production context of *Girlhood*. As noted above, its director is a successful white woman who benefits from very considerable cultural and ideological capital. In exercising this capital to make a film about young Black women, Sciamma manages to occupy a paradoxical and problematic relationship to power. On the one hand, as many critics have pointed out, in making a film in which the lead roles are played by four Black females, Sciamma innovates and challenges commonplace industrial practices and assumptions. However, she is able to do this, in part, *because* of her white privilege, and the notion of empowerment through patronage is unpalatable and discursively troubling despite the generally positive critical acclaim garnered by the film, which must, of course also be understood in terms of Sciamma's ability and talent. What is more, Sciamma also chose to recruit non-professional actors through a process of scouting, and there are uncomfortable connotations here around the use of cultural capital to enable aspirational shifts for the four young women selected in this way. For instance, blogger, Fanta Sylla (2015), has suggested that Sciamma's choices are indicative of and resound with debates about "the fallacy of solidarity" between women of colour, criticizing *Bande de filles* for its ostensibly universal representation of girlhood, without paying attention to the subtleties of distinction between women of colour. Sylla argues that

> Sciamma didn't have the experience, the imagination, the vision and empathy necessary to represent this girlhood in its complexity. If the film were a radical exploration of Black French girlhood in the *banlieue*, watching it would have been a novel, disturbing and alienating experience.
>
> (*Ibid.*)

Sylla's point here is that this was not the case for her (and therefore, presumably, for others). Other Black critics have hailed the film for providing a compelling narrative in "a movie landscape where there are so few depictions of Black girls getting to be Black girls" (Blay 2014) and describe the film as "uplifting" in its choice "to explore the bond between the girls, the power and confidence that they develop in their tight-knit group and how they support each other through their shared difficulties" (Anonymous 2015b).

The complexity of the production context demands much wider interrogation and goes beyond the remit of this chapter. However, the range of discursive positions and critical responses it evokes is indicative of apparently unspeakable dimensions of lived experience for Black women, and this is the focus of my chapter. In the discussion that follows, I explore how Sciamma's film succeeds in opening up space in which to notice the dynamics of power at work in the film, inviting critical reflection about its subject matter. Later, I will reflect further on what such analysis means for thinking through the psychological processes involved in the power relations that are in play, by deploying the image of "the girl-gang state of mind" as one that becomes useful in shaping a collaborative mode of solidarity between women that pays ongoing attention to structural and ideological forces.

Analysis

With all of this in mind, then, how might we make sense of the schema of adolescent Black femininity depicted in *Girlhood*? To think about this, we need to note several important elements of the film and its construction of both Marieme/Vic and her friends in terms of simultaneously split and bound experience, vulnerability and violence, dependence and defiance. What seems to be at stake are aspects of subjective experience that are communicable despite being unspeakable, writ large on the screen in deeply affective ways. In my work over a number of years now (Bainbridge 2008, 2014), I have argued that film provides a cultural arena in which to explore such experience, with a view to re-visiting our understanding of the containing dynamics of cinema and its power to allow us to work through complex, and often contradictory, emotional and psychological experience. Sciamma's film offers a fascinating evocation of these ideas in its invitation to grapple with the conundrum of subjectivity as experienced by young, Black, working-class women whose lives are shaped by institutional and ideological forces beyond their control. As Claire Mouflard has observed,

> In Sciamma's *banlieue*, teenage girls are constantly renegotiating their home and public life in accordance with gender and economic roles that appear to be culturally formatted by the state and conveyed to them both through the institutions and through the male figures in their lives . . . [inscribing them in] geographical, economic and social alienation.
>
> *(2016: 113)*

The film immediately invokes the lived experience of the constraints described by Mouflard in its depiction of the sharp contrast between the vibrant, chatter-laden freedom experienced by the girls on the football field and immediately outside the stadium and its rapid silencing on their entrance into the walkways of the *banlieue*, where masculinity dominates, as young men stare from top steps and elevated walls at the approaching group of young women, looming over the girls' shared sociality with a palpable sense of foreboding. The young women navigate their way through the high-rise landscape of home, and the lighting design of this sequence, with its emphasis on tall shadows and backlit silhouettes of seemingly faceless young men, hints at the oppressive atmosphere coded in the disparity of access to power between the young men and women who live there.[4] This also sets the scene for the atmosphere of Marieme's home in a fatherless family with a largely absent mother, an abusive older brother and caring responsibilities for two younger sisters. That Marieme's emotional experience is unspeakable is shown clearly in the scene where she meets with an unseen educational counsellor who advises her that she is to be displaced against her will into a vocational tier of education, rather than being allowed to progress to high school. High school was her best chance of escaping the tyranny of a future that will require repetition of her mother's experience and a lack of choice about this, no matter how strongly she might resist. Marieme cannot put this into words, although her pain is clear as we listen to the counsellor's disembodied voice thwarting her ambition and glossing over a fleeting opportunity to ask questions that might afford an opportunity to think differently about Marieme's future. It is this experience, alongside her burgeoning desire for her brother's friend, Ismaël (Idrissa Diabaté), that pushes Marieme into her transformational experience with Lady's (Assa Sylla) gang, an experience that enables her to explore both sides of the togetherness/splitting binary evoked in the opening sequences of the film and, I will argue, to discover that Black femininity is construed as a seemingly endless source of struggle that demands a disruptive relationship to hegemonic structures of subjectivity.

Binding and splitting in the girl-gang state of mind

In his account of "the seething flux" of adolescence, Donald Meltzer presents the adolescent world as a social structure, stating that its inhabitants are "the happy-unhappy multitude caught up betwixt the 'unsettling' of their latency period and the 'settling' into adult life" (1973: 51). Tracing pathways through adolescent development, Meltzer spells out very clearly that the journey is one from splitting to integration, albeit that the journey is not a smooth one, involving wild periods of instability. For the adolescent subject, the group becomes a crucial place of experience, providing what he describes as "a holding position in relation to splitting processes". Gradually, through the process of "disseminating parts of the self into members of the group", social processes are set in motion, enabling a shift from the persecutory and omnipotent terrors of the paranoid-schizoid psychological terrain of experience into the depressive arena of adulthood and the achievements fostered by it (ibid.: 54–55). However, as Hamish Canham observes, the problem with groups is that, in the contexts of any sense of perceived or real threat, they exert a very strong pull toward regressive infantile states of persistent anxiety, and where this is sustained, the "lure of the gang" becomes inescapable. For the gang "promises a life without many of the pains that recognizing difference, dependency, the inevitability of death, and vulnerability entails" (2002: 113–114).

Of course, the question of difference in this discussion by Canham is not coded with any specific reference to gender, sexuality or ethnicity, and we need to read further to understand how the state of mind at work in gangs is "used as a solution to the pains involved in having ambivalent feelings" as Canham argues, following Herbert Rosenfeld (1971 cited in Canham 2002: 116). Eventually, Meltzer returns to the theme of the gang, to explore the different textures of gang-related experience. Specifically, he formulates the idea of a "girl-gang state of mind", in which the struggle for "egalitarianism" is grounded in a refusal of the authority of the father, creating what Meltzer describes as its "anti-masculine, Amazonian quality . . . [in which] . . . the myth of feminine inferiority is vigorously denied, and yet its remnants seem affirmed by this very vigour" (2007: 447). Meltzer links this to "the injustice of the social order where femininity is not in itself obviously valued" (ibid.: 445), observing that this leads to girls being "strongly inclined to feel that only other girl-women can understand [the] dread [that this entails]" (ibid.: 446). In this way, then, the girl-gang state of mind simultaneously binds girls to one another, creating a form of shared sociality, while also paradoxically permitting them to express an ambivalent, schizoid mentality linked to the impossibility of their experience. These themes must surely be intensified for women of colour, and even more so for *young* women of colour who are also from underprivileged socio-economic/classed backgrounds. All of this is, I think, starkly on show in *Girlhood*, a film that therefore offers an important opportunity to consider the symbolic enactments at work in the story and the way that these articulate more usually unspoken dimensions of political and social experience.

The film narrative makes use of various tropes of splitting and binding to express the complexity of this inscription of identity. The importance of binding experience in adolescence accounts for the formation of gangs in the first place. It is no accident here that Marieme is seduced into Lady's gang shortly after learning that her education is to be abruptly re-directed into vocational training. The prospect of this is unbearable for her, and she sees the scope for rebellion and possible freedom in Lady's offer to join her gang. She negotiates her entry into the group by means of binding experiences linked to clothing, music, petty theft, dance and aggression, which is expressed toward rival girl gangs on "the other side of the tracks" as well as in Marieme's bullying of a younger schoolgirl for money. Marieme is finally "inducted" officially into the gang when Lady gives her the gift of a necklace announcing her gang name, "Vic – for *victoire*", and offers a piece of advice that will shape the rest of Marieme's journey in the film: "Do what you want".

The gift of the necklace and of the alternate name/gang moniker, "Vic – for *victoire*", also underscores the role of splitting in gang culture. Marieme has to continue to be the Marieme of her family life (caring for sisters, protecting them from an abusive brother, feeding them, washing up and deflecting all of the violent atmosphere of the family home on to herself). However, she is now also Vic, a young woman who dares to transgress, who shares unparalleled moments of joy with her gang mates when they closet themselves away in hotel rooms with cheap alcohol and marijuana, fleetingly escaping the pain of their everyday lives. Yet the split persona also invites envious rivalry and competition, enacted through both costume – Marieme's outfits often match those of Lady in ways that those of Adiatou (Lindsay Karimoh) and Fily (Mariétou Touré) do not – and when Lady gets "wasted" (i.e. beaten up) by the leader of a rival gang, an act that will be avenged by Vic, who takes a kitchen knife to the fight, cuts off her rival's bra and keeps it as a trophy. Of course, this induces painful competition between Vic and Lady, who is even more symbolically stripped of her authority thanks to her father cutting off her hair in punishment for the beating she took in the original fight. The overtones of struggle with and for phallic iterations of femininity in these sequences of violence deepen our sense that, for these young women, growing up girl in the 'hood is far from straightforward. Engaging in violent fights involving knives and the symbolic loss of long hair connotes the ways in which the violent residue of unspeakable intersectional experience struggles to find a cultural outlet, highlighting the familiar ways in which violence, which is more usually ascribed to masculinity, provides temporary respite for young women struggling to assert power. The masquerade of phallic femininity is palpable here. The resonances with debates about solidarity between feminists, and between women of colour and white women, also reverberate here, as the challenges around finding a means of political expression for both the individual and group experiences of women become overlaid with structures of dangerous competition and rivalry.

The film shows how young, Black, working-class, female experience simply cannot adequately be encoded. The matrix of overlaid schemas of difference is represented as impossibly complex, showing how the failures and silences of the hegemonic ideological value system cannot only be brought to light but also how they might be mined for clues to the texture of what goes unspoken. It is worth reiterating Canham's observations here: on the one hand, the gang "promises a life without any of the pains that recognizing difference . . . entails" (2002: 113). However, "when deprivation is coupled with abuse, it often leads . . . to a defensive internal manoeuvre designed to distance the ego from the pain of what it has been through" (ibid.: 125). In its evocation of these very dilemmas, *Girlhood* offers what I think of as "gestures of girlhood" in its play with what Richard Billow has characterized as a kind of striving for mutual recognition that takes place in gangs (2013: 141). Psychologically, this is an attempt to establish what he describes as "subject-to-subject relationships", and this, in turn, is a means of aspiring to an intrapsychic state that allows for the democratic integration of interpersonal and political or ideological experience. In *Girlhood*, this striving underpins some of the most emotive and affective scenes of binding between the members of Lady's gang, expressed through an embodied gestural politics that is echoed in Sciamma's cinematic style.

Gestures of girlhood

In her work on the psychoanalytic setting, psychoanalyst and philosopher Luce Irigaray explores the importance of gesture for communicating often dramatic dimensions of gendered subjectivity. Discussing the experience of the girl that goes unspoken in Freud's (1920) account of the *fort-da* game, Irigaray asserts that for the girl, gesture is also about staging and managing the psychic loss of the mother, which, she argues, is complicated for the girl-child because of their shared gendered experience, and because "the mother always remains too familiar and too close" (1987/1993: 98). For Irigaray, the importance of gesture is that it allows girls to express and explore aspects of their experience that are *not* inscribed in difference, but that rather depend on shared aspects of subjectivity in common. Reflecting on her experience of young women in the analytic setting, Irigaray suggests that the repertoire of such gestures includes whirling around in dance to signify abandonment (in both senses) and to attract recognition (ibid.: 97–98).

Irigaray's insight here shows how girls' experience can be articulated despite all the seeming prohibitions. This provides an interesting lens through which to read one of the best-known sequences in *Girlhood*, the scene in which Lady's gang clubs together to pay for a night in a hotel room, where they drink, get high and dance together to Rhianna's song, "Diamonds" (2012). This is a scene in which the sheer joy of the girls' shared "subject-to-subject" relationship dominates the mood of the film, eliding all the vulnerability and violence that encodes their experience of the walkways and stairwells of the *banlieue*, the domestic sphere, the exploitative workplace and the underground spaces of metro shopping malls and train tracks.

There are two notable stylistic aspects of this sequence that reveal how Sciamma uses not only narrative to explore experience but also the formal structures of cinema. First, the lighting design of the sequence has received critical acclaim for its achievement in successfully lighting Black skin for the screen (Ince 2017; McNeill 2017).[5] In what Kate Ince refers to as "an aesthetic of melancholy" (2017: 171), the sequence emphasizes the blue-black tones of both the actors' skin colour and their costumes. The aesthetic here does, indeed, connote melancholy, as Ince suggests, but I think it goes deeper than this. It also evokes the bruising experience of the lives of these young women, tinged as they are with violence and pain, both embodied and psychological.[6] The pain of their psychological experience stands in counterpoint to the embodied joy of their dancing together, suggesting something of the paradoxical and deeply complex signifier of the bruise, a mark on the body that bears witness to violent experience and that can bring the associated pain to life again through either the lightest accidental touch against an external object or through a self-harming, conscious prodding by one's own volition. The lingering, crushing effects of embodied and psychological experience are connoted here in the bruised aesthetic, adding to the paradoxically melancholic tone of this scene of apparent joy and speaking directly to the emotional complexity of the narrative as a whole.

Paradox is also at work in the second formal strategy I want to discuss here: the sound design of the scene. By overlaying Rhianna's original track on to the footage of the girls singing along, Sciamma effectively makes the music both diegetic and non-diegetic at the same time. The girls are both singing along (as we hear at the end of the scene) and apparently lip-syncing at the same time, thanks to the strategies of cinema.[7] This is a fascinating cinematic technique that simultaneously *disrupts* and *forges* identificatory processes. It heightens awareness of the distance necessary for us to feel ourselves to be *viewers* of the film, while also touching us, and speaking to our own real-word experience, in which Rhianna's song resonates with our own mnemic associations and, as discussed by Isabella McNeill (2017), with those evoked by Rhianna's personal stories of traumatic experience. The girls sing while not being heard while ventriloquizing – they invoke what we might think of as a karaoke rendition of gender, a performance that both embodies the possibilities of Black femininity and pushes at its boundaries, evoking the poignant search for a voice that such unspoken experience entails. Of course, in this scene, the girls also sing in a different language, suggesting that difference is experienced as another language, one that is not "known" but can nevertheless be sung through mimetic ventriloquism and performance. Like girls in a gang, then, as viewers we are both bound to the protagonists (and to one another) and divorced/separated at the same time, and this is enacted in the simultaneous use of Rhianna's song on the soundtrack and within the diegetic space of the narrative, mirroring the impossible, contradictory pulls exerted on female subjectivities inscribed in difference. There is also a palpable dimension of me/not-me experience for the viewer here that resonates with Kimberlyn Leary's assertion that "race, like gender, exists in transitional space. It is located in the tensions among biological distinction, sociocultural fact, and future possibilities" (1997: 63). While Leary herself does not refer to Winnicott here, his work nevertheless comes to mind. Winnicott's (1971) emphasis on the use of transitional me/not-me objects to negotiate separation from the mother in pursuit of a sense of mastery in the adult world speaks to the complex entanglement of embodied experience with psychological and emotional aspects of selfhood, as well as with broader sociocultural pressures and dynamics. Leary's observation can be deepened by thinking with Winnicott here. For Winnicott, feelings of mastery are closely tied to the sensory pleasures of the object, the kinds of pleasure writ large on the screen in this sequence of Sciamma's film, as we watch the sheer unbridled joy of experience manifest itself in terms of close bodily proximity, dancing with arms conjoined and so on. The affective qualities of this scene are deeply emotional, encouraging the introjection of a sense of the fleeting, binding sociality expressed within the group at this moment.

There are parallels, too, with the call made by Irigaray to establish what she describes as *parler femme* or "speaking (as) woman" in order to articulate aspects of feminine subjectivity that more usually go unspoken (1977/1985: 135). The terrain of *parler femme* is grounded in horizontal female relationships of sociality rather than occupying spaces of inheritance between generations. In *Girlhood*, the sequences involving dancing and singing are encoded in just such terms, showing how musical subcultures permit young women to find points of connection and commonality, when so much of the world cuts off any vision of their experience.

Irigaray's notion of *parler femme* is useful here insofar as it enables us to perceive how aspects of the feminine can be made explicit through cinematic strategies linked to gesture, embodiment, *mise-en-scène*, sound design and so on. The problem with Irigaray's work, however, is that it insists on maintaining a hierarchy of modes of difference in which gender is elevated about all other forms of experience. This means that, despite the assertions that I have made here and elsewhere (Bainbridge 2008), about the strategic value of working with Irigaray's logic, and despite the fact that the notion of *parler femme* opens up ways of viewing cinema that extract and exemplify how the feminine can indeed be put on show, it is nevertheless crucial to acknowledge that the strategic value of such an approach is limited because of the Irigarayan refusal to grapple with concepts of race and ethnicity. This insight is an important element of the work involved in this chapter, as I seek to reflect on my own methodological practices. I will return to this discussion below.

The gestures of girlhood in Sciamma's film go beyond the simple expression of binding experience expressed in and through the notion of *parler femme*. The limitations of ideological notions of femininity, and its raced and classed iterations often dominate the screen. We might think of the way a dominant hermeneutics of suspicion that surrounds young Black women is evoked in the shopping mall scene, for example, when a young white shop assistant indiscreetly follows Marieme as she browses the merchandise, or of the many different kinds of outfit, style and look tried on by Marieme/Vic as the film evolves. We variously see her wearing an American football kit, simple leisure wear and trainers, a tight-fitting, glamourous (stolen) dress, a leather jacket and, in later scenes, a high-end dress and platinum blonde wig as she plays the role of drug dealer and, later still, in scenes that show a distinct effort to erase all features of femininity, by binding her breasts and wearing loose-fitting sportswear with cornrow braids to give the illusion of short hair. Sciamma's visual and narrative strategies reveal the claustrophobic spaces of Black femininity but also open them up for scrutiny, throwing them into question. In the play with costume, for example, it is as though Marieme is experimenting at the margins of femininity, trying on guises of female subjectivity, trying to work out whether it might suit her or not. The sheer array of identity modes conjured in this dressing-up play can be read as a kind of refusal, an exposé of the constructedness of female identity and its lack of fit for young Black women of her background. The distinction drawn by Irigaray between masquerade and mimesis is instructive here (1977/1985: 220), and we might read Marieme as a purveyor of mimetic challenges to a set of ideological codes of femininity that exclude her on the grounds of ethnicity and social class.[8] Homi Bhabha's observation that mimicry is inscribed in ambivalence and therefore produces its excesses, slippages and differences at every turn is also important here (1994: 85).

However, there is an important difficulty in turning to Irigaray to grapple with the silences of the feminine inscribed in raced (and classed) difference. She has notoriously suggested that "sexual difference is an immediate natural given. The whole of human kind is composed of women and men and of nothing else. The problem of race is in fact a secondary problem" (1992/1996: 47). Here, as

Mary K. Bloodsworth-Lugo observes, Irigaray's ontology "relegates race to a subordinate position vis-à-vis sexual difference", thereby positing "sexual difference as unmarked by race" (2007: 55–57). As she goes on to argue, for women of colour, race is much more likely to be an organizing category of experience, and so the shameful politics of white liberal theory are exposed here. This observation is central to my attempt (and, indeed, to those of many other feminist scholars including, for example, Piotrowska [2017] and Ranjana Khanna [2003]) to move beyond the structuring absences of Irigarayan philosophy. As Bloodsworth-Lugo shows, it is imperative to bring into view the absent, structurally invisible dimensions of Black femininity, so that they become present despite the seeming impossibility of this.

I am reminded here of Bion's appropriation of Freud's imagery in a translation he made of a letter written by Freud to Lou Andreas Salomé: "when conducting an analysis, one must cast a beam of intense darkness so that something that has hitherto been obscured by the glare of the illumination can glitter all the more in the darkness" (Grotstein 2007: 12). Sciamma's film works, I think, do just this, so that we insinuate ourselves into the gaps opened up by the filmic strategies and start to comprehend the depth of silence enshrined within them. The claustrophobia of this experience is evoked in Sciamma's periodic use of cuts to black screen during the film so that the blackness resonates for the viewer at turning points in the plot. In the institutional space of the cinema, this technique deepens the darkness of the viewing environment for the spectator, and all the while foregrounding the importance of cinematic specificity, in a way that once again resonates with Bion's words. The oppressive, inescapable atmosphere invoked in these lingering moments perhaps translate a tiny part of the lived psychological experience of the subjectivity of our protagonists, showing how all iterations of performative identity become oppressive and thwarting in the end. We become shrouded in the unenveloped dereliction of subjectivity here, understanding how and why this experience simply cannot be spoken. This also provides valuable insight into how and why the girl-gang state of mind can provide much needed respite from the affective provocations inherent in the struggle to become both Black and feminine. There is an endless pursuit of fixity in a relay between embodied dimensions of identity that plays out psychologically and mires the subject in a logic of endless splitting, so that the apparent safety of feeling bound to others provides a degree of certainty at least, until the binding itself also becomes claustrophobic and unbearable as the individual is reduced to the whole, becoming unable to shake off the sense of the gang as an aspect of self experience that diminishes a sense of individual subjectivity while paradoxically seeming to provide a route toward it. Marieme's struggle with this leads her to abandon her binding to the girl gang as she strikes out in pursuit of life on her own terms, albeit the case that she needs to tread a path of criminality and obedience to men to get there. This section of the film opens up new perspectives on Marieme's struggle to discover herself as a subject.

Marieme goes to work for Abou (Djibril Gueye), an older man who runs a drug-dealing gang and who offers Marieme safety at least from the abusive relationship with her brother as well as space to live in what might feel like an independent existence in a flat in another *banlieue* that she shares with other members of Abou's gang. She has her own Playstation, a mattress on the floor, a kitchen to cook in, a friend (Monica) and her ongoing love relationship with Ismaël. Marieme lives as Vic in this segment of the film, abandoning her familial relations completely and "parking" her former life in doing so. She no longer wears stylish dresses unless she is on her way to work, when she also puts on a platinum blonde wig that allows us to pick her out as a mimetic paradox as she moves through a party scene populated with rich white people in the heart of Paris in order to deliver drugs. On her own time, Vic wears baggy sports clothing and cornrow braids, and she hangs out with the guys from the gang, joining in as they intimidate young girls. She cooks eggs for Monica (Dielika Coulibaly), and they exchange mutual criticism as they talk about their choices of "look". For Vic, Monica's conformity to the stereotype of the drug gangster's "ho" traps her in a code of behaviour that Vic herself refuses. For Monica, meanwhile, there is puzzlement about why Vic looks as though she is trying to "pass" as a man. This is, of course, to an extent, an effort to ward off unwanted sexual approaches from her fellow gang members and her boss, but we see that Vic pushes this to extremes, binding her breasts so that she looks even less womanly – a choice that leads her to fight with Ismaël, and, eventually, to refuse his offer of marriage as solution to her dilemmas and then to break up with him. Vic goes to a party with her crew, and toys briefly with desire for Monica as they dance close together and explore the frisson between them. This scene is rudely interrupted by Abou, who tries to force Vic to kiss him in a scene of devastating reinforcement of all that she has come to fear about the world: for Vic, men appear to impose their sexual expectations upon her, policing her preferences around her embodied identity and stripping her of any freedom of choice when it comes to sexual relationships.

What we see here is an extension of the play with identity and iterations of gender and difference in ways that move beyond the confines of heterosexual formations of femininity. Vic actively subverts the bodily codes of her gendered identity, toying with the release provided by inhabiting what Halberstam (1998)[9] refers to as "female masculinity" in scenes that can also be read as an attempt to insinuate herself into the spaces of masculine experience so as to explore exactly what it is that she is being refused access to. Vic places herself in the in-between spaces of experimentation, hyper-performativity and transformation in ways that thus articulate identity as queer, as I shall now briefly explore.

Breaking the frame

In their work on female masculinity, Halberstam has argued that "the categories available to women for racial, gendered and sexual identity are simply inadequate" (1998: 7). Halberstam also highlights the significance of naming in their work, showing how it articulates "the power of definition" (ibid.: 7); when names are changed, the power to reimagine identity is conferred on the individual, allowing a retreat from lived facets of identity, place, relationships and even gender.

For Halberstam, this constructs "a queer subject position" from which it is possible to challenge hegemonic models of gender conformity (ibid.: 9). It is easy to see how *Girlhood* puts this dynamic on show in its construction of Vic (who, at the same time, both is and is not Marieme) in the final segment of its story. What would it mean, then, to think of *Girlhood* as offering a queer representation of identity in order to highlight the politics of intersectional subjectivity?

Laura Alexandra Harris argued some time ago that working toward "queer Black feminism" can "disrupt the silences in feminism, Black feminism, and queer theories of race, class, and sexuality" (1996: 4), thereby opening up the intersection of sexual pleasure and the politics of race and class. As she suggests

> A queer Black feminist practice requires marking race and class in relation to desire and reveals that the telling of desire must always be a text written about race and class no matter how encoded with gender oppression . . . race and class [are] inextricable from . . . sexuality and feminist consciousness.
>
> *(Ibid.: 12–13)*

If we follow Harris' logic here, we might make interesting links to the importance of gang experiences for young women of colour. Meda Chesney-Lind and Katherine Irwin have observed that, while gang culture places girls in precarious positions because they do not have access to legitimate or illegitimate economic opportunities, it also enables girls to confront the hyper-masculine norms of ideology that surround them (2004: 49). Debbie Weeks has carried out research to show that because of the close imbrication of Black identities with sexualized connotations in the popular cultural imagination, young Black women are subjected to intensely sexualized othering in everyday life, leading to a great difficulty in finding space in which to explore their sexual identities because of the tension between deviance and hypersexuality in which their identities are construed (Weeks 2002: 252; 2004: 144–145). In this way, then, young Black women find themselves being interpellated as what Halberstam refers to as "in-betweenness" (2004: 210), a trope that resonates with the struggle portrayed by Marieme/Vic in *Girlhood* and that also reminds us of the double bind alluded to by Meltzer in his observations about the girl-gang state of mind and its evocation of femininity as paradoxically re-inscribed or trapped within the logic of patriarchy despite (because of?) its anti-masculine texture. Kimberley Roberts has shown how liminal figures of this type reveal the potential for the cultural subversion of gender norms (2002: 223, 230), and, for me, the institutional, figurative and imaginative spaces of cinema provide exactly the kind of containing environment needed for such apparently dangerous or difficult forays to be made. When we see on the cinema screen a girl protagonist who seemingly has no resources left to her, and no place to go, the audience is also left, I think, in a space of wondering, or perhaps in a state of being able to explore what Christopher Bollas describes as "unthought knowns" (1987: 4): this is, at least, my own experience of this film. The film offers space in which to think outside the frame of conventional practices of representation of gender and sexuality, in a way that is possible because of the containing function that cinema can have when it provides spaces for the experience and expression of emotion that lies beyond the scope of normal/conscious thinking processes.

For me, this strain of thinking offers a crucial lens through which to read the final scenes of *Girlhood*. Marieme returns fleetingly to the *banlieue*, ringing the buzzer to her family home but finding herself unable to speak when her sister asks who is there. She turns and stares at the view across Paris, bathed in sunshine and she leans against a pillar, crying. Her grief and sorrow speak volumes about her isolation in this moment, her desperate need to cut herself off completely in order to find freedom. The camera tracks in behind her, before zooming in on a strangely blurred shot of the distant cityscape, excluding Marieme from the frame for a moment, and connoting a closing shot. Suddenly Marieme rushes into view, crossing the frame from right to left. She pauses for a moment in a profile shot, placing herself as the object of focus, before running out of shot again. Her movement from one side of the frame to the other both speaks to her inscription in the margins of representability and gives voice to her struggle in the in-between spaces of representation in a way that feels full of life and hope.

Cinema itself is queered in this moment, as Marieme undoes its logic, highlighting the "off-screen" spaces of her identity and giving the spectator room to acknowledge these. Her flight into the unknown on her own terms becomes a site of cumulative learning, and one that is ripe with possibility. The bruised aesthetic that accentuated Marieme's vulnerability and her encounters with violence lifts in this scene to allow sunlight into the frame. The score consists of a track entitled "Where to Go?", a question posed in the active voice, connoting subjecthood. The cinema becomes a space of rupture, gesturing in and through girlhood to the spaces that lie beyond the girl-gang state of mind, spaces existing outside dominant modes of subjectivity so that girlhood becomes readable as a learning experience, a maturational process that does not only trap its subjects into the schizoid pursuit of safety in numbers (Waddell 2007: 202), but that can also lead to a profound capacity for resilience. Chiming with the sentiment of Rhianna's metonymic song, girlhood becomes a vision of ecstasy, something that is clearly alive, and full of hope – like Marieme's future, we hope, it shines bright.

Conclusion

Writing over 20 years ago, psychoanalyst, Kimberlyn Leary asked, "In which ways are gender and race comparable?" (1997: 161). Following the logic of postmodern debates about the role of sexuate difference in shaping subjectivity, she concluded, as discussed above, that race and gender exist in transitional space and are conceptually inscribed in the tensions of biology, society, culture and ideology (ibid.: 163). However, as Anita Biressi and Heather Nunn assert, the "tinderbox" texture of intersectional debates about race and lower socio-economic class inscriptions deepens a tendency toward the disparagement of working-class subjects (2013: 142). We could go further and observe that, when these dimensions of lived identity are shot through with questions of gender and sexuality, the quality of disparagement takes on an especially bruising tone, a feeling that is conveyed through the *mise-en-scène* of *Girlhood* and that also resonates with the struggle for Black feminist voices to be heard in a landscape of insistent colour blindness.

Sciamma's film encapsulates the fundamental complexity evoked by Leary's efforts to grapple with the apparent impossibility of conceptualizing race and gender *at the same time* – or rather, more specifically, the apparent impossibility of achieving such a task when the subject in question is both Black *and* female. With its focus on the contradictory and impossible silences of Black adolescent femininity, it shows us the importance of what Wilfred Bion calls "binding" (1965: 69), the principle by which aspects of experience are joined in constant conjunction, albeit that the meanings of each element might simply be unknown. Meaning is accumulated by dint of this ongoing conjunction, and I find this concept to be hugely interesting for thinking about what it is possible to say about Black femininity, a formation of identity that is laden with ontological complexity and psychological and sociocultural entanglements. As Patricia Collins has argued (1991/2000), Black female experience is situated within multiple intersecting sites of oppression, and these are not *additive* but rather *multiplicative* in texture.

Meltzer's notion of "the girl-gang state of mind" provides a useful analogy for the dynamic that underpins the competing, schizoid logic of different modes of feminist scholarship. As his work on this topic makes clear, the value of grouping together is that it provides a means of surviving scenarios of impoverishment and attack by dint of forging bonds *in spite of* the odds against this. Meltzer asserts that the "egalitarianism" in the girl-gang state of mind is linked to the social injustices of patriarchy and paradoxically allows women to bind themselves together while at the same time expressing ambivalence about doing so. This can be read as a gesture toward a temporary, strategic form of feminist politics aimed at uncovering the complex impossibilities of female intersectional experience. Perhaps this provides a way for us to comprehend the widespread critical appreciation of *Girlhood*, despite its challenging contexts of production, and to think anew about how the film invites us to think beyond familiar paradigms and to hold in tension the messy complexities of contemporary identity politics.

Notes

1 I would like to express my grateful thanks to Dr Karen Cross, Ms Judith Rifeser and especially to Professor Anita Biressi for their valuable feedback on early drafts of this work.

2 The notion of "cultural appropriation" has now become commonplace in popular commentary on social processes around ethnicity, identity and responsibility. Of course, the term is laden with assumptions, as well as a complex dynamic that is overlaid with textures of both guilt and reparative impulses. For a nuanced and deeply moving perspective on how the concept undermines efforts at collaborative learning and creativity, see Piotrowska (2017). See also Sciamma's own reflections on her engagement with this issue in the course of making this work (Blay 2015).

3 See also Piotrowska (2017) on how these issues are interrogated in the genre of documentary film-making.

4 Of course, the shadowy threat posed by the groups of young men in this scene fuels lazy cultural stereotypes about Black masculinity, and this is a frequent criticism of cinema that focuses on Black female experience.
5 Emma Wilson notes a comment made by the film's Director of Photography, Crystel Fournier: "We managed to do things we never could have done with white skins. The colour palette we used between blue and green can produce a gloomy effect and never enhances the actors. But our actresses, since their skin is warm, can handle these types of colours. We could push colours to a point impossible with white skins" (2017: 18).
6 *Precious* has also been analysed extensively for its treatment of pain as a key dimension of Black female experience. See, for example, Griffin (2013), Ordoñez (2010) and Regester (2015). The significance of unknowable pain experienced by people of colour must also underpin reflexive scholarship conducted by those who benefit from white privilege.
7 The majority of this sequence (2' 53") uses Rhianna's song as a non-diegetic soundtrack, depicting the girls as they seem to lip sync the words, before cutting to a 43" long passage in which the non-diegetic soundtrack matches the diegetic voices of the gang as they sing in their own voices.
8 As I explain elsewhere: "Masquerade is the term used to describe an alienated version of femininity which originates in a woman's awareness of a man's desire for her to be his other. The femininity of the masquerade is constructed by and for masculine desire, and thus does not allow woman to experience desire in her own right. Within masquerade, woman is permitted only to experience desire when man's desire permits (Irigaray 1977/1985: 220) . . . In mimicry, woman deliberately takes on the feminine style and posture attributed to her within dominant discourse in order to reveal the mechanisms of her oppression and exploitation (ibid.). Woman is then able to use these mechanisms to disrupt discursive coherence by deliberately taking on the role ascribed to the feminine to draw attention to the flimsiness of its construction within dominant discourse, and thus to seduce dominant discourse into revealing its repressed foundation" (Bainbridge 2008: 20).
9 In an effort to respect Halberstam's position on the importance of preserving "gender quandaries", I have opted here to omit their first names (Judith/Jack) and to use the gender-non-specific pronoun "their" when discussing their work. As Halberstam observes, in order to be politically dynamic, pronoun use "must categorically remain murky" (2012).

Bibliography

Anonymous (2015a) Karidja Touré discusses her acting debut in Céline Sciamma's Girlhood. *Film3Sixty*, 8 May. Available from: http://film3sixtymagazine.com/karidja-toure-discusses-her-acting-debut-in-celine-sciammas-girhood.(Accessed 25 January 2018).

Anonymous (2015b) *Girlhood*, directed by Celine Sciamma. *Shades of Noir*, 29 May. Available from: http://shadesofnoir.org.uk/girlhood-directed-by-celine-sciamma (Accessed 14 December 2017).

Bainbridge, C. (2008) *A feminine cinematics: Luce Irigaray, women, and film*. Basingstoke: Palgrave Macmillan.

Bainbridge, C. (2014) "Cinematic screaming" or "all about my mother": Lars von Trier's cinematic extremism as therapeutic encounter. In C. Bainbridge and C. Yates (ed.) *Media and the inner world: Psycho-cultural perspectives on emotion, media and popular culture*. Basingstoke: Palgrave Macmillan: 53–68.

Bhabha, H. (1994) *The location of culture*. London: Routledge.

Billow, R. M. (2013) The bully inside us: The gang in the mind. *Psychoanalytic Inquiry*, 33(2), 130–143.

Bion, W. (1965) *Transformations*. London: Karnac Books.

Biressi, A. and Nunn, H. (2013) *Class and contemporary British culture*. Basingstoke: Palgrave Macmillan.

Blay, Z. (2014) *Girlhood* captures the unique process of growing up that many Black girls must navigate. *Indiewire,* 5 September. Available from: www.indiewire.com/2014/09/tiff-2014-review-girlhood-captures-the-unique-process-of-growing-up-that-many-black-girls-must-navigate-158345 (Accessed 14 December 2017).

Blay, Z. (2015) Interview: *Girlhood* director Céline Sciamma on race, gender, and the universality of the story. *Indiewire,* 6 February. Available from: www.indiewire.com/2015/02/interview-girlhood-director-celine-sciamma-on-race-gender-the-universality-of-the-story-155800 (Accessed 25 January 2018).

Bloodsworth-Lugo, M. K. (2007) *In-between bodies: Sexual difference, race and sexuality*. New York: SUNY Press.

Bollas, C. (1987) *The shadow of the object: Psychoanalysis of the unthought known.* London: Free Associations Books.

Canham, H. (2002) Group and gang states of mind. *Journal of Child Psychotherapy,* 28(2), 113–127.

Chesney-Lind, M. and Irwin, K. (2004) From badness to meanness: Popular constructions of contemporary girlhood. In A. Harris (ed.) *All about the girls: Culture, power and identity.* London: Routledge: 45–58.

Chew-Bose, D. (2015) On Brown-girl exclusivity and writing our own narratives. *Buzzfeed News,* 8 March. Available from: www.buzzfeed.com/durgachewbose/on-brown-girl-exclusivity-and-writing-our-own-narratives (Accessed 25 January 2018).

Collins, P. (1991/2000) *Black feminist thought: Knowledge, consciousness, and the politics of empowerment.* Boston, MA: McGraw Hill.

Eddo-Lodge, R. (2017) *Why I'm no longer talking to white people about race.* London: Bloomsbury. Kindle Edition.

Freud, S. (1920) Beyond the pleasure principle. In J. Strachey (ed.) *The standard edition of the complete psychological works of Sigmund Freud,* vol. 18, London: Hogarth Press: 1–64.

Griffin, R. A. (2013) *Push*ing into *Precious*: Black women, media representation, and the glare of the white supremacist capitalist patriarchal gaze. *Critical Studies in Media Communication,* 31(3), 182–197.

Grotstein, J. S. (2007) *A beam of intense darkness: Wilfred Bion's legacy to psychoanalysis.* London: Karnac.

Halberstam, J. (1998) *Female masculinity*. Durham, NC: Duke University Press.

Halberstam, J. (2004) Oh bondage up yours! Female masculinity and the tomboy. In S. Bruhm and N. Hurley (ed.) *Curiouser: On the queerness of children.* Minneapolis, MN: University of Minnesota Press: 191–214.

Halberstam, J. (2012) On pronouns. Jack Halberstam: Gaga feminism and queer failure. Available from: www.jackhalberstam.com/on-pronouns (Accessed 14 December 2017).

Harris, L. A. (1996) Queer Black feminism: The pleasure principle. *Feminist Review,* 54, 3–30.

hooks, b. (2003) *Teaching community: A pedagogy of hope.* London: Routledge.

Ince, K. (2017) *The body and the screen: Female subjectivities in contemporary women's cinema.* London: Bloomsbury.

Irigaray, L. (1977/1985) *This sex which is not one,* trans. C. Porter. Ithaca, NY: Cornell University Press.

Irigaray, L. (1987/1993) Gesture in psychoanalysis. In *Sexes and genealogies,* trans. G. C. Gill. New York: Columbia University Press: 89–104.

Irigaray, L. (1992/1996) *i love to you: Sketch for a possible Felicity in history,* trans. A. Martin. London: Routledge.

Khanna, R. (2003) *Dark continents: Psychoanalysis and colonialism.* Durham, NC: Duke University Press.

Kyrola, K. (2017) Feeling bad and *Precious* (2009): Black suffering, white guilt, and intercorporeal subjectivity. *Subjectivity*, 10, 258–275.

Leary, K. (1997) Race in psychoanalytic space. *Gender and Psychoanalysis*, 2(2), 157–172.

McNeill, I. (2017) "Shine bright like a diamond": Music, performance and digitextuality in Céline Sciamma's Bande de filles (2014). *Studies in French Cinema*. Available from: www.tandfonline.com/doi/full/10.1080/14715880.2017.1345187 (Accessed 14 November 2017).

Meltzer, D. (1973) *Sexual states of mind*. London: Karnac Books.

Meltzer, D. (2007) *Sincerity and other works: The collected papers of Donald Meltzer*, ed. A. Hahn. London: Karnac Books.

Mouflard, C. (2016) "Il y a des règles": Gender, surveillance, and circulation in Céline Sciamma's *Bande de filles*. *Women in French Studies*, 24, 113–126.

Ordoñez, M.-B. (2010) Too precious for you. *Canadian Women's Studies*, 28(1). Available from: https://cws.journals.yorku.ca/index.php/cws/article/view/30790 (Accessed 14 December 2017).

Piotrowska, A. (2017) *Black and white: Cinema, politics and the arts in Zimbabwe*. London: Routledge.

Regester, C. (2015) Monstrous mother, incestuous father, and terrorized teen: Reading *Precious* as a horror film. *Journal of Film and Video*, 67(1), 30–45.

Rhianna (2012) Diamonds. *Unapologetic*. Def Jam Recordings.

Roberts, K. (2002) Pleasures and problems of the "angry girl". In F. Gateward and M. Pomerance (ed.) *Sugar, spice, and everything nice: Cinemas of girlhood*. Detroit: Wayne State University Press: 217–233.

Rosenfeld, H. (1971) A clinical approach to the psychoanalytic theory of the life and death instincts: An investigation into the aggressive aspects of narcissism. *International Journal of Psychoanalysis*, 52, 169–178.

Sylla, F. (2015) WoC versus Black women: Thoughts on the fallacy of solidarity and the erasure of Black women. Available from: https://medium.com/@littleglissant/woc-vs-black-women-bdd8a8cb7447 (Accessed 14 December 2017).

Tewolde-Berhan, A. (2015) *Girlhood* – A review: Fatally flawed examination of a young Black French girl's life. What's_On Africa, 28 July (Accessed 25 January 2018).

Waddell, M. (2007) Grouping or ganging: The psychodynamics of bullying. *British Journal of Psychotherapy*, 23(2), 189–204.

Weeks, D. (2002) Get your freak on: How Black girls sexualize identity. *Sex Education*, 2(3), 251–262.

Weeks, D. (2004) Where my girls at? Black girls and the construction of the sexual. In Anita Harris (ed.) *All about the girls: Culture, power and identity*. London: Routledge: 141–159.

Wilson, E. (2017) Scenes of hurt and rapture: Céline Sciamma's *Girlhood*. *Film Quarterly*, 70(3), 10–22.

Winnicott, D. W. (1971) *Playing and reality*. London: Routledge.

Filmography

Bande de filles/Girlhood (2014) Directed by Céline Sciamma, France.

Naissance des pieuvres/Water Lilies (2007) Directed by Céline Sciamma, France.

Precious (2010) Directed by Lee Daniels, USA.

Tomboy (2011) Céline Sciamma, France.

4

REVISITING JOAN RIVIERE

Vicky Lebeau

First published in the *International Journal of Psychoanalysis* in 1929, and reprinted in the influential *Formations of Fantasy*, edited by Victor Burgin, James Donald and Cora Kaplan in 1986, Joan Riviere's "Womanliness as a Masquerade" enjoys a unique, if now uneasy, place in the dialogue between psychoanalysis and feminism: from Ur-text attuned to the relations among sex, gender and identity to one of the most prominent examples of a silence – shared between psychoanalysis and feminism – on the question of racism in the formations of self and society. "Womanliness as a Masquerade" belongs to a moment in the relation between feminism and psychoanalysis dedicated to an ongoing exploration of the unconscious as a force to be reckoned with by the Left (academic and activist) in its attempts to secure a psycho-social understanding of political and personal change. The editorial Preface to *Formations of Fantasy* was explicit: the collection was a clarion call to engage psychoanalysis as a discourse – a theory, a practice, an institution – that, in its probing of unconscious life, seeks to transform our relation to ourselves and to the real world.

That call was in no way straightforward. As the editors attest, Riviere's article "conducts us to the promise and the problem of psychoanalysis in the arena of the social" – a summary that anticipates the subsequent criticism of "Womanliness as a Masquerade" as a missed encounter between psychoanalysis, feminism and a critical theory of racism (Burgin et al. 1986: 3). As Jean Walton was one of the first to point out, the fascination exerted by the spectacle of the masquerade may well have derived from the permission given by Riviere's text "to invoke, only to ignore, the cultural constructions of race that inform it" (1995: 800). "Riviere's indifference to the racialized components of her patient's fantasies," she continues, "is reproduced with a striking monotony by her feminist successors" (ibid.: 803).

Why revisit Riviere? This question has become a guide to my own perplexity in writing this chapter – perplexity that derives from a persistent intuition that something remains structural, but unthought, to "Womanliness as a Masquerade" and, by extension, to our continuing interpretations of it. Certainly, what is not in dispute here is Riviere's participation in what Frantz Fanon describes in *Black Skin, White Masks*, first published as *Peau Noire, Masques Blancs* in 1952, as the *imago* of the black man in European culture (1986: 169). Among other things, *Black Skin, White Masks* is an extraordinary exposition of the racist structure of feeling at work in European culture: "When we say," Fanon insists in on "The Negro and Psychopathology", "that European culture possesses an *imago* of the negro responsible for all the conflicts that may arise, we do not go beyond the real" (ibid., translation modified). The reality of the *imago*? The effects of the *imago* on the real world? The *imago* as a real event? We need that interpretative hesitation to grasp the full extent of Fanon's thought here, his challenge to psychoanalysis to think the origins of racism and hatred.

In what follows I want to suggest that if we read her concept of the masquerade alongside Riviere's less well-known "Jealousy as a Mechanism of Defence", published in 1932, we can open up a space between Riviere and Fanon that, while forcing psychoanalysis up against the real of racism, also challenges us to renew a psychoanalytic reading of "Womanliness as a Masquerade". That to read between Riviere and Fanon is to encounter psychoanalysis at the boundary between dream and culture, unconscious and ideology, is one of the starting-points of this chapter. That that boundary demands a different order of psychoanalytic reading is one of its provisional conclusions.

In the opening lines of her essay, Riviere introduces "Womanliness as a Masquerade" as her response to the typologies of female sexuality developed by Ernest Jones through the 1920s; her writing is clearly grounded in a need to describe a new "type" of woman: professional, intellectual, engaged in public life and "intermediate" (Riviere's term) in her relation to the divisions between male and female, masculine and feminine ("Womanliness as a Masquerade" belongs to the "great debate" about femininity and female sexuality in psychoanalysis through the 1920s and 1930s) (1929: 303). In fact, it is the pressure of such divisions that drives Riviere towards the enigmatic formulation at the heart of her essay:

> The reader may now ask how I define womanliness or where I draw the line between genuine womanliness and the "masquerade". My suggestion is not, however, that there is any such difference; whether radical or superficial, they are the same thing.
>
> *(Ibid.: 306)*

That formulation has sustained a rich exploration of femininity and identification, confounding any final congruence between a woman and her "womanliness". As Adrienne Harris has summarized: Riviere's essay is "a text beloved of Lacanians, feminists, and postmoderns alike as an early prototheorizing account of the performative border-living, liminal aspects of identity" (2012: 205). More anxiously, as a defence against a womanliness described as the primary mode of being sexual for a woman, the masquerade has been understood as a sign of women's alienation from themselves and their desires within a masculine and patriarchal social order. In Luce Irigaray's well-known statement, for example, masquerade is "what women do (. . .) in order to participate in man's desire, but at the cost of giving up theirs" (cited in Heath 1986: 54). Schematically, then, the masquerade – spectacle, performance, ruse – has been used to identify femininity with non-identity as such – "[A]uthentic womanliness", as Stephen Heath puts the point, "is such a mimicry, is the masquerade" – and then, by extension, to explore the impossibility of ever finally knowing, or achieving, an identification with any sex (male or female being only the inadequate, if ubiquitous, starting offer) (1986: 49).[1]

It is well known that Riviere based her analysis of the masquerade on the treatment of a successful, intellectual American woman "engaged in work of a propagandist nature which consisted principally in speaking and writing" (1929: 304). After every public performance, this woman experienced anxiety so acute that she was compelled to seek (sexual) reassurance from the men in her audience. Given its significance to what follows, it is worth quoting Riviere's account of her patient's symptoms in detail:

> Analysis then revealed that the explanation of her compulsive ogling and coquetting (. . .) was as follows: it was an unconscious attempt to ward off the anxiety which would ensue on account of the reprisals she anticipated from the father-figures after her intellectual performance. The exhibition in public of her intellectual proficiency, which was in itself carried through successfully, signified an exhibition of herself in possession of the father's penis, having castrated him. The display once over, she was seized by horrible dread of the retribution the father would then exact. Obviously it was a step towards propitiating the avenger to endeavour to offer herself to him sexually. This phantasy, it then appeared, had been very common in her childhood and youth, which had been spent in the Southern States of America; if a negro came to attack her, she planned to defend herself by making him kiss her and make love to her (ultimately so that she could then deliver him over to justice).
>
> *(Ibid.: 305–306)*

Further, Riviere observes that:

> In a dream which had a rather similar content to this childhood phantasy, she was in terror alone in the house; then a negro came in and found her washing clothes, with her sleeves rolled up and arms exposed. She resisted him, with the secret intention of attracting him sexually, and he began to admire her arms and caress them and her breasts. The meaning was that she had killed father and mother and obtained everything for herself (alone in the house), became terrified of their retribution (expected shots through the window), and defended herself by taking on a menial role (washing clothes) and by

> washing off dirt and sweat, guilt and blood, everything she had obtained by the deed, and "disguising herself" as merely a castrated woman.
>
> *(Ibid.: 306)*

"If a negro came to attack her . . ." At once acknowledged and ignored by Riviere, this imaginary scene agitates through "Womanliness as a Masquerade", opening on to the history of race murder in the American South: in particular, the "Southern white rape complex", its murderous fantasias of white woman and girlhood menaced by black men (Dowd Hall 1983). What matters in recent criticism of "Womanliness as a Masquerade" is what Riviere does not say as she moves from her patient's symptoms to her childhood phantasy, from phantasy to dream and, finally, from dream to its unconscious determinants located in a scene of intra-psychic attack on the parental imagoes of early infantile life ("The meaning was . . ."). A few pages later, Riviere makes that intra-psychic drama even more explicit: "The analysis showed that the origin of all these reactions (. . .) lay in the reaction to the parents during the oral-biting sadistic phase" (1929: 309).

Deriving her patient's symptoms, along with her fantasies and dreams, from infantile scenes, Riviere accounts for three different forms of representation in terms of a concealed "meaning"; or, symptom, phantasy and dream are here understood as forms via which something else – the infant's struggle with her primal drives, her relations to her earliest objects – can find expression. Either way, as Walton summarizes her criticism of Riviere's interpretative method,

> [I]t makes no difference in Riviere's account that the "man" in question here is black, that culturally sanctioned fantasies in which a white woman is sexually attacked by a black man form a significant component of dominant white racist hegemony in the United States.
>
> *(1995: 782)*

By contrast, drawing attention to the racist sexual imaginary structuring both Riviere's essay and her patient's psychic life, Walton argues for the necessity of exploring "local constructions of racialized identification and desire" to counter the displacement of the question of the relation between racism and the unconscious – more broadly, ideology and the unconscious – taking place in Riviere's writing (and, by extension, in the founding texts of psychoanalysis: Walton's essay includes a discussion of Melanie Klein's "Infantile Anxiety-Situations Reflected in a Work of Art and in the Creative Impulse" (1929) for its "quite astonishing (. . .) indifference" to the role of the portrait of a black woman in the material under discussion) (ibid.: 804, 794).

On one level, Walton is giving voice to an established suspicion of psychoanalysis as a tendentious hermeneutic, imposing its desire to rewrite the world in its own image – those bourgeois European dramas of sex, violence and incest – on the diverse materials that come its way. In the case of "Womanliness as a Masquerade", it is difficult to dispute the effects of that imposition (though my sense is that the silence often attributed to Riviere's feminist successors concerns the history of published readings of her essay rather than, say, the exploration of her work in more directly pedagogic contexts when, in my experience, the question of what Riviere is doing, or not doing, with her patient's fantasies of being attacked by a black man has been a prominent topic of discussion). But since the publication of Walton's "Re-Placing Race in (White) Psychoanalytic Discourse", feminist indifference (if that is what it is) has been displaced by a generative attention to what remains occluded in Riviere's essay: a "racial domain", in Walton's terms; the "African American presence", as Ai-Yu Niu puts it; or what Harris describes as the "presence of trauma unconsciously transcribed and repressed" (Walton 1995: 803; Ai-Yu Niu 2005: 135; Harris 2012: 206).

What remains to be said? I want now to suspend temporarily my reading of "Womanliness as a Masquerade" in order to take a brief detour through the closing paragraphs of "Jealousy as a Mechanism of Defence". With the exception of "Womanliness as a Masquerade", Riviere's writings remain largely unread outside the psychoanalytic institutions; thus to my knowledge, a telling coincidence between the race–sex fantasias invested by "Womanliness as a Masquerade" and the conclusion of "Jealousy as a Mechanism of Defence" has gone unnoticed. A key contribution to a psychoanalytic understanding of morbid jealousy, this essay tells another intriguing story of a woman suffering pains of jealousy at her husband's supposed affairs with other women (suspicions that, Riviere tells us, may not be without grounds) as well as the effects of a fantasy that dominates her life: namely, "seizing and obtaining from some other person something she greatly desired, thus robbing and despoiling him or her" (Riviere 1932: 416).

That unconscious dynamic, replayed variously in her patient's life, is explored with almost vertiginous diligence through Riviere's essay, leading inexorably towards her final comments on *Othello* – or rather, Othello – without which, as she puts it, a "psycho-analytic study of jealousy would be hardly conceivable":

> No detailed discussion of the play is needed: the unconscious motivation of jealousy that analysis reveals stands in the forefront of Shakespeare's plot, though he straightaway so cleverly discounts and glosses over it that we forget it forthwith. The first act of the play seems irrelevant to the subsequent story, yet it is vital in the depths. It shows us Desdemona's old father, his grief and fury caused by Othello's abduction of his daughter, his bitter reproaches and accusations, his threats and prophecies of disaster. Othello had won his loved object by seizure from her owner – the father. But more than this: to my mind the main expression of Othello's all-important psychic guilt (. . .) has been placed by Shakespeare where none can overlook it and yet again where none of us need see it for what it is – it is his blackness! "It is the cause, it is the cause, my soul" – the old tradition has it that with these words the actor spoke to his own image in a mirror, which he contrasts in the next breath with Desdemona's "whiter skin".
>
> *(Ibid.: 424)*

This is more than a conventional appeal to a shared cultural heritage, and to a celebrated poetic exploration of jealousy supposed to guarantee the value of a psychoanalytic insight. At this point, Fanon bears repeating: "In Europe the Negro has one function: that of symbolizing the lower emotions, the baser inclinations, the dark side of the soul" (1986: 190). Or, more bluntly: "Are they not forever saying that the niggers are just waiting for the chance to jump on white women?" (ibid.: 107). Riviere's language may be more decorous, but it is difficult to deny that that is indeed what she is saying when, in her tendentious description of the first act of Shakespeare's play, Othello is cast as Desdemona's abductor, and her father as a despoiled rightful owner, wrecked by grief and fury. In effect, Riviere is restating Iago's provocative description of Desdemona's secret marriage to Othello in which he casts their elopement as abduction, the white daughter as the legal property of her father, and the black man as a bestial thief:

> Zounds, sir, you're robbed; for shame, put on your gown;
> Your heart is burst; you have lost half your soul;
> Even now, now, very now, an old black ram
> Is tupping your white ewe.
>
> (Othello *Act 1, Scene 1, 86–89*)

The language is infamously brutalized (as is a world conceived in terms of rights to the ownership of people and of aggravated burglary). But Iago's logic structures Riviere's turn to *Othello*, her unthinking investment in being white and a concomitant massive de-idealization of blackness. Conjuring that imaginary scene of Othello gazing at his face in the mirror, Riviere finds only *his* guilt in *her* perception of his black skin:

> Does not Othello's blackness, also seemingly irrelevant, sum up in one symbol the whole story of his guilt, doubt, anxiety and his mode of defence against them? Iago the envious is but his alter ego. He cannot endure the evil in himself. He must make Desdemona black instead.
>
> *(1932: 424)*

Or, again: "It is his blackness!" It is difficult not to hear a note of excitement, a type of interpretative triumph, in Riviere's exclamation as she makes "blackness" the natural repository – Fanon might say the "predestined depository" – of those psychic pains belonging to us all: anxiety, hate, aggression, envy (Fanon 1986: 179).

In this context, part of the significance of "Jealousy as a Mechanism of Defence" is its unintended elaboration of Riviere's brief, but freighted, sketch of the racist fantasies and dreams at the heart of "Womanliness as a Masquerade". The pressure of the black *imago* becomes more apparent, more revealing, in that convergence between a patient's (day)dreams of being attacked by a black man, and Riviere's participation in the idea of Othello's seizure of a white woman from her owner-father. In "Womanliness as a Masquerade", that convergence is most obvious in a moment of textual repression, or internal exclusion, when Riviere brackets precisely that element of her patient's childhood phantasy that embeds a spectacle of lynching in the masquerade: "if a negro came to attack her, she planned to defend herself by making him kiss her and make love to her (ultimately so that she could then deliver him over to justice)" (1929: 305).

The parenthesis is crucial, a sign of Riviere's turning away from any elaboration of the meaning of the fact that her patient grew up in the Southern States, and the violence contained by this daydream of handing a black man over to a murderous mob ("Judge Lynch" in the parlance of the period). As Dowd Hall reflects on the persistence of lynching into the 1920s and 1930s, "even as white moderates criticized lynching in the abstract, they continued to justify outbreaks of mob violence for the one special crime of sexual assault" (1983: 344). In this sense, by fixing the idea of the masquerade as a fantasy of appeasement, Riviere invests a version of the feminine Oedipus complex negotiated through a cultural fantasy of racial violence: it is not the father who suffers castration and robbery, but the black man accused of rape or abduction. By extension, it appears to be possible to continue to aggress the father and his rights – in this instance, to make inroads on masculine privilege in the public domain – as long as you take a detour via the body of a black man. In other words, as a performance of appeasement, the masquerade is also embedded in a fantasy of vengeful sacrifice, legitimizing a murderous aggression by changing its object: the black *imago* is at work on both sides of the dream.

In this sense, Riviere anticipates, and confirms, Fanon's controversial analysis of the white woman's Oedipus complex – notably, its uses of the "free-floating aggression" that the father refuses to "take up" – in *Black Skin, White Masks* (Fanon 1986: 178). I have discussed elsewhere Fanon's commentary on feminine psychosexuality and feminist responses to it (Lebeau 1998, 2005). Suffice it to say here that his analysis emerges from his demand on psychoanalysis to think the origins and effects of racial hatred – the very demand foreclosed by Riviere as she displaces the problematic that comes right to the fore when she makes the connection (and it is she who makes it) between her patient's environment and the form taken by her childhood daydreaming: "This phantasy, it then appeared, had been very common" (Riviere 1929: 309). The ambiguity of Riviere's phrasing is apposite: the fantasy is common – typical, readymade, collective – in the Southern States (but not only there) and Riviere's patient is also said to daydream with it repeatedly. In other words, "if a negro came to attack her . . ." signals a type of recurring daydream, a child playing with a fantasy that preoccupies not only her waking life but her dreams: "In a dream which had a rather similar content to this childhood phantasy" (ibid.). Riviere notes, but does not pursue, that correspondence between ideology and dream, and the transfer from one to the other of an *imago* belonging not, or not only, to her patient's infantile unconscious but to the racist culture in which she lives.

What kind of dreaming is this? Riviere's occlusion of the racist *imago* structuring her patient's fantasy – and, of course, her own reading of *Othello* – leaves unremarked the coincidence between the forms of fantasy trafficked through public life and the intimate, and individual, process of dreaming. As Freud puts it, "each person is at liberty to construct his dream-world according to his individual peculiarities and so to make it unintelligible to other people" (1900: 241). What has happened to that liberty, and its creative freedoms, in "Womanliness as a Masquerade"? My point is not to attempt a "wild analysis" of Riviere's patient but to explore what remains unthought, unelaborated, by the analyst's rush to the depths, her pursuit of the infantile scenes supposed to be veiled behind the manifest content of her patient's symptoms, dreams and fantasies ("The meaning was . . ."). By the late 1920s, that method of interpretation – its privileging of what Freud describes as the "child's impulses still living on in the dream" – is well established; indeed, it has been exhaustively explored by Freud himself (ibid.: 191). But the curiosity of a dream that wears its heart on its sleeve bears further exploration, as Freud himself acknowledges when he uncovers a form of dreaming (if that is what it is) that appears to impose a limit on the wayward idiom of our dream lives. "There are a certain number of dreams," he writes, "which almost everyone has dreamt alike and which we are accustomed to assume must have the same meaning for everyone" (ibid.: 241).

Typical dreams, *typische Traume*: dreams of a type, belonging not, or not only, to an individual but to "everyone": a family, a community, a nation, a world (*Oedipus Rex*, that masterplot of murder and incest, is about to be introduced under the heading of "Dreams of the Death of Persons of Whom the Dreamer Is Fond"). Such dreams, on Freud's explanation, share two distinguishing features. On the one hand, there is a correlation between manifest content and feeling: in a typical dream, the death of a loved one will arouse a feeling of overwhelming grief (if that feeling is absent, then the dream is not "typical" and the manifest content must be treated as the usual façade). On the other hand, the dreamer of a typical dream either fails to produce any associations at all, or those associations become obscure and meagre. "Our art disappoints our expectations precisely in relation to this material," Freud concludes – as if psychoanalysis is initially paralysed by a form of dreaming that calls into question the idea of the dream as a world apart, the privileged symbol of the right to a mind of one's own (ibid.).

The implications of this form of dreaming remain to be thought. To track the editorial history of "Typical Dreams" (Section D of Chapter V) and "Representation by Symbols in Dreams – Some Further Typical Dreams" (Section E of Chapter VI, "The Dream-Work") is to find oneself in the throes of Freud's attempts to work through the significance of such dreaming to psychoanalysis and its evolving techniques of interpretation. What does the "typical dream" do to hard-won psychoanalytic insights into the individual poetics of dreams? What kind of dream is it that can have the same form and meaning for everyone? What does that homogeneity mean for the new technique of free association as one of the privileged routes to the unconscious mind?

That such questions quickly become entangled with the role of symbolism in dreams is perhaps inevitable. Symbols, as Freud puts it in 1916, are "stable translations", enabling a form of dream interpretation that, at once ancient and popular, is also likely to generate the most violent resistance to psychoanalysis and its insights (in "The Theory of Symbolism", also published in 1916, Ernest Jones described its interpretation of symbols as "the centre of the strongest opposition to psycho-analysis in general") (Freud 1916: 153; Jones 1977: 87). Theoretically, part of what is at stake here is the distinction between the manifest and latent contents of the dream so central to Freud's development of dream interpretation. It is one of the founding tenets of his theory of dreams that the dream-work is there to effect the transformation of one thing into another – the latent thoughts into the manifest surface of the dream – via the mechanisms of the primary process: condensation, distortion, displacement. The dream-work mangles and distorts; it makes unintelligible the (latent) wishes that we cannot bear even in our dreams (Freud 1900: 506). That work is the very essence of dreaming, Freud insists in a footnote added in 1925: "dreams are nothing other than a particular *form* of thinking" (ibid.). In other words, the dream-work is reducible neither to the manifest nor to the latent contents of the dream; the mistake of many analysts, Freud continues, is to attempt to find the essence of dreams in the wishes concealed behind their bizarre appearances (ibid.).

It is in the course of his lengthy discussion of the mechanisms of the dream-work that Freud introduces a concept that may offer an account of the production of the typical dream: secondary revision, that part of the dream-work charged with turning the dream into an intelligible experience. Secondary revision is something like an act of interpretation – of making the manifest content make sense – that takes place within the dream itself. It manufactures an appearance of meaning, and sustains the distinction between the manifest and latent content. But there is one crucial exception to that distinction:

> [T]here is one case in which it [secondary revision] is to a great extent spared the labour of as it were, building up a façade for the dream – the case, namely, in which a formation of that kind already exists, available for use in the material of the dream-thoughts. I am in the habit of describing the element in the dream-thoughts which I have in mind as a "phantasy". I shall perhaps avoid misunderstanding if I mention the "day-dream" as something analogous to it in waking life.
>
> *(Ibid.: 491)*

The implications of this passage are potentially far-reaching, with the concept of *Phantasie* radically disrupting both the distinctions between manifest and latent content, surface and depth, and the boundary between culture and the unconscious. Secondary revision describes a process not only of re-making the dream but of appropriating a ready-made fantasy inhabiting the dream-thoughts – a form of continuity, a type of repository, which Freud encounters too in his explorations of the typical and the symbolic in dreams. His "special interest" in such dreams derives, in part, from the fact that they appear poised to extend the reach of psychoanalysis into cultural and social life (thus extending what Freud calls its "practical applicability") (ibid.: 241). Equally, as we've seen, both the typical and the symbolic threaten to bring free association, and with it psychoanalysis, to a halt, obliging Freud to adopt what he describes as a "combined technique" that, by "fill[ing] the gaps from the interpreter's knowledge of symbols", can be used to counter that stalling of free association (ibid.: 353).

The significance of Freud's discussion of the typical dream, and the ready-made *Phantasie*, is its encounter with the possibility that what is there, and waiting to be discovered, in the dream is not a wishful-shameful fantasy belonging to our infantile selves but a symbol, an *imago*, possessing us all. It is as if the dream can be occupied by something in profound conformity with, rather than resistance to, the domain of social intelligibility. On the cusp between culture and the unconscious, *Phantasie* emerges in the mode of the typical, the common, the symbolic; it inhabits, and disrupts, the mobility of the primary processes, their creative idiom; it is a type of fixation, interfering with, and thereby limiting, the creativity of dreaming – and, thus, the patient's capacity to freely associate, to *think*, in the presence of it. "It will be observed," writes D. W. Winnicott in "Dreaming, Fantasying, and Living", "that creative playing is allied to dreaming and to living but essentially does not belong to fantasying" (1991: 31). Fantasying – at least in its fixated, stereotypical forms – interferes with both dreaming and living, inflicting a loss of individual symbolization that Winnicott casts in terms of repetition and redundancy: "A dog is a dog is a dog" (ibid.: 33).

"If a negro came to attack her": what is this if not a form of typical dreaming? What Riviere appears to have encountered with her patient – what her readers encounter in "Womanliness as a Masquerade" – is a form of dreaming in which the dream-work does not take place: a typical dream, a dream preoccupied by the black *imago*, by the fantasy of the black man as a lascivious violator of paternal rights. "The negro," as Fanon puts it, "is firmly fixed at the genital; or at least he has been fixed there (. . .) whoever says rape says negro" (1986: 165–166, translation modified). Beyond reason, this racialized sexual imaginary is not, as Fanon points out, susceptible to fact; what is at stake is meaning, and how it is made or unmade (ibid.: 168). Reading across from Fanon to Riviere, it is possible to glimpse the mind of a child, and a woman, stalled by the presence of an *imago* that brings the possibility of making meanings – the transformation of one thing into another in dream, in fantasy, in interpretation – to a halt. "No detailed reading of the play is needed": nothing more to be said here, as Riviere succumbs to the lure of the stereotype, its capacity to fix meaning – however scrambled, however destructive – in place.

In terms of a return to Riviere, finally, the challenge is not only how to make psychoanalysis attend to racism and history, but how to sustain its capacity for thinking and dreaming in the face of whatever that attention uncovers: in this instance, a murderous coincidence between culture and dream. Not until the publication of *Black Skin, White Masks* was psychoanalysis confronted, and potentially supported, by a writing that puts the convergence between unconscious fantasy and cultural life at the heart of its enquiry. It is that commitment that turns *Black Skin, White Masks* into a transformative object for psychoanalysis in its attempts to keep the mind alive in the face of racist hatred and aggression – the space at once foreclosed and made available by "Womanliness as a Masquerade".

Acknowledgements

A Research Fellowship from the Leverhulme Trust supported the completion of this chapter. I would also like to thank Vincent Quinn and Agnieszka Piotrowska for their generous and patient comments on earlier drafts.

Note

1 In light of what Jacqueline Rose has recently described as the "coercive violence of gendering" exposed by some of the current discussions around feminism and trans-politics, Riviere's essay continues to find its purchase. "What is a woman?" "Who *counts* as a woman?": so often framing those encounters, such questions recall the enigmatic formulation at the heart of Riviere's analysis (Rose 2016).

Bibliography

Ai-Yu Niu, G. (2005) Performing White Triangles: Joan Riviere's "Womanliness as a Masquerade" and *Imitation of Life* (1959). *Quarterly Review of Film and Video*, 22, 135–144.

Burgin, V., Donald, J. and Kaplan, C. (1986) *Formations of Fantasy*. London and New York: Methuen.

Dowd Hall, J. (1983) "The Mind that Burns in Each Body": Women, Rape, and Racial Violence. In A. Snitow, C. Stansell and S. Thompson (eds.), *Desire: The Politics of Sexuality*. London: Virago.

Fanon, F. (1986). *Black Skin, White Masks*. Trans. C. L. Markmann. London: Pluto Press.

Freud, S. (1900). The Interpretation of Dreams. In J. Strachey (ed.), *The Standard Edition of the Complete Psychological Works of Sigmund Freud*, Vols IV and V. London: Hogarth Press.

Freud, S. (1916) 'Symbolism in Dreams'. In J. Strachey (ed.), *The Standard Edition of the Complete Psychological Works of Sigmund Freud*, Vol. XV. London: Hogarth Press.

Harris, A. (2012) The House of Different, or White Silence. *Studies in Gender and Sexuality*, 13, 197–216.

Heath, S. (1986) Joan Riviere and the Masquerade. In B. Burgin, J. Donald and C. Kaplan, *Formations of Fantasy*. London and New York: Methuen.

Jones, Ernest (1977). *Papers on Psycho-Analysis*. London: Maresfield Reprints.

Lebeau, V. (1998) Psychopolitics: Frantz Fanon's *Black Skin, White Masks*. In J. Campbell and J. Harbord (eds.), *Psycho-Politics and Cultural Desires*. London: UCL Press.

Lebeau, V. (2005) Children of Violence. In M. Silverman (ed.), *Frantz Fanon's Black Skin, White Masks: New Interdisciplinary Essays*. Manchester and New York: Manchester University Press.

Ogden, T. H. (2016) *Reclaiming Unlived Life: Experiences in Psychoanalysis*. London and New York: Routledge.

Riviere, J. (1929) Womanliness as a Masquerade. *International Journal of Psycho-Analysis*, 10, 303–313.

Riviere, J. (1932). Jealousy as a Mechanism of Defence. *International Journal of Psycho-Analysis*, 13, 414–424.

Riviere, J. (1991) *The Inner World and Joan Riviere: Collected Papers 1920–1958*. Ed. A. Hughes. London and New York: Karnac Books.

Rose, J. (2016) Who Do You Think You Are? *London Review of Books*, 39(9), 3–13.

Walton, J. (1995) Re-Placing Race in (White) Psychoanalytic Discourse: Founding Narratives of Feminism. *Critical Inquiry*, 21, 775–804.

Winnicott, D. W. (1991) *Playing and Reality*. London and New York: Routledge.

5

SUPPLEMENTARY JOUISSANCE AND FEMININE SEXUAL RAPPORT

Bracha L. Ettinger

I. Supplementary jouissance

Introduction: inscriptions of supplementary femininity beyond the phallus[1]

The more Lacan establishes the "woman" within the phallic scope, the more a supplementary space, subversively insisting on undermining the founding of "woman" in the phallus, is in my view disclosed. I have called this space beyond the phallus: matrixial borderspace. In this space I link the unconscious memory traces of the part and partial objects – the *objet a* – to "supplementary" feminine jouissance.[2] The later Lacanian theory lays, from a certain elusive angle – in a manoeuvre described by J. A Miller as "Lacan against Lacan" – the hypothesis of the primacy of the register of the Real with its jouissance, in contrast to a net composed of the domination of the Symbolic over the Imaginary and the subordination of the Real to them both. Lacan turns to his inverted theoretical side when he wishes to touch, in his late teaching, a face of the Real that is not cut by, shaped or descended from a symbolic function; when he looks for a sense that vibrates and resonates straight from the Real and not for signification emanating from the Symbolic's pre-established reason. Lacan emphasizes the importance of finding a different mode of inscription that is not dependent on the signifier, by which something of the supplementary feminine experience might find inscription and not *just happen*. An inscription such as this is bound up with art, or else it is bound up with mysticism and psychosis.

If the "woman", as Lacan says in 1973, does not exist and does not signify anything, this statement can be placed in line with his later thoughts from 1975–1976, and we can say that this may be so only in the phallic arena, while *beyond-the-phallus*, a space Lacan hints at in 1973, from the angle I have called matrixial, if "woman" ex-sists with her *jouis-presence* then not only is *she* not orchestrated by the Oedipal model of sexuality and identification, but also *she* excavates tunnels of sense and draws a zone of difference which is indeed paradoxical for the phallus.

I propose that a female *swerve*[3] and a rapport in a Real connected to the womb are wound around a feminine jouissance. Affective swerve and rapport are for me the incidents in the Real at the basis of a feminine-matrixial difference that is supplemental to the feminine-phallic difference that relates, to begin with, to "penis envy" and to its lack. The feminine originary swerve is not occupied during the split of the subject that occurs in agreement with the castration model nor is it dissolved inside relations to the Other qua "treasure of signifiers". The swerve is captured in an originary rapport, and both create and engrave passages and means of transport towards the Symbolic through which traces of jouissance, sensations, affects, feelings and fantasies are channelled; means that do not converge in a process of castration. The matrixial swerve and rapport inscribe a "supplementary" difference and create supplementary *feminine-Other-desire*, transported, transformed and transferred within the matrixial borderspace, beyond metaphor and metonymy, by what I have termed *metramorphosis*.

In the context of Lacan's late theory but moving forward on, I will relate to connections between the female specificity in the Real and its swerve, the *feminine/prenatal* co-existence and the fantasy of prebirth incest of *I* with the archaic *m/Other-to-be*, a fantasy that I call matrixial and connect to the *Mutterliebesphantasie* that Freud suggested in the aesthetic experience of the *Unheimlich* (1919: 244, 248–249), and to the "envelopes" between mother and infant that get lost in birth according to Lacan (1961–1962). A matrixial fantasy bursts forth in each individual in jointness within a composite subjectivity. It is entwined between I and non-I from different directions: it appears as a fantasy of the becoming-subject (male or female) in relation to a woman as a *becoming-archaic-m/Other-to-be*, as a fantasy of a return to the womb, as a fantasy of the woman as potential *m/Other* or as an actual becoming-mother who relates to the becoming-subject she carries – all concerning the partial dimension of relations between partial subjects and partial/part-objects. I suggest that singular qualities of this cluster of fantasy testify that the feminine/prenatal[4] encounter doesn't melt away retroactively into an Oedipal "castration" model and is not constructed, subjugated or destroyed by the phallus, but remains beside it in the field of the unconscious. A connectionist web, knitted by *metramorphoses*, a web of knots and links, borderline relations and rapports between several partial subjects and partial/part objects in co-emergence and co-fading in a non-conscious borderspace creates a *feminine-Other-sense* and embroiders a feminine-Other-desire linked to a *beyond-the-phallus jouissance* and to an assembled *speak/through-being* (*parl'être*). Feminine sex-difference from the matrixial angle doesn't depend on essence but is contrived via "webbing" links to the invisible female specificity in the Real.

The phallic arena

The phallic arena is based on the mechanism of castration, and hence its processes of subjectivization are characterized by cuts from the corporeal, separations from

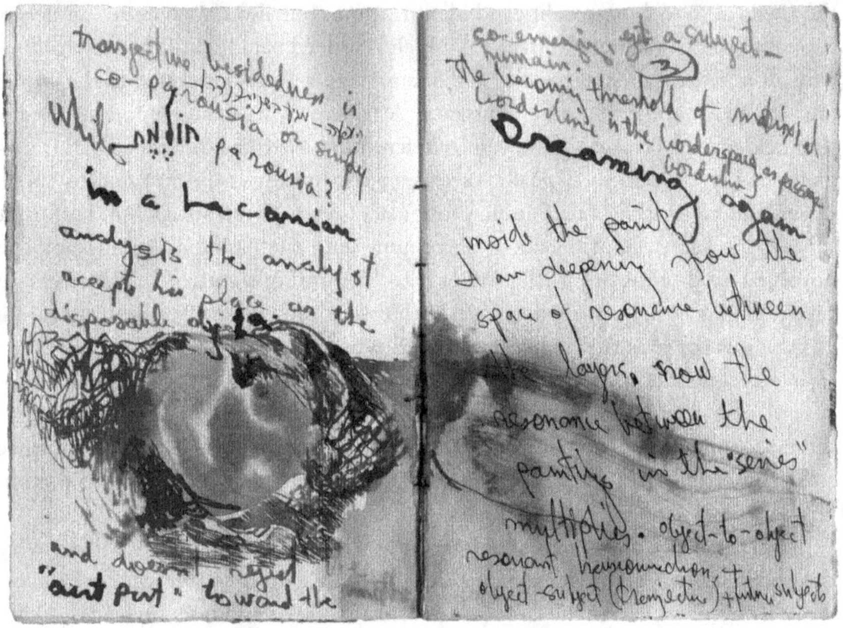

FIGURE 5.1 Bracha L. Ettinger, notebook, 2011–2012 (16 × 22 cm, double page).

Source: Courtesy of the artist.

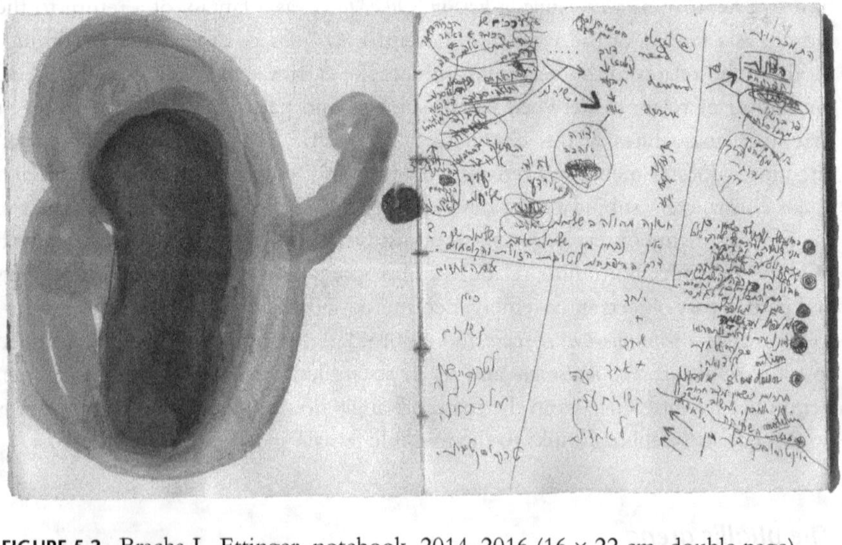

FIGURE 5.2 Bracha L. Ettinger, notebook, 2014–2016 (16 × 22 cm, double page).

Source: Courtesy of the artist.

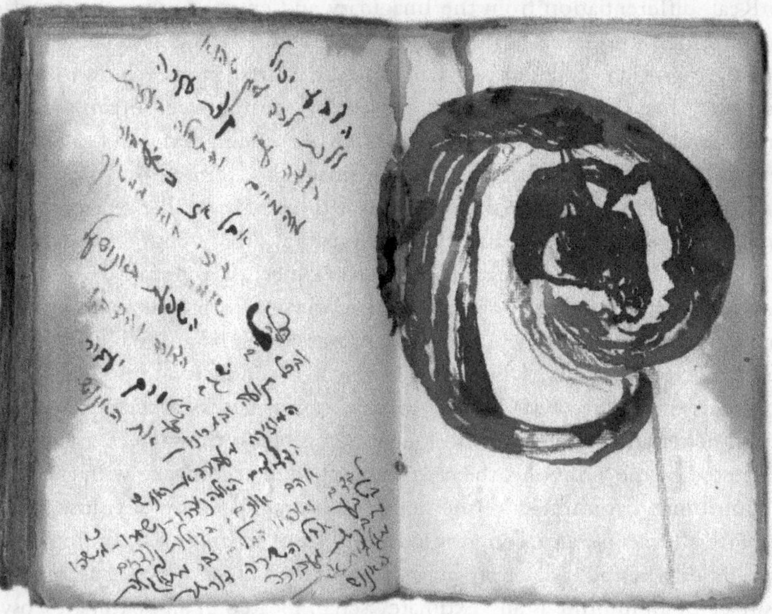

FIGURE 5.3 Bracha L. Ettinger, notebook, 2008 (16 × 22 cm, double page).
Source: Courtesy of the artist.

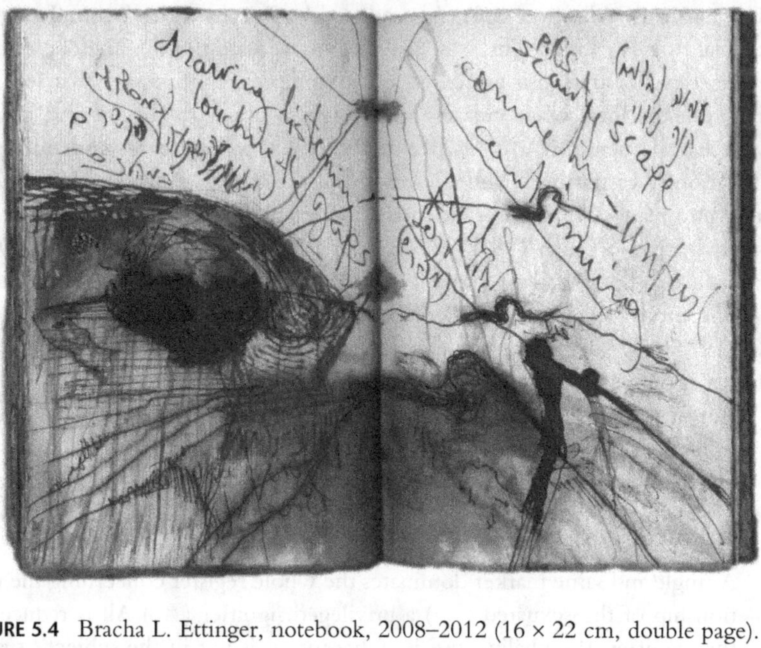

FIGURE 5.4 Bracha L. Ettinger, notebook, 2008–2012 (16 × 22 cm, double page).
Source: Courtesy of the artist.

the Real, differentiation from the Imaginary and entrances into the specifically human dimension – the Symbolic – by means of the signifier as it gels split from the signified[5] and through language articulated in speech and knitted in discourse.[6] The cuts from the Real and the schisms between organ and object, signifier and signified create a psychic surplus, a residue that is not digested into the Symbolic or incorporated inside the Imaginary, termed by Lacan the *objet (petit) a*. The *objet a* is a trace of an imprint, a primary trace that replaces an originary imprint which has remained from the partial drive's engagements with the archaic part object and the archaic mother-as-object or as primordial-Other that I call *m/Other*. The *objet a* is issued in the course of a primary schism through which the subject itself emerges as well as splits, when language blurs the archaic modes of experience and when discourse, which conducts and presents the laws and orders of society, nests in their place and restructures archaic processes and modes, materials and events as no longer accessible to the subject. Even though undigested by the Symbolic, the *objet a* is clipped in accordance with the pageant of significance determined by the signifier and regulated by discourse, and it is therefore a *border-phallic* inscription of remnants of separation from impulses and from "bodily samplings" of *my-corpo-reality* and of *my-m/Other*. Lacan refers to this trace of an imprint as an "extimate" scrap, located in an "extimate" psychic space in the Real. The *objet a* and its site are "holes" hidden from the expanse of signification. The *objet a* is an index that something has happened in its hollowed site, and indicates the libidinal event as extimated to the subject and linked to *the Thing (Das Ding)*.

The entire "Oedipus complex" is reduced by Lacan to the "castration complex", claims J. A. Miller. This echoes Freud's conception of the libido as entirely *masculine/One*. Castration is presented as the sole process of passage that separates events from the Real while creating the subject as divided. "The *objet a*, if taken only in Lacan's sense, is a container of the effect of castration. containing the signification of castration" (Miller 1982–1983: 4/5/1983). And sexuality, since it "comes into play (. . .) through the mediation – paradoxical as that may seem – of the partial drives" (Lacan 1981b: 193) is therefore shaped, like the *objet a*, by the pair: phallus/castration. Lacan himself remarks in the 1970s that his is a one-sided, masculine model where both subject and object are structured "in a male way only" (1975a: 58); moreover not only the split subject and the lacking object but also what is outside subject and object – the *jouissance* for example – still dwells in the realm of the phallus that from the outset appears as an intermediate concept that commands all three domains of the psyche: it is symbolic, it is also imaginary, it is also between the Symbolic and the Imaginary, it has a correlate in the physical male Real[7] – the penis, and it also marks sexual jouissance:

> A single and same marker dominates the whole register concerning the relationship of the sexuated (. . .) a privileged signifier (. . .) All is reduced to this signifier: the phallus, precisely because it is not in the subject's system since it does not represent the subject but (. . .) sexual jouissance as outside

> the system, which is to say, absolute; sexual *jouissance* in so far as it has this privilege over all the others.
>
> (*Lacan 1968–1969: 14/5/1969*)

Furthermore, desire is also phallic par excellence, for any release of something from a *jouisssance* and from the real partial dimension on to the symbolic register occurs as tearing by means of the castration mechanism and inlaying inside pre-established discourse. "The desire is certainly antinomic in relation to the *jouissance* since it supposes, this desire, to be established, it supposes (. . .) a rupture of *jouissance. Castration is even the only liberator of desire that may be conceived of.*" But there is something more (. . .) We can nevertheless conceive of *another sexual jouissance*, a feminine one, in addition to the masculine one: "*Jouissance* behind castration (. . .) the unthinkable *jouissance* [that] is the *jouissance* of the subject before the mark of the signifier (. . .) would be inconceivable without feminine sexuality" (Miller 1982–1983: 2/3/1983, original emphasis). The "supplementary" feminine sexuality is connected to a *jouissance* that occurs on the plane of the partial relations before or behind castration, and we have some idea of its existence even though the symbolic system is incapable of reporting on it.

Something of the erotic antennae of the psyche transmits to, and receives from the other, through the fantasy mechanism, an echo of "holes": of an archaic sexual rapport unappropriated retroactively by the phallus and of an *objet a* that diffracts and assembles traces by borderlinks and escapes the phallus as well.

Feminine swerve as a site of rapport

Echoes of psychic unconscious "holes" and knots sprout through art and re(a)sonate meaning. *Matrix* and *metramorphosis* are concepts by which I have proposed to display and organize a particular spectrum of opaque trans-individual mental events, sensations, affects and fantasies bounded with traces of archaic rapport with the feminine-Other, with her body, her trauma, fantasy, sensations, emotions and even desires. In the matrixial apparatus and by metramorphic processes this spectrum can weave its holes and knots, unconsciously get organized and arise at the horizons of appearance. Matrix supplies a symbol by which a psychic register that doesn't take shelter under the wings of the phallus may be identified and recognized. The womb in this model is not a passive conceiving recipient and the mother is not the pre-symbolic origin that must be replaced by a symbol. The womb here represents a swerve which is *a site of rapport* alongside the almost-lost envelopes between *I* and *non-I* – between partial subjects and between them and their shared part objects and archaic m/Other – which is inscribed as a feminine beyond-the-phallus almost-missed-encounter in the Other (A).[8]

The basis of subjectivity-as-encounter in the rapport between the becoming-subject and the *becoming-m/Other-to-be* with-in her originary *swerve*-site should not lead us astray to look for the matrixial almost-missed-encounter in natural biology, just as the phallic structure and the process of castration do not present the father/son relations as endangering the real male organ. Metramorphosis is a passage-route through which matrixial affects, events, materials and modes infiltrate and diversify on to the margins of the Symbolic.

Matrix is an unconscious space of simultaneous co-emergence and co-fading of the *I* and the *uncognized non-I*, which is neither fused nor rejected. Matrix is based on feminine/prenatal rapport and is conceived of as a shared psychic borderspace in which *differentiation-in-co-emergence* and *distance-in-proximity* are continuously reattuned by metramorphosis created by, and further creating, accompanied by matrixial affects, *relations-without-relating* on the borders of presence and absence, subject and object, me and the stranger. In the unconscious, the matrixial borderline dimension involved in the process of creating *feminine-Other-desire* and sense coexists with the phallic dimension and alternates with it in terms of approaching the thresholds of the conscious.

Metramorphosis is a process of inter-psychic trans-individual communication and transformation that transgress the individual subject, between several entities in a matrixial borderspace. In joint marginal awareness, perceived boundaries dissolve to become new boundaries; forms are transgressed; borderlines surpassed and transformed into thresholds; links are conceived, transformed and dissolved. A contingent borderlink of rapport and a borderspace of swerve and encounter emerge as a sex-difference and as a creative instance which engraves traces that may be revealed/invented in *with*ness-in-differentiation. In the matrix, rapport-without-relating transforms the unknown other and me and turns both of us into partial subjects – still unknown to each other – in *subjectivity-as-encounter*.

Lost envelopes and diffracted objet a

I will propose an analysis from a matrixial perspective of some of Lacan's ideas, which in the phallic perspective are paradoxical and like the "woman" beyond the phallus are "impossible." In the matrixial perspective something from the feminine rapport can be communicated in "dialogue" produced by and producing an assembled "*speak/through-being*" (*parl'être*).

From: J. Lacan, *Le sinthome*:

> The libido, as its name indicates, can only be a participant of the hole, which moreover goes for all other modes through which the body and the Real are presented, and it's obviously through this that I'm trying to get back to the function of art.
>
> *(1975–1976: 9/xii/1975)*

From: J. Lacan, *L'identification*:

> One of the first possibilities concerning a hole is becoming two holes. I've been told: What do you not refer to, what do not refer your images to embryology? Understand that they are never very far away.

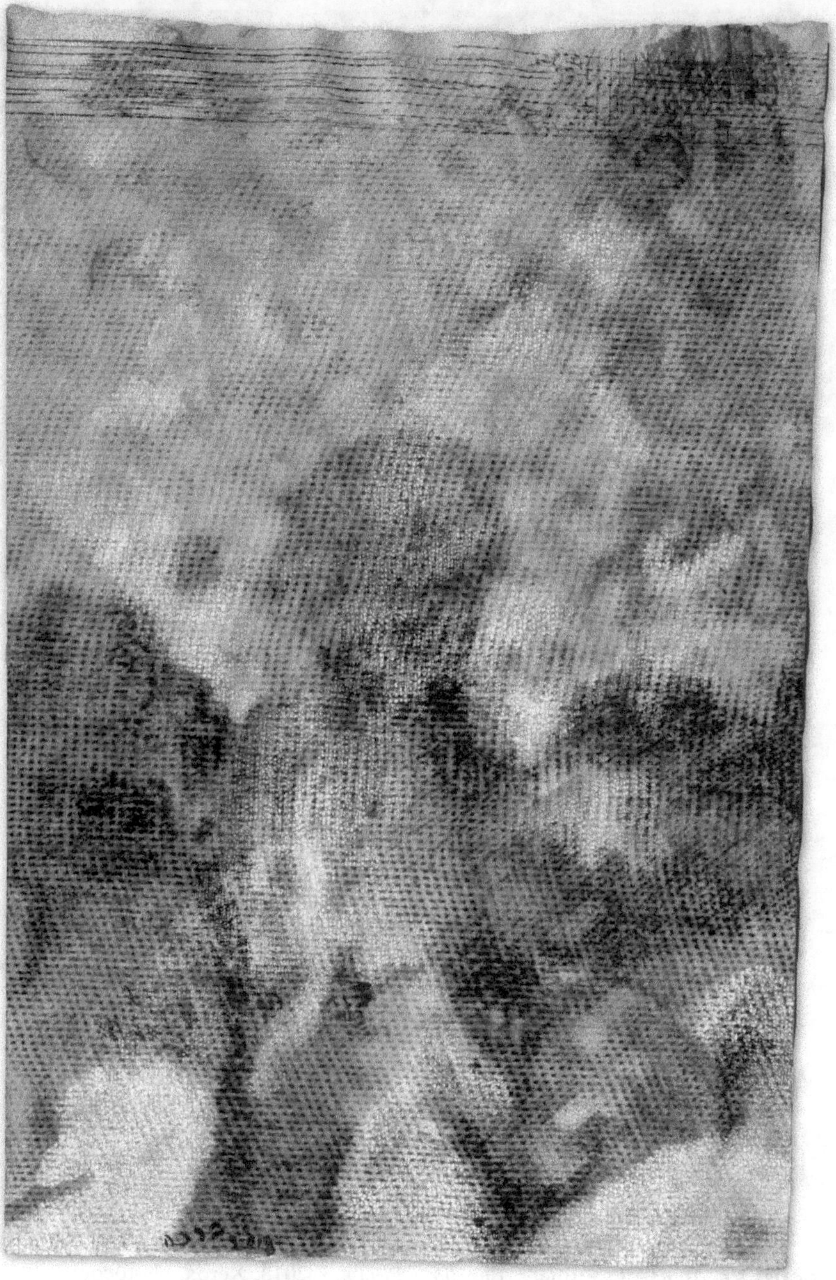

FIGURE 5.5 Bracha L. Ettinger, *Eurydice – Pieta n.1*, 2018. Photocopic pigment and ashes, Indian ink on paper (36 × 24.5 cm).

Source: Courtesy of the artist.

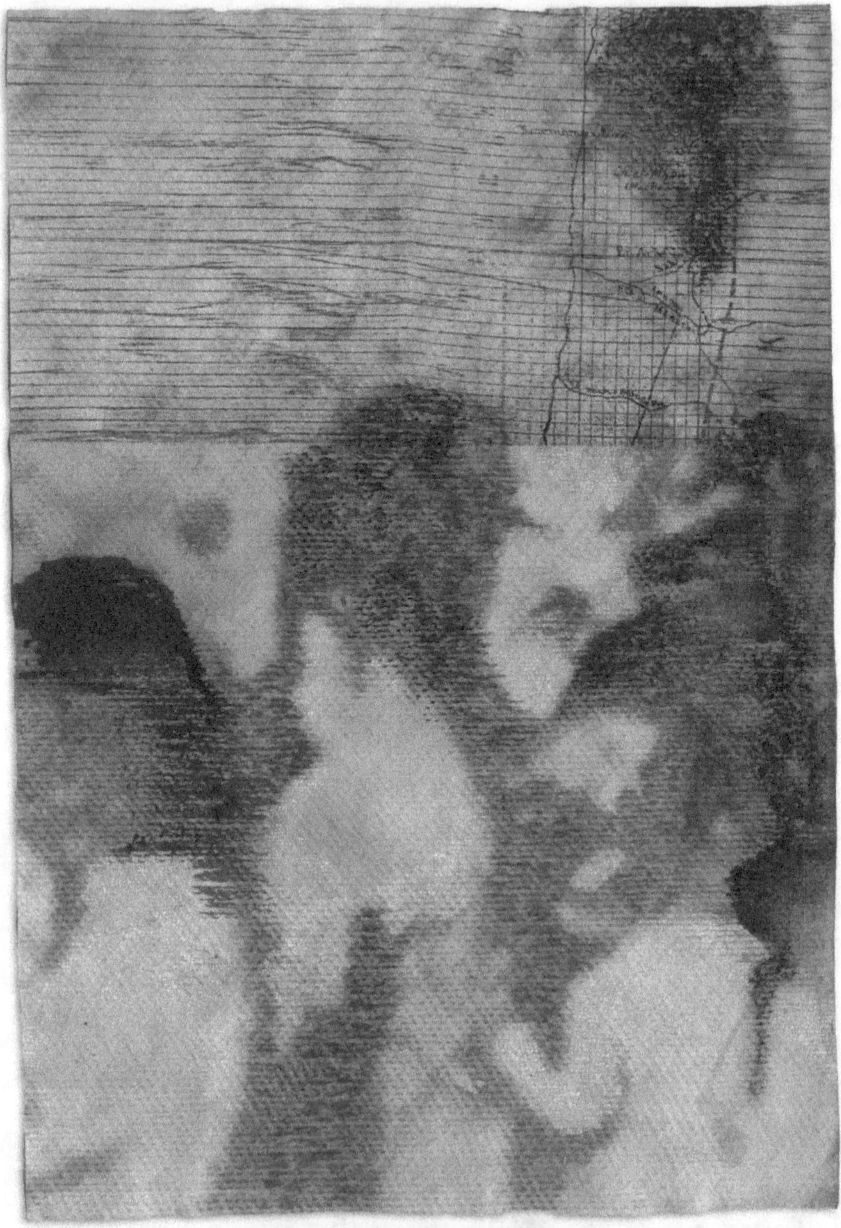

FIGURE 5.6 Bracha L. Ettinger, *Eurydice – Pieta n.3*, 2018. Xerox, photocopic pigment and ashes, Indian ink on paper (35.3 × 24.7 cm).

Source: Courtesy of the artist.

> If there is something that permits us to conceive of it as a carrier of (. . .) I-don't-know-what primary narcissism, it is assuredly the reference to the subject, not so much as the body of the parasite mother, but to those lost envelopes where the continuity between the interior and the exterior is so easily read (. . .) there is something where the rapport to the body [*corps*] must be accentuated, to incorporation, to the *Eiverleibung*, that is, we must look from a side *in which the father would be left entirely aside* (. . .) I left it completely to the side.
>
> The whole dialectic of these past few years up to and including the Kleinian dialectic which is yet the closest, remains falsified because the emphasis has not been placed on the essential deviation ["mother" distinct from "father" as a deviation and not as an opposition].
>
> *(1961–1962: V/1962)*

From: J. Lacan, *D'un autre a l'Autre*:

> It is not for nothing that place evokes the buried-up-against [*placage*] which is essential in defining the bosom as analogous to placenta, inasmuch as it defines the subjective relationship which is appropriate to institute it in the mother–child relationship. The ambioceptor role of the bosom between the child and the mother is in reality the prevalent role. It is as the *objet a*, in being buried-up-against-her-insides, that the child-subject is articulated, that its message is received by the mother, and that it [the message] is given back to it.
>
> *(1968–1969: 14/IV/1969)*

The hole of the knot with no interiority or exteriority, the extimate space or tunnel, place of archaic events and site of their originary traces, is described by Lacan following Merleau-Ponty like a reversible glove or like a fabric and its hidden lining. I suggest developing the idea of the "hole that turns into two holes" in a matrixial perspective in the direction of *severality* in a few ways: as *diffraction* of the *objet a* between two – or several, not infinite, not one – entities, as sharing of the *objet a* by two – or several – individuals, as composing the *objet a* by several components and as *dispersing* and *divergence* of "grains" of subjectivity between several different individuals, where the *objet a* becomes a *borderlink* between them: an *a-link*. All of this takes place in the subject insisting on becoming a subject, the "subject in insistence" already while becoming a subject in the womb and co-emerging in prebirth incest (a non-sexual incest) together with the mother-to-be, with neither fusion nor rejection. The becoming-subject-to-be is a presubject in the desire and the discourse of the m/Other-to-be who transgresses her own individual psychic boundaries and takes part in the pre-subject's Real that stretches "between trauma and fantasy". The feminine swerve participates in any trauma of the *I* and the *non-I* in the matrixial stratum. The traumatic rapport is articulated in connectivity and the fantastic link is retroactively embroidered into sense. The postnatal relations (breast/bosom) contain functions and structural elements borrowed from the prenatal apparatus (bosom/placenta), and the matrixial angle illuminates the borderspace between inside and outside in subjectivity-as-encounter, where a *continuity* between interior and exterior rather than a *split* comes to light.

Lacan asserted that be didn't develop the side from which the father moves aside; and leaving such a side aside demanded a price. Lacan also confessed having prohibited those around him from daring to advance the issue of the prenatal mother and also argues for both a difference and a link between "woman" and "mother". Indeed here, in the matrixial borderspace, in the zone of the "lost envelopes" where a hole becomes several boles, it is not motherhood nor mother/child *relations* that are intended, but a "before" as "beside" or "beyond" the Phallus, that concerns the "woman" before post-natal motherhood and before becoming the archaic future-mother for a becoming-subject. We are dealing with the singularity of each psychic matrixial encounter between *I* and *non-I* which is analogous to the intrauterine feminine/prenatal encounter. We are dealing with a site that indicates hidden female specificity that creates a feminine originary swerve, and with the possibility of inscribing traces of the *encounter* in the Other, as a web, in an enlarged-Other which thereby contains unconscious sub-knowledge which is not conditioned by repression of signifiers. Furthermore, I suggest that such an assembled *speak/through-being* can discern and transmit the matrixial rapport via art and work it through in psychoanalytic transference/countertransference relations.

Pre-birth incest

It is impossible to deal with the "lost envelopes" from the side of "the Name of the Father": the side of the phallic Symbolic, the site of the network of signifiers with the social-cultural principles inscribed in the Symbolic and transmitted by discourse. But in psychoanalysis since Freud they do not get to be processed from an-other side either, because the hole they perforate in the symbolic Other is dangerous: it endangers male sexuality and narcissism. (Freud 1908/1959: 205–226). The woman *only* ought to develop the other side, hints Lacan in the 1970s, since there are matters that concern *only* the woman.[9]

The matter of the womb as a sex-difference first appeared and later was rejected by Freud from the question of sexuality. It was rejected in the service of male narcissism since narcissism is founded, in Freud, upon a libidinal investment in a corporeal object – i.e. the penis, which the male subject has in reality and owns in imagination. Assigning a first-rate importance to a corporeal object which the male subject doesn't have would represent an affliction to narcissism: its imaginary and symbolic significance and importance had therefore of necessity to be denied. The "universal" and "neutral" concept of narcissism that is supposed to serve both sexes is built upon libidinal investment in one's own male organ even if the subject (she) doesn't have it. If the sex-difference represented by the womb is presented by Freud to begin with as the first sexual question for boys and is later rejected on the ground of its threat to male narcissism, the question of the womb as a sex-difference that is significant for girls is rejected even right from the start, on the threshold of any possible serious consideration. For Lacan, as we have elsewhere discussed,[10] it is not the male organ that is the focus of the notion of the phallus, and castration mechanism is first of all symbolic. Still, the phallus and its principles empty the beyond-the-phallus field of any possible signification. Lacan, however, does suggest to examine, from the side where the father remains outside, some kind of primary narcissism linked to the lost envelopes that stretch between interior and exterior and are related to the maternal body – even though he himself sticks to the phallic model and will not do this research himself. Lacan even hints that he (any-man) shouldn't touch upon matters that concern women only and claims that what he did develop concerning the woman is already *too much* (1975a) and stems from his own psychotic side (1975–1976).

When we divert the focus towards the zone of feminine/prenatal encounter beyond-the-phallus and examine its significance for the woman, we are touching upon a basic taboo left unarticulated in psychoanalysis. Language disavows this encounter's jouissance and does not transmit it through itself; human social law and order are constructed upon its foreclosure since it indicates a forbidden rapport for the post-Oedipal male subject: the incestual rapport with the Other-"woman" as an *archaic-becoming-m/Other-to-be* – and not just with the m/Other. This rapport is dangerous; its encounter in the Real for the man/boy threatens to stand only as the return to the womb, a regression towards an archaic Real. Its value in the Symbolic is that of regression, since this rapport cannot wear another, supplementary, future incarnation in the Real, such as gestating and giving birth via one's own body. For the post-Oedipal female subject this rapport is a regression towards an archaic Real as well as a possible imaginary projection towards embodied future; it thus also has *a value of potentiality* on top of the value of regression in the Symbolic. It is also, sometimes, a painful and joyful present: a "*jouis-present*".

While Freud develops the narrative of the archaic father and treats the taboo of boy/mother incest that is structured by/for it, there is no similar structure concerning the archaic future-mother and no prohibition that is parallel to that of the Oedipal incest. Indeed the prebirth (non-sexual) incest cannot be forbidden – it occurs to give life. Yet, for its highly psychotic potential for the male subject in the phallic paradigm it cannot be elaborated but only silenced; not even excluded from the Symbolic by repression (from which it could then come back as the return of the repressed and produce an-other desire) but only marginalized as unthinkable. And whatever of it which escapes this destiny, is thinkable, and hastens to find shelter inside the phallic model under the wings of "the Name of the Father," is reduced to its measures and called upon to serve, in terms of fertility and procreation in the framework of heterosexuality within patriarchal legacy.

A passage to the partial dimension in the sharing with the intimate stranger

Another narrative, feminine and supplementary, has been sacrificed in order to preserve and protect the phallic integrity of the subject (whether male or female).

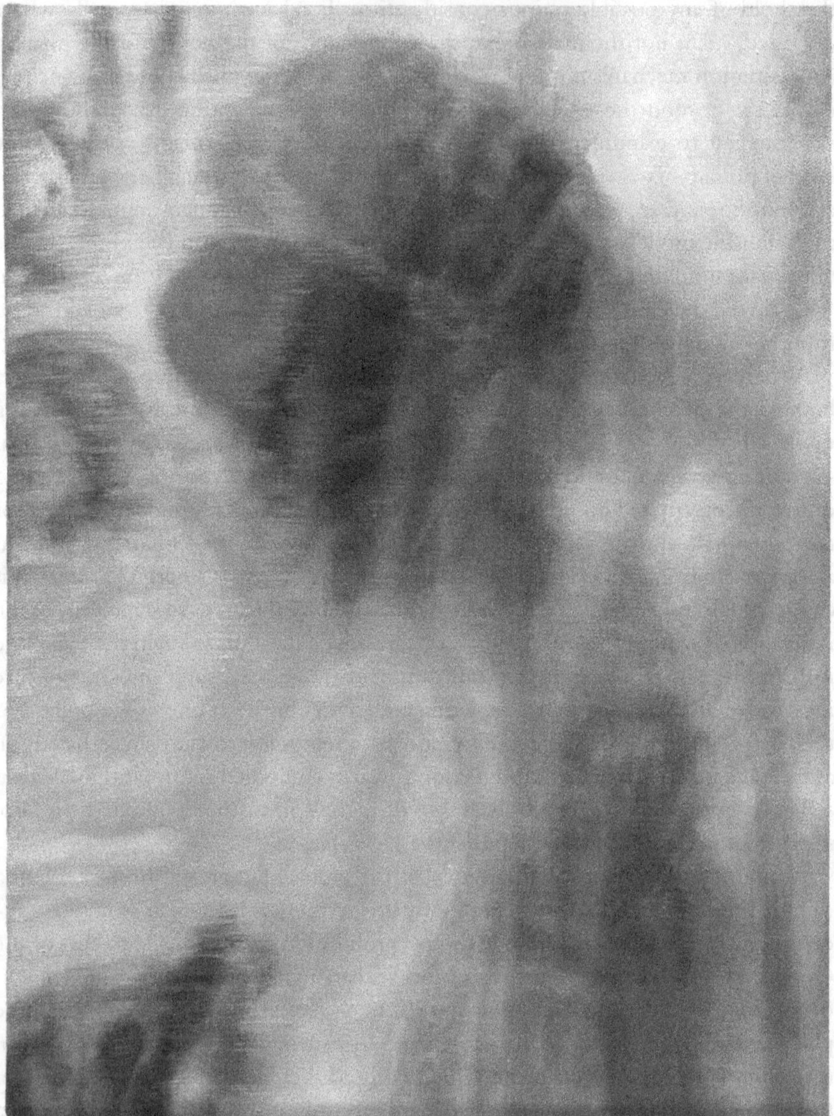

FIGURE 5.7 Bracha L. Ettinger, *Eurydice n.54 – Mothers and a Child.* Collection: Castello di Rivoli, 2018. Oil on canvas (40 × 30 cm).

Source: Courtesy of the artist.

The sacrificed feminine possible narratives touch upon diffraction, multiplicity of severality, dispersal and partiality, shareability and hybridity, with-ness and conductivity, passability and potentiality. This ensemble of ideas together touches upon a rapport with the unknown other, the unknown yet intimate stranger, a rapport that threatens the patriarchal kin-relations since it is unappropriated by the

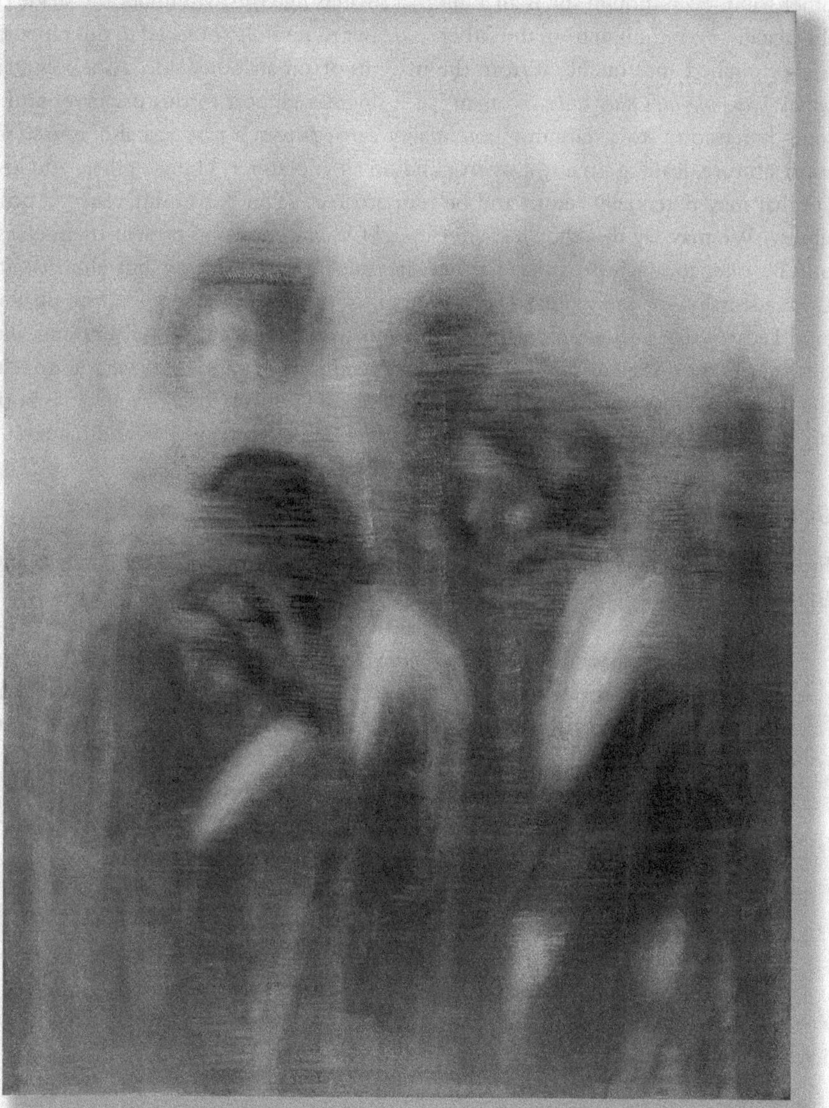

FIGURE 5.8 Bracha L. Ettinger, *Eurydice – Medusa – Pieta n.2*, 2015–2018. Oil on canvas (40 × 30 cm).

Source: Courtesy of the artist.

phallus. A rapport where the subject is not One or All but is a potential intersection whose *objet* is both half-lost, partly shared and hybrid.

Indeed the route of a post-Oedipal non-psychotic adult man, who accepts the servitude, the burden and the benediction of the phallus, is forever blocked to the feminine-matrixial rapport in the traumatic level of the Real. The woman, on the other hand, even though she is an adult that shelters like the man under the shade of the phallus, even though from the father's side her route is also blocked to this rapport, is also touched and touches it from the margins of/on an-other side. As a potential *archaic-becoming-m/Other-to-be*, woman has a singular rapport to this originary feminine dimension,[11] to a feminine potentiality carried from a past and also aspired to from a future, leaning on a real swerve and on an encounter-Thing, archaic and lost yet that may potentially return and be reincarnated, again but in difference; a possibility. We may say that the "lost envelopes" Other-return and present themselves, one by one, to a woman; that for her they are not entirely lost but almost-lost. Coincidentally, for the woman, both the lack of the sexual rapport – in the phallus (and Lacan's repeated expression: "there is no sexual rapport" is well known) and this same rapport itself *co-exist* on the levels of trauma and fantasy and even desire – in the matrixial dimension beyond the phallus. And the subject, male or female, is born in "misunderstanding" into a double-sphered feminine desire: phallic and matrixial.

Birth in misunderstanding in a beyond-the-phallus sphere

From: J. Lacan, *Le malentendu* [The misunderstanding] (translated by J. Simas and Bracha L. Ettinger):

> I do not say that the word is creator. I say something altogether different because my practice obliges me to: I say that the word is unconscious – that is, misunderstood. If you think that all can be revealed about it, well, you are fooling yourselves: not all can be. That means a part of it will never be revealed. This is precisely where religion goes wrong. And it also serves as a rampart around Revelation – which religion prides itself on in order to exploit. As for psychoanalysis, its exploit is to exploit misunderstanding. With, as its end result, a revelation which is fantasy (. . .) Otto Rank came close to this when he spoke of the trauma of birth. As for the trauma, there is no other trauma: Man is born misunderstood.
>
> *(1980, n.p.)*

Lacan elaborates:

> Since I've been asked about what's called the status of the body, I reach this point to emphasize the fact that it can only be grasped from this point. The body only makes its apparition in the real as misunderstanding. Let's be radical about it: your body is the fruit of a *lineage* [legacy, heritage] – and a large number of your troubles are due to the fact that this lineage had already been swimming in misunderstanding as best it could. It was swimming for the simple reason that it would speak/through-being to whoever happened to be around at the time. That is what it has transmitted to you by "giving you Life", as we say. It's from this that you inherit. And this explains your being at odds with yourself, when that is the case.
>
> *(Ibid.)*

He continues:

> The misunderstanding is already present from before. Inasmuch as from before you are part of this wonderful legacy, or rather you have a stake in the babble of your ancestors. No need for you to babble yourself. From before, what sustains you in the name of the unconscious, i.e. misunderstanding, is rooted there.
>
> There is no other trauma of birth than that of being born desired. Desired, or not – it's all the same since it is speaking-through-being. The speak/through-being in question is generally divided into two speakers. Two speakers who do not speak the same language. Two who do not understand each other speaking. Two who just don't get on together. Two who conspire for reproduction, but from an accomplished misunderstanding, which your body will carry through the said reproduction.
>
> *(Ibid.)*

And concludes:

> I admit that language can be useful for sensible communication (. . .) sensible communication is dialogue (. . .) Dialogue is rare. As for the production of a new body of speaker, it is so rare that it is *de facto* absent. It is not absent in principle, but the principle is inscribed only in the symbolic. This is the case of the so-called family principle, for example. No doubt, there has always been some apprehension of this. Enough for the unconscious to be considered as the knowledge of God. What nevertheless distinguishes the knowledge called unconscious from the knowledge of God is that the latter was supposed to be for our good. That is what is untenable. Hence the question I have raised: Does God believe in God?
>
> *(Ibid.)*

My clinical experience shows that not only the negation of the phallus but also a total identification with it at the expense of a space beyond it, and an inability to communicate inside and from the matrixial sphere, lead lo a dead-end. This is testified to, in my view, by post-partum psychoses which are bound up with the impossibility to get in touch with a matrixial experience in the Real and with the difficulties in the passage from it to a mother/infant relationship. Infantile autism and the way it is bound to the mental state of the mother before the birth of the infant (Tustin 1990) is in my view misunderstood by psychoanalysis. Certain psychoses in adolescence are bound according to our findings to the stage of intra-uterine existence (Ettinger et al. 1991) but are projected by analysts on the mother's character and her post-natal motherhood. Hence we can conclude that something in a Symbolic that will be perceived as wider than the phallic-Symbolic can permit even in non-pathogenetic circumstances a certain non-conscious accessibility to the matrixial stratum. Even if this wider-Symbolic, or rather the feminine supplement to the Symbolic, is to be revealed/invented/formulated in/for each encounter anew, and is contingent and unforeseen. A total blockage of the matrix may be no less pathological for women than its total invasion.

Assembled speak/through-being and an-Other feminine desire

Matrixial femininity is unpredictable precisely because trans-subjectivity is delivered in it as a potential in the encounter with the stranger, and since its *objet a* is dispersed, shared and hybrid. In the light of the matrix I interpret Lacan's speak/through-being in "*Le malentendu*" as the being of a "woman" which is unlimited to one individual and is charged with affect and desire in *withness* – in jointness-in-differentiation – is an assembled being of severality in the partial dimension, a being of encounter between *I* and *non-I* in the Real "between trauma and fantasy", a potential being that communicates in transference relationships through dialogue, although rare, nonexistent in actuality perhaps and yet not impossible: a dialogue inscribed as a potentiality in the Other, unconscious inscription but such that is not reduced to the repressed chain of the signifier.

If the matrixial encounter may wear the form of a potential dialogue in a trans-subjective speak/through-being, then through speaking, something of the matrixial sphere of being may find expression, beyond art and psychosis, in the psychoanalytic meeting. And maybe that's what Lacan is aiming at when, while transporting the analyst from his status of a subject who is supposed to know (*sujet-supposé-savoir*) to his status of relics in the form of *objet a*, he somewhat subversively says:

> I have said and done enough to stop anyone from daring – at least anyone from my neighboring circles – from daring to advance the idea that one can be the mother [as an analyst in a didactic analysis]. Yet this is precisely what this is all about.
>
> *(1961–1962)*

For me, in parallel to the passage from positioning the analyst as a *sujet-supposé-savoir* to his positioning as an *objet a*, a passage occurs from a masculine to a feminine position, as well as a move from transference as repetition to transference as "impossible" encounter – impossible in the phallus yet potential in the matrix – between the subject and psychic traces that are incarnated in objects.

Since woman is both subjected to the phallus, censured by it and also escapes it, the feminine-matrixial sex-difference is not equal nor opposite to the masculine difference, but is something else. The "woman" is "and-and," the "woman" bypasses the phallus and connects to "the rare dialogue" that is "*de facto*" – but not "in principle" – absent from the Symbolic, to a dialogue that contains what may potentially each time otherwise become inscribed, inscription of traces of swerve and rapport, traces where matrixial trauma and fantasy arise as connected to the female corporeal specificity and related to a feminine-Other desire, composite from a phallic desire plus something else. The feminine-Other-desire vehiculed by an assembled speak/through-being linked to a "double-opening" wider-Other creates in misunderstanding the inheritance transmitted to the becoming-subject in co-emergence with her. Indeed, her desire does include traces of unconscious communication "in the Name of the Father" with desires and messages that infiltrate from discourse through the family lineage which includes desires and messages from whoever took an unforgettable unconscious part in the parental "babble". But it also includes, I suggest, traces of archaic incestual rapport, m/Otherly and non-sexual, partially *foreclosed* with-in-side the feminine, traces inscribed not by signifiers but in a sub-symbolic connectionist mode and included in a wider-Other, enlarging the margins of the Symbolic. A borderspace of inter-with-ness and of transgression of the individual's borders seeks ways to become known and thinkable.

II. Feminine borderlinking

Sexual rapport in the "matrix" and non-rapport in the "phallus"

Up until the end of his teaching, Lacan repeatedly claimed that there is no sexual rapport, that psychoanalysis itself attests to that, and that this lack of rapport is the basis of psychoanalytic discourse, but that if such rapport were to exist, it would be feminine. Logical and topological considerations mainly, but also aesthetic-poetic ones, led Lacan, if only in brief passages in some of his very late seminars (1973–1974; 1975–1976), to imply enigmatically a psychic zone in which feminine sexual rapport that the signifier has not appropriated and exploded and castration has not cut-out and kicked-away might occur. A "supplementary" feminine non-conscious zone is stretched out of – and retreats back into – art, separated from psychosis, if at all, by less than a hair's breath. Yet, even though Lacan speaks of supplementary femininity and – albeit rarely – raises the possibility of the existence of sexual rapport on the woman's side only and in psychosis, mysticism or art, it is important to emphasize that the assertion that "there is no sexual rapport" resides at the centre of his teaching: there is no sexual rapport in the "phallus" (the unconscious informed by the phallic mechanism); no rapport to the real experience of the woman; no contact with the feminine-Other in sexual relationships based on the phallic model of *jouissance* for both sexes; and, above all, there are no ways to report on a feminine sexual rapport if/where it does occur, no inscription of it by signifiers in the Symbolic: "*there is no sexual rapport*" signifies exactly this rapport's "lack of the signifier" (Miller 1985–1986), a "deficit in knowledge" (Miller 1982–1983).

The phallic sexual jouissance, based on what Freud described as organ-pleasure, whose privileged position in the mental structure of both men and women is shown by psychoanalytic experience, relates to an organ of the subject itself or to the other treated as an object that represents an organ, and not to the other as an-other subject; it is therefore "an obstacle to sexual rapport" (Lacan 1973–1974). Significating an event from the Real by means of the signifier "kills" the libidinal event, and is therefore an obstacle to the inscription of sexuality as a rapport. First, jouissance of an organ cannot be jouissance of a relation; and, second, the value of the emergence of castration is that of a sexual non-rapport (cf. Miller 1982–1983).

Trans-subjective web

However, there exists a jouissance of a totally different order, which is not an obstacle to sexual rapport but its culmination; such jouissance is exposed despite the fact "that language in a way sanctions" it (Lacan 1973–1974). Feminine sexuality testifies to a sphere where an-other jouissance exists and inscribes traces, where the non-conscious is wider than the unconscious structured as a language, where the Other is different from the Other that is a container of the repressed chain of signifiers.

In a series of essays I proposed that feminine jouissance, which Lacan describes as enveloped in its continuity as unthinkably is knowable and *transcripted*, though not (yet) inscribed in and by the signifiers. It aspires to release itself as *an-other* gaze via supplementary aspects of the psychic object that participate in the shaping of a *feminine dimension of desire*; but as long as all desire is formulated as a castration of this continuity, the phallic vicious circle traps it in its net and prevents its passability into culture (see Ettinger 1992; 1996b [added for the 1998 publication of "Supplementary Jouissance"]). In the transformational processes that language allows, termed metaphor and metonymy, "the *jouissance* is reduced to the phallic signifier" (Miller 1994–1995), and there is no other possible sublimation or passability of the "woman" and her rapport into the Symbolic. Lacan suggests, however, looking for a possible different inscription for the supplementary feminine sexuality: "something that is other than the Symbolic (. . .) that which already from three appears in any and all writing" (1973–1974), whereby he distances himself from language in order to approach what he calls "lalangue".

Inscribed in a mode of webbing that privileges Severality over the One or All, I suggest that matrixial desire sprouts, not from a phantasm about sharing, but from a border shareability in trauma and phantasm that re(a)sonates meaning and creates feminine-Other-desire via metramorphosis. In the matrix, there grow originary relations of proximity-in-distance that cannot be reduced to fusion or split, and these awaken specific affects. Metramorphosis is a transformational process that is not reduced to the phallic signifier and "makes sense" already from the several. It creates and covenants directly knots in a trans-subjective non-conscious web and touches upon the "sinthome"[12] from a feminine psychic zone in the joint border-space, at the site of shared and partial, assembled and diffracted subjectivity. This feminine zone in the woman, I add, does not indicate a psychotic site. Moreover, psychosis in a woman may rather relate to its total foreclosure or to the melting of the matrixial stratum inside the phallic stratum.

The other sex is supported by sinthome

Feminine sexual rapport and non-rapport co-exist. What could be another mode of inscription that would fit the non-rapport? How can what Lacan describes (following

Merleau-Ponty) as a "glove" be inscribed and described as a basis for an "impossible" rapport? What would be a mode that would enable the passage of feminine *jouissance*, its swerve and its sexual rapport towards culture following their unforeseen incarnation, so that such a swerve and rapport would not be either just enacted in the Real or realized in psychosis? What would discover their passage as an-other knowledge, a knowledge that would not imply their foreclosing split from the subject? What would evade their constitution as a deficit in knowledge?

From: J. Lacan, *Le sinthôme*:

> The sinthôme (. . .) something that allows the Symbolic, the Imaginary, and the Real to go on holding together (. . .) what I call, what I designate (. . .) of the sinthôme, which is marked here with a circle (. . .) of string, is meant to take place at the very spot where, say, the trace of the knot goes wrong. [It's a] "slip of the knot".
>
> It is inasmuch as there is "sinthôme" that there is no sexual equivalence, which is to say there is rapport; for it is obvious that if we say that non-rapport derives from equivalence, it is inasmuch as there is no equivalence that the rapport is structured.
>
> Where there is rapport, it is inasmuch as there is sinthôme, which is to say where, as I've said, it is by sinthôme that the other sex is sustained. I allowed myself to say that the sinthôme is precisely speaking the sex I don't belong to, which is to say a woman. Because a woman is a sinthôme for every man, it is perfectly clear that there needs be found another name for what becomes of man for a woman, since for that very reason the sinthôme is characterized by non-equivalence. One can say that man is for a woman all that you like, such as an affliction worse than a sinthôme; you can articulate it as you please: even as devastation. But if there is no equivalence, you are forced to specify what becomes of "sinthôme".
>
> *(1975–1976)*

Lacan adds:

> There is no equivalence, that's the only thing, that's the only recess where what the speak/through-being, the human being, sexual rapport is sustained (. . .) the sinthôme's direct link, it is this something which must be situated in its doings with the Real, with the real of the unconscious (. . .) it is the sinthôme we must deal with in the very rapport Freud maintained was natural – which doesn't mean a thing – the sexual rapport.
>
> All that subsists of the sexual rapport is that geometry which we alluded to in relation to the glove. That is all that remains of the human space of a basis for the rapport.
>
> *(Ibid.)*

In his late theory. Lacan describes the intra-psychic registers (Real, Symbolic, Imaginary) as rings, linked to each other by a Borromean knot. This knot is a kind of triangular warp-and-woof weave, a kind of braid made of three stems, where the stem of the Real is inseparable in principle, structurally and primarily, from the stems of the Imaginary and the Symbolic. In a braid such as this, where interior and exterior can be turned inside out like a glove, the Real itself already stores some kind of knowledge: "there is knowledge in the Real" that can be articulated, "something that is written and should be read in deciphering it" (Lacan 1973–1974).

Knowledge of the Real and supplementary feminine sex-difference

I want to propose that if the Real, and not only the Symbolic, harbours already some knowledge, we may suppose that a feminine difference occurs already in the Real. A rapport – for me a movement of borderlinking between several partial subjects – and an affective swerve based on "dehiscence" and "bursting"[13] in the field of affects, germinates directly from/with-in and in contact with a real female bodily specificity. These swerving and borderlinking movements comprise a sexual-feminine difference. We may conceive of an alignment of a sexual difference independently and in difference from the phallic organization of difference. The matrixial difference is created from the beginning as a feminine dimension of potentiality in a weave of affects and information interwoven in an inter-psychic and even trans-psychic web.

According to my interpretation of *The "Uncanny"*, a differentiating potential on the level of affection is indicated by Freud when he discusses the anxiety that accompanies the experiencing of art. The matrixial affects as primary differentiation, introduce a difference on the level of the Thing as they give signals that some-Thing happens, and that a transition from Thing to object takes place, without a total separation from the Thing. Matrixial affects index a transformation and an exchange, and matrixial phenomena testify that such a passage takes place and a minimal meaning is created. A tremolos of meaning of differentiation-in-togetherness is tracing itself. Thus, the matrixial affect is the affect of the Thing inasmuch as it inscribes traces in I and non-I. The differential affectivity is at this level inseparable from this passage. Their co-incidence is fatal; it works for meaning through the work of art.

> She [a "woman"] manages to succeed at sexual union. Only this union is the union of one with two, or of each with each, of each of these three strands. The sexual union, if I may say so, is internal to its weave. And that is where she plays her part, in really showing us what a knot is.
>
> *(Lacan 1973–1974)*

In the Borromean knot, the unconscious is disharmonious; the knot leads us to deal with knowledge which is not only independent of the signifier, but also advances us towards the "pure" Real even more than does the phantasm when the latter is articulated inside the phallic field. "The desire to know meets obstacles. In order to embody the obstacle I have invented the knot" (Lacan 1975–1976). Lacan clearly looks for ways of knowing "woman" beyond mere affirmations of her existence. The "woman" beyond-the-phallus exhibits the intra-psychic knot, but remains a radical Other. But further to that, in the matrixial stratum, she exhibits intersections of knots in a trans-psychic web, and therefore "woman" is a border-Other. The knots enigmatically account for the failure to inscribe feminine desire in Lacan's still (and until the very end) phallic paradigm. However, with the concept of the "knot" it already becomes clear that for Lacan the possibility of describing the "supplementary" femininity within the phallic framework has reached its limits. In the passage to a matrixial apparatus, metramorphosis that may be thought of as a co-poietic activity in a trans-psychic web remembers, inscribes and transfers the feminine *jouissance*, swerve and borderlinking via art across the threshold of culture. If knowledge stored in the Real is not a host of data awaiting decoding by means of signification that will also constitute a cleft in it and a split from it, but is an "invention, that's what happens in every encounter, in any first encounter with sexual rapport" (Lacan 1973–1974), then a metramorphic process of webbing and with-nessing, a metramorphic process of exchange of affect and phantasm based on conduction of/in trauma in jointness and a metramorphic process of transmissions-in-transformation of phantasm, initially between a becoming-subject and a becoming-m/Other-to-be, but more generally between I in co-emergence with an uncognized non-I (which can be considered a plural-several, partial and diffracted "woman"), can release knowledge from "holes" in the Real. Swerving and contacting become themselves a kind of knowledge; they are the inscriptions of traces of borderlinking. We can consider them as manifestations of the "sinthome" that releases/creates/invents/reveals, from a feminine side, a potential desire whose sense does not depend on the signifier.

Passions of the (a)

The register of phantasm in psychoanalytic theory enables one to conceptualize a connection between a mental object and a desiring subject at the level of the Thing before originary repression and before it was emptied and erased by the symbolic Other, before the Other was empowered via the phallus. But more than such a conceptualization is possible! In order to overcome the limitations of the split created by the pair phantasm/desire, and approach what is even "closer to us than phantasm" and "brings us closer to the pure Real", we may rather speak, together with J. A. Miller, of the "passions" of the (a) itself (1985–1986). These dwell in the matrix in an aggregated, enlarged-Other in whose constitution they also take part when acting directly as unthought sub-knowledge in a sub-symbolic connectionist web.[14]

If a subjective supplementary sex-difference is possible. experiencing its traumatic event and exhausting its jouissance are not enough. Conceptualizing a level of an-Other feminine difference and of non-equivalence between the sexes promoted by feminine jouissance, swerve and borderlinking is possible only if whatever of it that escapes pre-established discourse is yet unthoughtly known and not only ex-sists with-in, inside and in connection with female corpo-reality. An originary feminine difference is possible only if it is traced, if it can be "written", become somewhat aesthetically thinkable, yet not by distinct symbols, and receive or give sense.

The encounter between trauma, phantasm and desire is the domain proper of working art. It is making art that enables me to articulate something of – and about – the feminine swerve and its borderlinking via concepts issued by/in/from the work. If psychoanalytic discourse leans on the feminine difference as lack or absence, on the impossibility of elaborating what is beyond the phallic field, on the impossibility of feminine rapport and on the othering of "woman" to the point of her foreclosure, art may be a site from which some light may be shed on "woman". This site is not available for "therapy", but it allows psychoanalytic research to extract something from whatever is imprinted in it for the first time and "use" it as its proper material.

Encounter between trauma and phantasm

Following the originary tissue of I and non-I in the womb, a traumatic/phantasmatic encounter occurs in the non-conscious matrixial channel. This encounter is a covenant with the unknown, a borderlinking in the Real which is sexual according to the Freudian definition of partial sexuality (sexuality before Oedipus). Intra-psychic knots are connected to trans-psychic borderlinks. "Inventions" that are inseparable from their inscription as unconscious sub-knowledge are created and shared between several individuals. This articulation of a matrixial borderspace brings us back, but differently, to the early Lacanian assumption of intersubjectivity, which he renounced following his later theoretical inversion. Intersubjectivity re-infiltrates Lacan's late teaching in a way that may, to my mind, be understood anew in the light of the feminine matrixial difference. For the early Lacan of the 1950s, the assumption of intersubjectivity is condensed in the formula, "the subject's desire is the desire of the Other": relations towards significant others take place in terms of the symbolic satisfaction brought about by recognition of the subject stemming from the Other and reaching the subject through speech. The passage through significant others happens only inasmuch as the Other vehicled by them is represented by signifiers and represents society, history and law entwined in the cultural discourse and in language. What can be the meaning of my reintroducing the matter of intersubjectivity in the context of late Lacanian theory, and what significance may we suggest for a feminine-Other-desire in it? Where, theoretically speaking, could an encounter occur between the Other's desire and the trauma of the I? In what sense may the Other's desire be articulated in a direct, positive relation to the subject's *jouissance*, if desire is what "kills" *jouissance*, according to Lacan, and if the Other is considered by him an alienated network of the signifier's chain? Where can the subject's trauma and phantasm meet with the Other's phantasm? What, if any, can be the meaning, for the I, of the phantasm of the Other? How does the phantasm of the Other connect with the I's phantasm and desire?

Indeed, in classical Lacanian theory, the desire of the subject, not its phantasm, corresponds to, or reflects, the desire of the Other – not its phantasm; trauma is always individual (both in the early and in the late theory), and phantasm is in correlation to a *jouissance* that the subject assumes in the realm of the Other.

Thus, an Other who would be larger than "the treasure of the signifiers" is to be hypothesized in order for all these encounters to become possible or valid. Likewise, we have to conceive of differentiating moves like swerving and borderlinking that are not based on an absence or lack (in relation to which both sexes are considered equal in the kingdom of the Phallus), but on co-emergence and co-fading in transformation that produce and modify the partial dimension of wit(h)nessing. In the passage from intersubjectivity to subjectivity-as-encounter, wit(h)nessing-in-differentiation of I with non-I takes place in the site of the relations between symbolic subjects without replacing or erasing them.

An enlarged Other, analogous to a double-opening matrice, in which the chain of the signifier, on the one hand, and the *objet a* in discordance with it on the other hand, dwell together, is described by Lacan in his late teaching; it is an Other which I find in concordance with an I, described by Miller, which is larger than the subject. "There are subjective positions that are wider than those of the subject of the signifier; that's what one studies with the phantasm" (Miller 1982–1983), for phantasm is not subordinated to the retroactivity of signifying. Phantasm exposes archaic ways of introjecting external objects and projecting internal ones (M. Klein), modes of treating archaic internal objects that are "mental representation of the impulse" (S. Freud), as well as psychic routes of search after the archaic object as lost or as a lack (Lacan, Bion).[15] If the I is the subject as containing the vital function of *jouissance* (Miller 1985–1986), then something of the libidinal energy is not entirely lost in the process of symbolization. In order to speak of the I, there should be added to the subject "that which is found at its origin, namely, jouissance" (Lacan 1968–1969).

In face of the I and non-I defined in the matrix as an assembled and diffracted partial subjectivity that contains, shares and transmits its jouissance, I will posit such an Other which is not only the complex of the signifiers' chain, but contains the (*a*) that will never have a perfect concordance with the One. And it is for such a lack of concordance, as well as for the potential with-nessing with the stranger, that "misunderstanding" in the trauma of birth and, even more so, of prebirth can be said to go on forever. The subject emerging in relation to the Other defined as the network of signifiers replaces the traces of the part-objects; the I, by contrast, and likewise (I suggest, by means of the same parameters) the non-I co-emerging in relation to a wider-Other with several openings, include them. An "extimate" borderlinking makes it possible to locate traces of the subject's "lost envelopes" as *objet a* and an *a-link* in the I and non-I ensemble, as a kind of in-(me)side outside(me) and as an intimate outside that dwells in the m/Other, but is hidden in me, and to place in a composite Other the erotic traces that are inscribed in the non-conscious psyche, but not by distinct signifiers.

Jouissance of encounter as a basis for an-Other desire

An uncanny insinuation that something strange, deviating from the phallus and bound to intersubjective relations might take place in the field of symbolic desire can, I believe, already be found in this exceptional expression: "phantasm as the desire of the other" (Lacan 1966: 825). In the context of Lacan's classical theory, such a connection between phantasm and desire rings like a slip of the tongue. I connect it to the possibility of a linkage in "misunderstanding" between the trauma and phantasm of the becoming-subject and the trauma, phantasm and desire of the woman who is a real archaic becoming-m/Other-to-be, towards whose desire the subject is attuned in phantasm, in whose phantasm and desire the subject, even before s/he was born, was already playing a part. "This desire with which the child is invested", says Lacan – connecting again, by the way, phantasm and desire – "starts off always as the result of subjective interpretation, as a function of the maternal desire alone, of her own phantasm".[16] The subject is invested both in and by the desire and in/by the phantasm of the m/Other, and this has effects, positive or negative, according to each case. Considerations of early pathology must relate to the prebirth stage: The first amputation the psychotic is subjected to occurs, according to Lacan, before his/her birth [when] for the mother, s/he is the object of her own metabolism [and] paternal participation is denied, unacceptable. S/he is, from this moment on and throughout pregnancy, the part-object that comes to fill a phantasmatic lack on the level of her body. Yet, in contrast to this phantasmatic projection of a part-object as a "cork" of this kind on behalf of a mother who denies the father, there may emerge in the mother-to-be's phantasm, and may be projected towards her co-emerging-subject, *an objet a* that relates to the Thing, yet is brought about "not so much as lacking" (as "absence" in contrast to "presence") but as "to be" (Lacan 1961–1962), where I find an indication to an intermediate position and a potentiality.

I suggest that the *jouissance* that emerges in the hollowed tunnel of encounter on the level of prebirth incest, and a web of connections between the trauma and phantasm of the prenatal becoming-subject (I), male or female, and the trauma, phantasm and desire of the "woman" as becoming-archaic-m/Other-to-be (non-I) that relates to the I, both of them in co-naissance as partial subjects and partial objects of/for each other – "grains" of I and non-I and not yet "mother" and "infant" – constitute a rapport from a feminine to-be-side that seeps into later systems and stages. I propose that this encounter, which for psychoanalytic theory is sexual in the partial pre-Oedipal dimension, which constitutes a sexual, or rather libidinal rapport or psychically invested rapport, is inscribed to make sense. An im-pure, composite, hybrid object diffracts and penetrates into a matrixial subjectivity made of covenants between several potential entities, unknown to each other, but carrying a potentiality to be revealed to each other when transformed by the encounter. This "rapport" is forever invested through transconnecting with a feminine-maternal body-psyche.

Feminine *jouissance*, which "does not wait for phallic organization to enter into play, will take on aspects of revelation which it will keep forever" (Lacan 1961–1962) – a revelation that marks in the matrix the singularity of each encounter as a unique creation of borderlinking with the unknown as co-poiesis. The matrixial co-poiesis appears to be in concordance with Lacan's idea that a "woman" is accessible "one by one" in the sense of a sequence of unique cases, but the idea of the unique encounter is here added. Inasmuch as the matrixial stratum is a weave that emerges in the Real – in the psychic register that is most closely linked to libido and to corporeal event, and first of all to the experience related to the womb as inside or outside me and as outside and inside us – it spreads out between trauma and phantasm of each becoming-subject together with the trauma and the phantasm of its specific m/Other-to-be, and a potentiality is inscribed in it, a possibility of unexpected revelation in some kind of dialogue.

The feminine-Other-desire as an assembled speak/through-being within a singular series of encounters is already a networked desire. Her desire is both phallic from the *Name of the Father*'s side and matrixial from its be-side. An exclusively phallic desire in such a meeting, which would have designated the reduction of the libido as masculine (only) to the signifier at the price of the destruction of supplementary feminine eroticism, could only have deepened the misunderstanding into which the subject is born and reduced its feminine potentiality.

The traumatic desire of the archaic becoming-m/Other-to-be

The enigma of femininity that touches upon originary repression, the *Urverdrängung*, the primordial unconscious as connected to sex and death beyond/before the separating line of castration, beyond/before the threshold of language, is foreclosed in the phallus and emerging-by- and fading-by-transformation in metramorphosis. And something of this co-emergence and co-fading in the Real is delivered into the Symbolic's "margins" via matrixial covenant(s) experienced in transference and counter-transference and hidden in art. We must beware of understanding from all this that the archaic m/Other-to-be – linked to the Thing that undergoes originary repression, which passes through foreclosure, dispersal or emerging-by- and fading-by-transformation – is simply the mother that was, or a part of her body. Melanie Klein, according to Lacan, assumes in the extimate site of the Thing the mythological body of the mother. In a similar way, seemingly the archaic father in Lacan's own work is not the actual father of past times. Raising the *objet a* as "woman" in art to the level of the Thing, the site of primordial extimity does not designate a regressive step like in the Phallus. And linking with an inter-with Thing via art does not indicate a return to the womb in the Real or a psychosis, but a realization of unforeseen potentiality of borderlinking, where "original" and "ready-made" intersect without fusion or rejection in artworking.

The I's phantasm of Origin is involved with that of his/her singular feminine Other, of his/her uncognized non-I, which is also linked to her own other non-I(s), all hovering together in a singular matrix. An encounter occurs at the limits of language, which are included from the outset in Lacanian theory (as E. Laurent says), for at the horizon of any possible language are carved the question of the mother, the phantasm of the Origin, the trauma of the subject and the meeting with the Other. These arise together with the enigma of the desire of the m/Other-to-be, bounded in a sexual borderlinking that will get lost in the future and become an archaic shared layer. "The first desire is the desire of the mother whose value is traumatic" (Laurent 1995), for it is incestual. Incest is "only the return to the maternal womb" (Lemoine 1995). To this I add: Only if the becoming-subject that already shares and participates in the m/Other-to-be's phantasm and trauma is already *differentiating what is* shared, can something be traumatically lost in birth and give birth to *birth as trauma.* The desire of the m/Other (non-I) meets the I's trauma and phantasm and in-forms sexual borderlinking.

> I stated by putting it in the present tense that there is no sexual rapport. That is the basis of Psychoanalysis (. . .) There is no sexual rapport except for neighboring generations; namely, parents on the one band, and children on the other. That's what the interdiction of incest wards off. I talk about sexual rapport.
>
> *(Lacan 1978)*

As I have proposed elsewhere (Ettinger 1995a), in the experience of the matrixial uncanny the sublimation of feminine/prenatal existence bursts forth as covenantal in the artwork. If Freud's aesthetic "uncanny" buds both from intrauterine life or womb fantasies (1919), from what I have called a matrixial complex as well as from the childhood castration complex, these two complexes indicate, to my mind, two different clusters, apparati and functions, and not simply two different organs, female and male (Ettinger 1997b [reference added for the 1998 publication]).

In the no-place of the Thing in art, Lacan identifies via the sinthome something of the dimension of the revelation of "feminine" rapport – and not necessarily as psychosis. I see in the feminine sinthome possibilities of matrixial sublimation in/from different aspects of the feminine sexual difference. By means of metramorphosis, something of the matrix arises to the surface in art as a shared hybrid gaze "between absence and presence", just as something of the horror of castration emerges through the phallic gaze that indicates the *either* absence *or* presence.

A border-Other in becoming-together between presence and absence

I will end with a matrixial interpretation of a short passage from Lacan's seminar, where he speaks of "woman" not as an absence, as in his classical theory, but as between presence and absence.

From J. Lacan *Ou pire* (translated by J. Simas and Bracha L. Ettinger):

> [T]he between involved in sexual rapport but displaced and precisely Other-imposed. To Other-impose, and it is curious that in imposing this Other, what I advanced today concerns only the woman. And it is she who, in this figure of the Other, gives us an illustration within our reach to be, as a poet has written, "between center and absence,"[17] between the meaning she takes from what I've called the at-least-one, between the center as pure existence or jouis-presence and absence (. . .) which I could nor write but to define as "Not-all", that which is not included in the phallic function, yet which is not its negation (. . .) absence which is no less *jouissance* then being jouis-absence.
>
> *(1971–1972: 8/3/1972)*

If one possibility of an archaic "nothing" is the focus of the interdiction of the elusive feminine sexual rapport based on prenatal incest, if this "nothing" is a lack created by foreclosure, the archaic "centre" is precisely the focus of such an-other rapport, in the intersection of its jouissance as "presence." Beyond the originary feminine/prenatal real stage, if "man" is either at the centre of such a rapport – and then also inside psychosis – or cut away from it, in the "nothing" and then also in the arms of the law that structures desire as masculine (i.e. if man is either in "centre" or in "nothing"), the woman traverses paradoxical between-instants that are not either/or between these oppositions reproduced by the phallus, but are "and-and" or neither/nor. These between-instants where we wit(h)ness are impossible in terms of the phallic dimension. A composition of contradictions, an "and-and" is each time a revelation in the feminine dimension. Is not revelation "what happens in any first encounter with sexual rapport" (Lacan 1973–1974)?

If, for Lacan, the "woman" between *jouis-presence* and *jouis-absence* is Other, even when she is a between, in the matrix she is not Other, but a border-Other becoming[18] between in wit(h)nessing. Lacan's feminine "and-and" beyond-the-phallus position receives its full significance in a covenant which is not only created in contingency, but also dissolved in relations with the stranger and only in a partial way. A matrixial dissolving is not a parting/cutting by either repression or foreclosure, but a transformation with-in-ter others inscribed in metramorphosis. Something of the impossible position of and-and and in-ter-with the Other that secretly drips from the Real to the Imaginary and the Symbolic wounded in a knot, is interlaced in subjectivity-as-encounter in a severality which lies before and beside the subject as One. Something is interwoven between several elements into a tissue whose connections are accessible to sublimation. Something, but not-All.

Border-Other as wit(h)ness: conclusions

The matrixial desire is composite; it includes a matrixial alongside a phallic desire. It allows an assembled and partial speak/through-being which is not the individual to be described. The matrix which supplies a "supplementary" sexual difference is a borderspace of co-birth in originary differentiation linked to a female swerve and borderlinking in the Real. The feminine/prenatal encounter that is linked in male and female to the feminine swerve served me as a basis for devising a model for a stratum of subjectivization in which co-emerging and co-fading I and non-I, sharing a psychic borderspace and hybridized *objet a*, discern each other by conductible borderlinks, interlink to each other while transmitting affects and pathic information, and address one another in a borderlinking-without-relating that takes place in the course of alternations in distance-in-proximity in a reciprocal non-cognition, in a non-cognitive discerning. This borderspace is created both by a swerve and by encounters with the stranger on the level of trauma and phantasm in the Real, by unconscious connections shaped on a sub-symbolic level that in-forms a wider-Other, and by deposits of the feminine-Other-desire which relates to her phantasm and is already involved in earlier matrixial and phallic circles. Opening from severality and contingency, me and the stranger, the I and the intimate yet unknown non-I share an ephemeral, unpredictable, and singular alliance, in which each participant is partial and relational, is not a centre/entity nor absence/nothing, but a between entity/centre/presence/pure existence and lack or nothing, in wit(h)ness. The matrixial object is composite and hybrid; the feminine-Other participates in several specific covenants. The "woman", which is not confined to the contours of the one-body with its inside versus outside polarity, the "woman" which is inter-with the Other, leans on a sexual difference based on borderspacing and webbing links, and not on essence or negation. The "woman" is not a foreclosed Other, but a potential border-Other which is becoming-between and with. The woman is an in-ter-becoming, wit(h)nessing her partial I and Other. Between centre and nothing, she is a border-Other as wit(h)nessing.[19]

Notes

1 "Supplementary Jouissance and Feminine Sexual Rapport" was first published in Hebrew in a limited edition of ten exemplaries by BLE Atelier, Paris, 1995. Translations from French to English of J. Lacan are by Joseph Simas and Bracha Lichtenberg Ettinger. Passages from this text were presented on two occasions: *Los Poderes de La Palnbra/ Les pouvoirs de la parole*, IXe rencontre internationale du Champs freudien, Buenos Aires, 18–21 July 1996; and *The Clinical Limits of Gender*, EEP Conference, London, 22–23 March 1997. This text was subsequently published in English, in two parts, as: Lichtenberg Ettinger, B. (1998) Supplementary Jouissance [1995]. *The Almanac of Psychoanalysis*, I, 162–176; and Lichtenberg Ettinger, B. (2000) Feminine Borderlinking [1995]. *The Almanac of Psychoanalysis*, II, 152–169.

2 In the late Lacanian theory, feminine jouissance is "supplementary" and "there is no sexual rapport".

3 I am thinking of Merleau-Ponty's "*écart*" meaning deviation and digression. While M.-P. relates to a deviation in the sensory field, I relate to the psychic field of affects.

4 I refer to late pregnancy when the infant, according to Winnicott, is "post-mature" and we assume the beginning of phantasmatic life.

5 This is the Lacanian classical position. From the angle of the superiority of the Symbolic and the Imaginary upon the Real resonates relations of exclusion or rejection: "it's either

he or me" since "speech is already trapped in a network of symbolic couples and opposition" (Lacan 1981a: 107, 126).

6 On this matter, see Ettinger (1990).
7 On the expansion of the concept of the phallus, as commanding the three realms, see Ettinger (1992).
8 In *Encore* Lacan refers to the Other as a "site" that may be described by a letter.
9 She ought to, but she can't, adds Lacan in *Encore*, for since she is not-All, her sex says nothing to her.
10 See Ettinger (1992) and (1997a).
11 It is possible to speak of a dimension that belongs to the side of "woman" in the schema of sexuation. Likewise the archaic father is a dimension in masculinity, different from yet related to the Name of the Father.
12 Ancient way of writing *symptome* – playing on the expressions, among others, of "saint man" and "sinner man".
13 Speaking of the ontogenesis of the aesthetic world, Merleau-Ponty draws in terms of the "*écart*" – a space of bursting and dehiscence before the bifurcation into object and subject on the level of sensorial perception. By "swerve" I intend an analogous differentiating potential on the level of affection and sensing beyond the senses (cf. Merleau-Ponty, 1964: 169).
14 For further discussion of these matters, see Ettinger (1996a).
15 For an extensive discussion of the difference between objects in the different theories, see Ettinger (1995b).
16 Cf. "Lacan says: Desire is the desire of the Other. And now I say: if desire is the desire of the other, phantasy is not the phantasy of the Other", etc. (Soler 1989: 43).
17 An expression borrowed from the poet H. Michaux.
18 In this expression, the word "becoming" echoes G. Deleuze and F. Guauari's expression "becoming-woman" (1980).
19 [Editorial notes, 1998] With the concepts of *matrix* and *metramorphosis* BLE turns to the womb as a conceptual basis for hypothesis concerning an originary supplementary feminine sexual difference.

Matrix is defined by the author as an unconscious borderspace of simultaneous co-emergence and co-fading of the I and uncognized non-I – or partial subjects – neither fused nor rejected, which produce, share and transmit joint, hybrid and diffracted objects via conductible borderlinks. The matrixial apparatus proposes a specific perception of feminine/prenatal borderlinking, where the womb stands for a shared psychic borderspace in which *differentiation-in-co-emergence, seperation-in-jointness* and *distance-in-proximity* are continuously reattuned by metramorphosis created by, and further creating – together with matrixial affects – relations without relating on the borders of presence and absence, subject and object, among subjects and partial subjects, between me and the stranger, and between those and part-objects or relational objects.

Metramorphosis is a process of intra-psychic and inter-psychic or trans-individual exchange, transformation and affective "communication", between several matrixial entities. Co-emerging and co-fading I(s) and non-I(s) interlace their borderlinks in metramorphosis. It is a passage through which affected events, materials and modes of becoming infiltrate and diversify on to non-conscious margins of the Symbolic through sub-symbolic webs.

Bibliography

Deleuze, G. and Guattari, F. (1980) *Capitalisme et schizophrénie: Mille plateaux*. Paris: Editions de Minuit.

Ettinger, B. (1990) The Woman Doesn't Exist and Doesn't Signify Anything. *Catalogue: Feminine Presence*. Tel Aviv Museum of Art.

Ettinger, B. (1992) Matrix and Metramorphosis. *Differences*, 4(3), 176–208.
Ettinger, B. (1995a) *The Matrixial Gaze*. Leeds: FAHN Leeds University Press.
Ettinger, B. (1995b) Woman as Objet a Between Phantasy and Art. *Complexity – Journal of Philosophy and the Visual Arts*, 6, 57–77.
Ettinger, B. (1996a) Metramorphic Borderlinks and Matrixial Borderspace. In J. Welchman (ed.) *Rethinking Borders*. London: Macmillan.
Ettinger, B. (1996b) The With-In-Visible Screen. In C. De Zegher (ed.) *Inside the Visible*. Cambridge: MIT Press.
Ettinger, B. (1997a) Feminine/Prenatal Weaving in Subjectivity-as-Encounter. *Psychoanalytic Dialogues*, 7(3), 367–405.
Ettinger, B. (1997b) Reply to Commentary. *Psychoanalytic Dialogues*, 7(3), 423–429.
Ettinger, B., Telerand, A., Kronenberg, Y. and Gaoni, B. (1991) Verbal Hallucinations in Psychotic Patients. *Israel Journal of Psychiatry*, 28(2), 39–49.
Freud, S. (1908/1959) On the Sexual Theories of Children. In J. Strachey (ed.) *The Standard Edition of the Complete Psychological Works of Sigmund Freud*, Vol. IX. London: Hogarth Press.
Freud, S. (1919) The "Uncanny". In J. Strachey (ed.) *The Standard Edition of the Complete Psychological Works of Sigmund Freud*, Vol. XVII. London: Hogarth Press.
Lacan, J. (1961–1962) *L'identification*. Unpublished seminar.
Lacan, J. (1966) *Écrits*. Paris: Seuil.
Lacan, J. (1968–1969) *D'un autre à l'Autre*. Unpublished seminar.
Lacan, J. (1971–1972) *. . . ou pire*. Unpublished seminar.
Lacan, J. (1973–1974) *Les non-dupes errent*. Unpublished seminar.
Lacan, J. (1975a) *Le Séminaire de Jacques Lacan, Livre XX: Encore*. Paris: Seuil.
Lacan, J. (1975b) Seminar of 21-1-75. *Ornicar?* 104–110.
Lacan, J. (1975–1976) *Le sinthome*. Unpublished seminar.
Lacan, J. (1978) *Le moment de conclure*. Unpublished seminar.
Lacan, J. (1980) *Le malentendu*. *Ornicar?* 22.
Lacan, J. (1981a) *Le Séminaire de Jacques Lacan, Livre III: Les Psychoses*. Paris: Seuil.
Lacan, J. (1981b) *The Four Fundamental Concepts of Psycho-Analysis*. Ed. J. A. Miller, trans. A. Sheridan. New York: Norton.
Laurent, E. (1995) *Soiree Paris*. Unpublished discussion.
Lemoine, E. (1995) *L'envers de Paris*. Unpublished discussion.
Merleau-Ponty, M. (1964) *Le visible et l'invisible*. Paris: Gallimard.
Miller. J. A. (1982–1983) *Du symptome au fantasme et retour*. Unpublished seminar.
Miller. J. A. (1985–1986) *Extimité*. Unpublished course.
Miller. J. A. (1994–1995) *Silet*. Unpublished course.
Soler, C. (1989) *Hysteria and Obsession: A Seminar of the Freudian Field*. Tel Aviv: GEP.
Tustin, F. (1990) *The Protective Shell in Children and Adults*. London: Karnac.

6

SELF-RECREATION THROUGH THE UNCANNY ENCOUNTER

Reading the feminine close-up in cinema

Nava Dushi and Igor Rodin

In this chapter we examine the phenomenon of what we term the feminine close-up in cinema[1] with the aims of theorizing its relation to the feminine and questioning the principle of indexicality, that is, that of an image as an implied "signifier of",[2] with relation to the representation of femininity. Starting with and against the background of the phallic, "made-to-be-fetishized" close-up, our discursive itinerary circles around the varying levels of potentiality of what Bracha L. Ettinger (2006) defines as *matrixial*, that is, beyond-the-phallus, a-structural readings of the image. Proposing the concept of the *matrixial gaze*, Ettinger engages with new textures of the plane of representation/vision/gaze as she delves into the problematics of the dialectics between the visible and the Real. For Ettinger, the function of the Lacanian gaze as *objet a* – that is, that of exposing the fundamental gap between *the visible* and *the seen* for the speaking being – cannot exhaust the scopic field of subjectivity. She states: "when *beyond appearance* we search for a 'lack aspect', a lacking 'something', separated, fragmented, and lost, this lacking something is not just any no-thing! It is a particular no-thing" (ibid.: 44, original emphasis). In other words, Ettinger organizes her theoretical discourse not around the entrance into language (the symbolic castration), which inevitably prioritizes castration as a guiding principle for approaching subjectivity, but around the intrauterine experience of the fetus: the co-emergence of the *I* (the fetus) and the *non-I* (the body of the (m)Other). The latter, thus, is regarded not only as that which *precedes* the subject-object/intersubjective relation chronologically, but also *preconditions* it, and in that sense, challenges the post-Kantian/Cartesian anthropocentric logic of the cogito as the core element of subjectivity, which still dominates the psychoanalytic discourse in general, and its place in the theoretical study of cinema in particular. In this light, the feminine close-up, as we see it, should be withdrawn from the constrains of representation, that is, from its reduction to a close-up on a face of a human being whose exterior view supposedly hints at some physiological and psycho-cultural givenness.

Hence, our discussion departs from the classification of the close-up in seminal works of film theory as a technical and/or semantic device of cinematic enunciation, whether it is Rudolf Arnheim's cognitive study of the close-up, or, "apparent size" manipulation, and its connotated effects, such as thematization, emphasis, surprise and suspense (1957: 128–129); Béla Balázs' emphasis on physiognomy, his theorization of the close-up as a catalyst for "the mood of a scene", the poetry of film, or an abstraction, by means of which "time as well as space can be dislocated" (2010: 39–41); or, on a broader social scale, Walter Benjamin's scrutiny of the increasing cultural significance of cinema that assigns to the close-up the capacity to accentuate the "hidden details in familiar objects", or the tendency to expand the space of "[o]ur bars, city streets, our offices and furnished rooms, our railroad stations and our factories [which] seemed to close relentlessly around us" (1968: 230–252). In later theoretical accounts, we find that the close-up is assumed as given and incorporated into the discussion of cinematic form, continuity, dramatic emphasis, and point of view (Bordwell and Thompson 2008), or alternately, associated with the manipulation and subjection of the female body to the objectifying hegemonic "gaze" of its male viewer (Mulvey 1999).[3] Against these prevalent approaches, we argue, the understanding of the feminine close-up in cinema should be re-approached and re-aligned with what the, late teaching of Lacan, theories of deconstruction,[4] the matrixial theory of Ettinger, the artistic and the cinematic image have taught us about femininity. What is common to all these is their departure from seeing the relationship between Being and the Symbolized as causal, as well as the self-ontologization of their theoretical perspectives.[5]

In tracing the borderline between the fetishistic close-up and the feminine close-up, which transgresses the imaginary/symbolic representational field, what we seek to explore is the range of the feminine close-up in resonance with the realm of the Ettingerian *encounter-event* (Ettinger 2006: 86–87), that is, a non-regressive, re-constituting encounter with the image, in relation to thresholds of visibility. We align our inquiry with the sensibility of the matrixial reading by avoiding two critical shortcomings. The first concerns the possible application of the Freudian *uncanny* in the analysis of cinematic images, an approach that inevitably results in a semiotic discourse. In order to apply the concept of the *uncanny* to the cinematic image, it has to be located, or sought, on the side of the *encounter* with the image, rather than that of the *image* itself. The *uncanny*, therefore, is not an *immanent trait* of the image, but a trait of a possible encounter with a specific subject, the *potentiality* of which stems from a certain "alignment of forces" among the different components of the image. The *uncanny* manifests itself through the *syntax* of the image that "mocks" the syntax that lies at the basis of a pro-regressive reading. The gaze for Lacan, as Ettinger sums up, "is a model of a purged *objet a* because it is not 'polluted' by the *demand* of the subject, but rather reflects *desire* in its distilled form" (ibid.: 42, original emphasis). Therefore, endowing an image with a priori traits contradicts the very nature of the gaze in that this endowment calls for the universalization of its meaning rather than confront the idiosyncrasy of its reading. The second shortcoming involves the temptation to categorize, annex and re-territorialize the range of the feminine close-up. As our theorization takes off from an existing theoretical glossary that is deeply grounded in a hermeneutic tradition, a special accent should be put on the effort to untie this tradition's connotative knots in order to shed a new theoretical light on the phenomenon of the feminine close-up in cinema as a de-gendered category that is not to be (re-) constructed through the imaginary identification.

Our appeal to the *uncanny* is in search of a hazy territory that opens up in an encounter with the image, in an encounter that produces two kinds of potentialities for the viewer. On the one hand, there is the Freudian *uncanny*, which he defines as "what arouses dread and horror", the unfamiliar that blurs the boundaries between the animate and the inanimate, "the idea of being robbed of one's eyes", as he puts it (1997: 193, 205). Whereas the latter formulation in itself allegedly stands in a strict opposition to the phallic gaze as *objet a*, it stumbles on itself as Freud refers the uncanny effect to the anxiety belonging to the castration complex of childhood, that is to say, to the very epicentre of the phallic structuring. The interconnectedness of different modes of castration – in this case the symbolic and the imaginary – stems from the construction of the symptom-desire through language and *object a* as its residual.[6] Therefore, by subverting the psychic structure, the *uncanny* reveals its nature as that which opposes inscription into language, that is, into the boundaries of the symptom-desire. Thus, the intrusion of the uncanny marks the limits of the area within which the symptom-desire operates. On the other hand, there is the Ettingerian *uncanny* (Ettinger 2006: 157–161), which brings back the womb-fantasy, its primary, pre-castration status, tying it to an originary feminine difference, as opposed to residual effects of oedipalization. By distinguishing the Freudian *uncanny* from the Ettingerian *uncanny* this chapter lays the ground for an exploration of the feminine close-up not on the basis of a pro-regressive identification of its function as a technical and/or semantic device of cinematic expression, but as an emerging/withering potentiality for self-recreation. Furthermore, while we recognize the contribution of recent works to the study of the relevance of the late Lacan and the contingency of that which remains beyond the scope of the visible, namely, the gaze as *objet a*, our discussion advances a move from those post-structuralist approaches – which continue to be informed by the oedipalized perspective that by the very nature of its theorized male/female division assumes a transcendental position – to a pro-matrixial theoretical position that undermines the gulf propagated by the Phallus in search of immanence, in the Deleuzian-Guattarian sense (Deleuze and Guattari, 1994).

The phallic close-up

Our discussion of the phallic close-up issues from the concept of *facialized consciousness* coined by Félix Guattari in referring to the "the facializing eye-nose-forehead triangle that collects, formalizes, neutralizes, and crushes the specific traits of the other semiotic components" (2011: 75). This faciality remains "in constant resonance with social roles and the capitalistic Imaginary" (ibid.: 77), mandating the translatability of the visible (ibid.: 79), that is, its applicability to the "or . . . or . . ." phallic paradigm. In this case, the image is grounded in its orientation toward self-specification. Thus, when the triangle of the face is fully exposed, it lends itself to objectivization: of the face, to its ethnic, gendered, racial, sexualized, definition. Consider the soft focus, centred, evenly lit, eye-level close-ups of the loving and loved Ingrid Bergman in *Casablanca* (1942): each instance of their calculated insertion in a sequence of shot-reverse shot codifies her iconic representation. On the other end of the spectrum, we find the no less iconic close-ups of Maria Falconetti in *The Passion of Joan of Arc* (1928), which, nevertheless, progressively transitions from evenly lit, centred close-ups of horror and suffering, to extreme close-ups of low-/high-angled, off-centre and fragmented images, a series in which:

> Dreyer avoids the shot-reverse shot [*champ-contrechamp*] procedure which would maintain a real relation between each face and the other, and would still be part of the action-image. He prefers to isolate each face in a close up which is only partly filled, so that the position to the right or to the left directly induces a virtual conjunction which no longer needs to pass through the real connection between the people.
>
> *(Deleuze 1986: 107)*

In that, Dreyer tears the close-up from its symbolized transferability, from the coded objectification of the face. The intensive commingling of faces, bodies, objects, expressions and affects assume a collective enunciation – a passion.[7] Hence, our exploration of the cinematic manifestations of the feminine close-up traces the range that opens between the aforementioned phallic triangle of the face and the site at which the unfolding representation brings about the dissemination of the triangle as a gendered and essentialized category.[8]

In its adherence to the facial triangle as a point of reference for the symbolic codification of the face, the phallic close-up includes both men and women as long as they are pushed to be read and *are* read as gendered entities. The departure from the phallic close-up begins as the *uncanny* starts to infiltrate the representation. It begins where motion of the parts decomposes the quasi-*gestalt* of the frozen image calling for the phallic gaze to occur, bringing about the total eclipse of regression where the ontology of the viewer collapses into the lost object, the need and oedipality. As the *uncanny* seeps in, the phallic triangle eludes the focus of the gaze and destabilizes the well-established mechanisms of regression, pushing the viewer to *seek* meaning-bearing points rather than *surrender* to that which is obtrusively imposed on her/him. The situation of seeking, though, is not the *result* of a decision made on the part of the viewer, but an affect of decentralization and loss of grounding that seeks creative openings in order to work through its frustration. The image is that which is active and activating, while *decision* is the reflex of symbolization, the trace of the phallic structure that works in a concurrent manner. Decision is always a posteriori in relation to affect, invariably subject to *belatedness*.

Being associated with the work of the drive, decision is always secondary in relation to the encounter-event.

The fading of the phallic close-up begins in the banal site at which some intrusion does not allow one to fix the attention on the triangle: a movement of the head, the coincidence of other activity in the frame, an extreme and distorted close-up, a loss of focus or ambiguous framing. When the face is blurred, corrupted, is seen in movement, magnified or commingles with another face, the imaginary/symbolic annexation of the close-up is violated and traversed. A close-up of a metallic-blue candy wrapper fluttering in the wind waved by a tiny hand extended out of a window crack of a moving vehicle against a pale blue sky and flying out of the frame; a close-up of a child leaning against the back seat of a moving vehicle, laying her head on her arms gazing through the rear window at the passing traffic in a dark tunnel, the lights of the tunnel and the vehicles passing through it reflected on the rear window obscure her image, the lights of moving vehicles inside the tunnel generate strokes of colour smearing against the black background, the vehicles move toward the camera the camera moves away; an extreme close-up of the child's face increasingly obscured by the movement of the vehicle and by the reflecting yellow and red lights of the moving vehicles (Kieslowski, *Three Colors: Blue*, 1993). These opening close-ups proceed to the horizons at which the human image falls out of visibility. An unidentifiable feather-like foregrounded focalized speck is made animate by a movement induced by a regulated flow of air, its background is hazy and out of focus, a figure enters the right side of the frame approaching the camera then seen reflected in a dark pupil of a seeing magnified eye (ibid.). The feminine close-up produces a crisis of identity, as its propagated proximity radicalizes this crisis leaving a taint of claustrophobia on the texture of the encounter.[9]

The element of repetition of de-focalization, de-centralization and contingency, as the precondition of the encounter with the image, forges what Guattari (1995) defines as *transversalist subjectivity*: ever-becoming, idiosyncratic and open to extralinguistic, affective, corpo-Real investments. In Lacanian terms, it could be related to as a *sinthomatic*, as opposed to a *symptomatic*, subject. For Lacan, the *sinthomatization* of the subject is associated with his identification with the symptom that, for example, in the case of James Joyce, results in *writing* as a solution for holding the Borromean knot of subjectivity together (Verhaeghe and Declercq, 2002). This points to the privileged position of the "aesthetic state of mind" as that which, as opposed to the over-oedipalized subjectivity, can incorporate "all the suffering in the world" in a creative, and non narcissistic-martyric manner.

The *cross-cutting close-up* exemplifies the possible implications of this pro-transversalist self-recreation, displaying a sequence of close-ups that cuts across and runs through multiple locations and temporalities generating intensities that abstract the spatiotemporal grounding of the seen.[10] Zooming in to the figure of a red-headed girl seated by a fire who turns her head and her look toward the camera, which makes a sharp pan to the left that wipes off the image; a close-up of a hand held against a burning piece of wood lit by its flickering flame; a close-up of a young boy turning his head from left to right his face lit by a warm flickering light; a lantern flickering, turning off and on as the camera dollies toward it; a close-up of a female figure emerging from the dark, walking toward the camera, then followed by the camera in a pan to the right as it passes behind another female figure, whose face is half lit by a light emanating from the left, putting turquoise earrings on and looking toward an unseen mirror and toward the camera that abruptly pans back to the left to a close-up of the young boy standing by the entrance, his figure barely made visible by the fading of the last, or first, sun rays (Tarkovsky, *The Mirror*, 1975).

The *cross-cutting close-up* inspires a transition from the gender-driven category that postulates the binary relations man/woman where the symbolic/imaginary register is oxymoronically detached from the immanence of the Real, to a sexual Phallic/Matrixial system of axes that prioritizes contingency and movement in opposition to regressive repetition and fixedness. While gender is governed by imaginary/symbolic construction, the sexual is related to the drive and *jouissance* as its idiosyncratic manifestation in a form of libidinal investments in erotogenic zones, partial objects and speech. Thus, gender and the Matrixial/Maternal appear to us as a *dichotomy*, that is, in this specific context one of its subsets should be put aside, obviously that which is grounded in the symbolic.

One of the implications of the resolution of this dichotomy between gender and sexuality is the non-binary relation between the Phallic and the Matrixial. As opposed to the gender discourse, that tends to present them as oppositions, it should be emphasized that due to their being associated with the drive(s) they appeal to *different* formations of the psyche and do not contradict one another. While the Phallus stands for the male phantasy and its extrapolations, the Matrix does the same for the female/maternal phantasy, inscribing such a non-translatable-to-the-phallic-language experience as pregnancy into the theoretical discourse.

Deleuze's conceptualization of the *affect image*, that is, the close-up, resonates with the aforementioned beyond-temporality of the proximate moving image. The *affect image*, as he states, is

> independent of all determinate space-time; but it is nonetheless created in a history which produces it as the expressed and the expression of a space or a time, of an epoch or a milieu (this is why the affect is the "new" and new affects are ceaselessly created (. . .) by the work of art).
>
> *(Deleuze 1986: 99)*

For Deleuze – as opposed to the psychoanalytic perspective, which is understandably restricted to the needs of one-to-one treatment – history is neither one's property, nor a cultural convention, but an ontological phenomenon the approach to which demands thinking not in terms of units of meaning but in intensities. The *cross-cutting close-up* embodies such an intensity that tends to overshadow the settings and persons, thus carving a space for another reading of the image.

The feminine close-up

Jean-Luc Nancy's concept of the *distinct* (2005) presents a view, one can argue, that ranges between the pro-regressive disjunction and the Ettingerian *encounter-event* with regards to the encounter with the image, which we consider as equally relatable to the moving image, as both can be understood in terms of *untouchability*. The *distinct*, as Nancy puts it, is the sacred in a sense of that which signifies "the separate, what is set aside, removed, cut off, or that which one cannot touch, which one can approach only by a touch without contact" (ibid.: 1). With that, both the phallic pro-regressive and the matrixial pro-creative potentialities find their way into this concept, unconsciously underscoring the ambivalence of the encounter with the visible. On the one hand, the common ground between the image as *distinct* and the Freudian-Lacanian Thing is established as it is defined in terms of being *desirable*, thus alluding to the phallic partial object, *objet a*. The image, says Nancy, "is desirable, or it is not an image (but a *chromo*, an ornament, a vision or representation)" (ibid.: 6). On the other hand, Nancy proceeds by articulating the state of mind of the viewer when "he enters into [a kind of] *self-coincidence*, [as] he enters into the image, he no longer looks at it – though he does not cease to be in front of it. He penetrates it, is penetrated by it: by it, its distance and its distinction, at the same time" (ibid.: 9–10). There is a sense, says Nancy, "that [the image] is non signifying but not insignificant" (ibid.: 11).

Nancy's further grapple with this ambivalence argues for the necessity of art,

> the sense in which it is (. . .) disquieting, and can be threatening: because it conceals its very being from signification or from definition, but also because it can threaten itself and destroy in itself the images of itself that have been deposited in a signifying code and in an assured beauty.
>
> *(Ibid.: 13)*

This "threat of the art" points to a traumaticity that is immanent to the encounter-event, to a traumaticity as the royal road to self-recreation. The traumaticity of self-recreation of the post-Oedipal creature is that of *cohabitation* – between *Heimlich* and *Unheimlich*, as "the prefix 'un'- is the token of repression" (Freud 1919/1955: 245). Ettinger adds:

> A center-less *heimlich* affect silently ascends behind the "*unheimlich*" aesthetic experience (Freud), anguishing and soothing, tearing and stitching the wounds of a nomadic place, opening in it a rhythm of interval for an exile, suspended like a rotating sea-wave between its fading and a next birth.
>
> *(2006: 161)*

The feminine close-up inhabits the phallic image, and yet it is neither primary nor secondary to it. It transgresses the triangle's imaginary/symbolic trappings and hence has no permanent identifiable loci: the feminine close-up is in a perpetual state of emerging and withering away. Thus, the feminine close-up as the image that is "unsure of itself" creates a space for identification not at the level of *ideality* but at the level of *incoherence*, bestowing legitimacy to the fragility of the one who is looking in the mirror, in other words, shifting the focus from the Father, who calls for the subject to satisfy his expectations through the symbolic/imaginary identification, to the Mother, whose sole precondition for acceptance is the fact of one's existence, not his formations.

Due to this, the close-up, in our view, is feminine, as long as it is inclusive of both men and women, animals, plants, objects, overlappings and smearings, movements and flows, while not allowing the viewer enough time and audio-visual formalization to be "robbed of his eyes". The light wind ruffles the surface of the shallow water making the algae pulsate and oscillate. A lonesome leaf crosses the frame as the camera pans parallel to the current of the river from right to left. After the cut, the camera changes directions: now it pans from left to right as different elements of the streamside vegetation fall into its focus. A man's knee area enters the frame upon which the camera starts to tilt up until it stops on the man's face. The man cannot fix his gaze, so he depresses his eyes. The camera comes back to contemplate the contingent pulsation of the algae as it zooms in until the end of the scene (Tarkovsky, *Solaris*, 1972). The antinomy of different temporalities (the leaf, the algae/water, the man) and vectors of movement (of the camera), the man's inscription into the ecosystem of the sequence – all these tend to deconstruct the self-containment of forms the most clear-cut of which is the human body. Thus, what permeates the sequence through the dynamic and fluidal *cross-cutting close-up* is the feminine close-up par excellence, that which defies anthropocentricity, that is, genderization and oedipalization of the seen. The algae, the flecks of sunlight, the man's knees, hands and face are brought under the same common denominator at the level of intensity, inner rhythm and *co-emergence.*

Self-recreation through the uncanny encounter

Freud writes:

> The uncanny as it is depicted in *literature*, in stories and imaginative productions, merits in truth a separate discussion. To begin with, it is a much more fertile province than the uncanny in real life, for it contains the whole of the latter and something more besides, something that cannot be found in real life.
>
> *(1919/1955: 245)*

Thus, the discussion of the *uncanny* is directly related by Freud, among other things, to the provision of the aesthetic encounter. Resonating with his notions of primal repression, the navel of the dream and other vanishing points of symbolization,[11] Freud's "something more", here, points to the possibility of some *long-term* effect of the uncanny encounter, that which goes beyond the boundaries of the transient affect and is conditioned by the irreversible inscription of new layers into the subjective structure.

As opposed to the Freudian vision of the *uncanny* as a phantasmatic atrocity to be escaped from – in the sense that disturbing images are to be repressed – the Ettingerian matrixial paradigm provides a pathway to traumaticity as that which opens up a space for one's self-recreation through identification with the invisible and the unspoken, thus appealing to the *immanence* of traumaticity in self-recreation. Within the cinematic context, the maternal connotations of a feminine image inscribed in the feminine close-up render the encounter with a disturbing proximity to gestures, holes and textures of the female body, partial bodies, objects, etc. insistently uncanny. As Jacques-Alain Miller remarks, within the intersubjective realm *proximity in space* and *accessibility* stand in an inverse relation to one another (2008: 13–15). In fact, he says, this is the essence of the Oedipal Complex: the family figures that are accessible in space turn to inaccessible figures from the libidinal point of view. This is what he relates to as the *erotic of space*, when the Eros deconstructs metric relations. The Phallic Eros, we emphasize.

Thus, the presence of the Maternal within the image bears the stamp of death, as representation is always Janus-faced, oscillating between the matricide of representability and the nostalgia for the intrauterine *co-poiesis*,[12] in terms of Ettinger. The matricide as a metaphor for the fundamental feature of the entrance into language stands for irreversible detachment from the m/Other that continues to perpetuate itself through her demonization and exclusion from the language. In this sense it is possible to put the equal sign between the matricide (Woman-does-not-exist), the incest taboo and what Lacan calls "the fading of the subject", meaning that where language starts the subject ends. Hence the barred S that signifies the subject ($). As opposed to this, the Ettingerian *co-poiesis* proposes to look at subjectivity through the lens of the intrauterine experience where the co-existence is not grounded in a fundamental exclusion and detachment, but at the level of a psychical co-resonance: what she calls co-emergence between *I* and *non-I*. It is precisely this kind of traumatic-and-too-intimate encounter with the feminine image that opens up a space for transformative and creative reading.

Yet, articulating the problem of matricide is associated with the danger of slipping into patricide. Still, it is due to the Father that we create concepts. Without him we would find ourselves in an asylum, and the Father who would put us there is not the same Father as that which gave us the syntax in order to turn the water of speech-jouissance into wine of a clinical or philosophical concept. Creative work is based on resistance, but resistance is by no means negation. It is an outburst of energy that emerges at the epicentre of intercrossing vectors of energetic/material flow and creates life and a long-term momentum for a living being on the planet Earth. While negation reproduces the same vector of flow reinforcing it with the repression of the "no", creation is by definition *ex nihilo*, that is, its primary goal is not coming into conflict with the existing signifier but to spot a locus where no signifier has gone before.

Still, the dive into the *uncanny* may turn the possible encounter-event into a Mariana Trench, as it is, according to Ettinger, "open-ended, at the cost of a catastrophe of identity, and even at the risk of the collapse of the fragile matrixial gaze itself – at the risk of the disintegration of its screen" (2006: 160). Therefore, reading as one's openness to self-recreation is about a *certain level* of traumaticity of the encounter necessary for the signifying chain to stretch and to intensify – to contain new signifiers and meanings. Thus, reading is about *timing* and *contingency*: having fallen into a too compulsive slot it may not-soon or never be inscribed into one's language; other times, it may hold the potentiality of the encounter in abeyance, opening up one that more, or less, begs to occur, which, under these or those circumstances will seek and/or find the encounter-event.

The slipping of the visible into invisibility

In this chapter, we presented an alternative view of the feminine close-up in cinema. Departing from the constraints that categories of gender and the imaginary identification impose on the concept of face, reducing it to a physiological and psycho-cultural givenness, we sought to synchronize the concept of the feminine close-up with the psychoanalytic understanding of femininity as beyond-representational entity, following Jacques Lacan and Bracha L. Ettinger. In this light, within the context of the cinematic language, we argued, the full exposure of the face-nose-forehead triangle of the female body cannot be regarded as that which *stands for* femininity.

Through supplementation of Freud's and Ettinger's conceptualizations of the *uncanny* we formulated the encounter with the proximate image as opening up a twofold potentiality for the viewer, that of regression and self-recreation, the latter stemming from a transformative encounter with the feminine layers of the image, the *encounter-event*. The latter, as we showed, is conditioned not only by a historical readiness of the subject-viewer, but also by contingency and timing, as well as a certain level of traumaticity, immanent to the process of self-recreation.

To conclude, the feminine close-up, as we see it, resonates with the way Andrei Tarkovsky sees black-and-white cinema as having more access to the truth, the aspiration to which is immanent to every art form.[13] For Tarkovsky, it is actually black-and-white cinema that is more realistic, not colour cinema, and it is because the latter draws all of the viewer's attention to its seemingly neutral resemblance of the outer world. Yet, "truth in life does not resemble truth in art" (Tarkovsky 2016). The colour film presents itself in the form of an imposed succession of "postcards" making one *look* but not *see*, which refers directly to the phallic gaze as *objet a*. In the case of black-and-white cinema, one is drawn into the world of expressive means, rather than that of mimicry. Similarly, we say, in order to *see* a face it should be put into motion, make us chase it and never catch it, just like femininity that *does not exist*. It is precisely this slipping of the visible into invisibility that makes a close-up feminine.

Notes

1 In this chapter we conceptualize the feminine close-up as inherent to cinema. That is, our discussion attends to the potentiality of the cinematic image to affect a creative encounter with its viewer.

2 Our use of the term indexicality is consistent with Peirce's semiotic theory, which implies a direct causal relationship between signifier and something that is perceived as signified. We refer to this relationship as implied since the signifier does not exist in the form that can be caught by means of language.

3 The gaze theorized in the early applications of Lacan's terminology by scholars such as Laura Mulvey and Christian Metz was based in an erroneous interpretation that placed undue emphasis on the Lacanian mirror phase and the imaginary. Mulvey's influential essay "Visual Pleasure and Narrative Cinema", as we see it, presents a phallic approach to femininity, which intermixed the scopic *jouissance* with a politically informed agenda. Since the former is primary to the latter their discussion as existing on the same plane should be qualified. As such, the use of parenthesis in the context of Mulvey's work is to emphasize its difference from references to the gaze made throughout the paper. It is important to note that while David Bordwell is commonly associated with the post-theory turn in cinema studies, one cannot ignore the fact that in his scholarly oeuvre he developed a formalist and cognitivist theory of cinema. In that sense, as D. N. Rodowick observes, his work cannot be considered a retreat from theory, for "no one's commitment to good theory building is greater or more admirable" (2007: 95).

4 Implying not only the work of Jacques Derrida but also that of Jean-Luc Nancy.

5 What we imply here is their theoretical evolvement that appears to have been guided by questioning the structure of language, inscribing into their philosophical praxis the problematic of the failure of the oedipalized/phallocentric language on the one hand, and the impossibility of a meta-language on the other.

6 See, for example, relevant sections in *Anxiety: The Seminar of Jacques Lacan, Book X* (2014).

7 Dreyer's use of what Deleuze conceptualizes as "affective cutting", is linked with the rise of what he terms "flowing close-up": "This is, undoubtedly, a continuous movement by which the camera passes from the close-up to the medium or full shot, but it is primarily a way of treating the medium shot and the full shot *as* close-ups" (Deleuze 1986: 107).

8 In a segment titled "The Two Poles of the Face" Deleuze conceptualizes the close-up in similar terms. When the face is grasped as an outline that traces the nose, the mouth, etc., it produces a "surface of faceification" (1986: 88). Yet, when the close-up "works through dispersed features taken globally; fragmentary and broken lines which indicate here the quivering of the lips, there the brilliance of a look, and which involve content which to a greater or lesser extent rebels against the outline" we find the traits of "faceicity". Yet, for Deleuze, these poles are not mutually exclusive: "it is a matter of two poles, sometimes one prevailing over the other and appearing almost pure, sometimes the two being mixed in one direction or another" (ibid.).

9 Propagated proximity can be read as corresponding with Laura U. Marks' theorization of "haptic visuality", which, in congruence with Vivian Sobchack's phenomenology of the cinematic experience, appeals to the embodied synaesthetic union of intellect and the senses. While both Marks and Sobchack theorize the capacity of cinema/video to overcome the limits of visuality and its modes of expression by way of a dialogical approach to the viewing experience: "the act of viewing, seen in terms of existential phenomenology, is one in which both I and the object of my vision constitute each other" (Marks 1998: 339), our discussion conceptualizes the feminine close-up as a rupturing event, which rather than effect an embodied synthesis of the senses, deploys a psychoanalytic/ontological/materialist approach with the aims of contemplating the slipping of the visual into invisibility.

10 The *cross-cutting close-up* differs from Dreyer's *flowing close-ups* only in that it involves the cutting across locations and temporalities. Thus, it deconstructs the whole logic of applying the phallic syntax to reading the cinematic image. This logic implies perceiving scenes

as basic "blocks of meaning" and cuts as boundaries that they cannot not transcend, but only through the imaginative/interpretative bridging that is made by the viewer. The main problem consists in that such a segregative approach represents a projection of the logic of the Symbolic as that which denies the flexible and nomadic essence of the Real. This kind of logic imbues the cut with powers of the ultimate law and cannot be applied to dealing with the feminine core of the image.

11 Under the term *vanishing points of symbolization* we understand not only literally taking Freud's inability to narrativize that which lies beyond what *he himself* defined as beyond interpretation but, in a broader sense, moments of clash between the Real and the symbolic where language fails to (re-)produce itself. In fact, it can appear in a variety of inconspicuous forms when compared to a post-traumatic speech and other forms of paroxysm where the "splash" of *jouissance* is too obvious. In a routine-like manner the aforementioned clashes can be "resolved" by the speaking being in a "peaceful" manner, such as mockery or labelling the subversive event as nonsense. The symptomatic opposition to *nonsense* on the side of the phallocentric culture points, in turn, to something that can be called *the vanishing point of the Phallus*.

12 See, for example, Ettinger (2005).

13 See *Meeting Andrei Tarkovsky: Cinema Is a Mosaic Made of time*, a lecture given by Tarkovsky in Rome in 1982. www.youtube.com/watch?v=4JRfeshEboI&t=1211s

Bibliography

Arnheim, R. (1957) *Film as Art*. Berkeley, CA: University of California Press.

Balázs, B. (2010) The Close-Up. In *Béla Balázs: The Early Film Theory: Visible Man and the Spirit of Film*. New York: Berghahn Books.

Benjamin, W. (1968) The Work of Art in the Age of Mechanical Reproduction. In H. Arendt (ed.) *Illuminations: Essays and Reflections*. New York: Schocken Books.

Bordwell, D. and Thompson, K. (2008) The Shot: Cinematography. In *Film Art: An Introduction* (8th ed.). New York: McGraw-Hill.

Deleuze, G. (1986) *Cinema 1: The Movement-Image*. Minneapolis, MN: University of Minnesota Press.

Deleuze, G. and Guattari, F. (1994) *What Is Philosophy?* New York: Columbia University Press.

Ettinger, B. L. (2005) Copoiesis. *Ephemera*, 5(X), 703–713.

Ettinger, B. L. (2006) *The Matrixial Borderspace*. Minneapolis, MN: University of Minnesota Press.

Freud, S. (1919/1955) The Uncanny. In J. Strachey (ed.) *The Standard Edition of the Complete Psychological Works of Sigmund Freud*, Vol. XVII. London: Hogarth Press.

Freud, S. (1997) *Writings on Art and Literature*. Stanford, CA: Stanford University Press.

Guattari, F. (1995) On the Production of Subjectivity. In *Chaosmosis: An Ethico-Aesthetic Paradigm*. Sydney: Power Publications.

Guattari, F. (2011) Signifying Faciality, Diagrammatic Faciality. In *The Machinic Unconscious: Essays in Schizoanalysis*. Los Angeles, CA: Semiotext(e).

Lacan, J. (2014) *Anxiety: The Seminar of Jacques Lacan, Book X*. Oxford: Polity Press.

Marks, L.U. (1998) Video Haptics and Erotics. *Screen*, 39(4), 331–347.

Miller, J.-A. (2008) *L'érotique du temps (Ha'Erotika Shel Ha'Zman)*. Tel Aviv: Resling.

Mulvey, L. (1999) Visual Pleasure and Narrative Cinema. In L. Braudy and M. Cohen (eds.) *Film Theory and Criticism: Introductory Readings*. Oxford: Oxford University Press.

Nancy, J. L. (2005) The Image – The Distinct. In *The Ground of the Image*. New York: Fordham University Press.

Rodowick, D. N. (2007) An Elegy for Theory. *October*, 122(1), 91–109.

Tarkovsky, A. (2016) *Meeting Andrei Tarkovsky: Cinema is a Mosaic Made of time.* [Video]. Available at: www.youtube.com/watch?v=4JRfeshEboI&t=1211s.

Verhaeghe, P. and Declercq, F. (2002) Lacan's Analytical Goal: "Le Sinthome" or the Feminine Way. In L. Thurston (ed.) *Essays on the Final Lacan: Re-Inventing the Symptom.* New York: The Other Press.

Filmography

Casablanca (1942) Directed by Michael Curtiz. Los Angeles, CA: Warner Bros.

Solaris (1972) Directed by Andrei Tarkovsky. New York: The Criterion Collection

The Mirror (1975) Directed by Andrei Tarkovsky. New York: Kino International

The Passion of Joan of Arc (1928) Directed by Carl Theodor Dreyer. New York: The Criterion Collection.

Three Colors: Blue (1993) Directed by Krzysztof Kieślowski. New York: The Criterion Collection.

7

RIVER'S EDGE

The ebb and flow of feminine ex-sistence

Allister Mactaggart

Psychoanalysis and detection

It is reported that before his death Sigmund Freud apparently enjoyed reading detective novels, particularly those of Agatha Christie and Dorothy Sayers, much to the confusion of his daughter, Anna, and the Welsh psychoanalyst Ernest Jones (Kristeva 2002: 239). Yet should Freud's reading matter late on in his life really appear so remarkable? Slavoj Žižek, for one, has remarked upon the close links between the figure of the detective and the psychoanalyst as the Lacanian "subject supposed to know" (1992: 57) via the concept of transference that comes into play in the analytic situation. The analyst behind the couch is conjured into the position by the analysand as this "subject supposed to know", and for whom the analysand, as the "murderer", "produces the truth for this supposed subject by virtue of their very attempts to cover it up" as Ian Parker puts it in his discussion of Žižek's formulation (Parker 2004: 71). Detectives and psychoanalysts thus both seek out and learn from the clues that lead to the "truth"; both of crimes, for the detective, and of the innermost "kernel" of the subject for the analysand. Furthermore, in analysis it is the analysand who produces that truth in the safety of the consulting room, and thus provides links between the private and the public, the I and the Other, our individual psyches and the social link that binds us together.

Femininity in/as fiction

Julia Kristeva also remarks that "the detective novel, a popular genre that keeps the possibility of questioning alive, basically tells the reader, 'You can know'" (2002: 4). What is it that the reader can know? In a new world order of globalised neoliberal power and corruption, only an intimate revolt seems possible, she argues, especially in a European culture: "a culture fashioned by doubt and critique – [which] is losing its moral and aesthetic impact" (ibid.). Kristeva notes that when people no longer read "serious" literature they may still read detective fiction, and asks whether this remains our "only remaining defense against the 'banality of evil'". (ibid.). Using Hannah Arendt's phrase to encapsulate how we are now all immiserated within the current global power structures, Kristeva considers both her books on this subject to be "a low form of revolt" (ibid.), but questions whether "higher" forms are any more effective in a new world order of diffused yet totalising technocratic power structures. While her comments relate to the novel form of detective fiction, they may well apply, I would suggest, to the detective genre as such, which is equally dominant in film and television, the latter of which forms the basis of this chapter.

The detective genre on television has, indeed, perhaps become, in recent years, the pre-eminent site for culturally investigating some of the pressing issues that demand further investigation. The epithets "Nordic Noir" or "Scandi Noir", applied fairly loosely to such programmes as *The Killing* (*Forbrydelsen*, Denmark, 2007–2014), *The Bridge* (*Bron/Broen*, Sweden/Denmark, 2011–2018), *Trapped* (*Ófærð*, Iceland, 2015–), and *Follow the Money* (*Bedrag*, Denmark, 2016–), together with other series "beyond Nordic Noir" such as *Witnesses* (*Les témoins*, France, 2014–), *Marcella* in Britain (Britain, 2016–, written by Hans Rosenfeldt, the man behind *The Bridge*) and others, have all helped to bring to the fore a widespread and creative questioning of key issues that affect us in the twenty-first century in relation to, inter alia: crime, detection, mental health, politics and corruption. In his Marxist analysis of detective fiction Ernest Mandel remarks that, "The history of the crime story is a social history, for it appears intertwined with the history of bourgeois society itself" (1984: 135). I would argue that this widespread fascination with detective fiction, in all its guises, would appear to reflect to some degree the impact of global neoliberal capitalism whereby the spectacle is a central part of the mechanism of our isolation and alienation, yet, at the same time, unceasingly speaks about what ails us and demands further investigation.

In this chapter I will seek to address what the British six-part television series *River* (2015) permits the viewer to put into question and to seek to know in respect of issues surrounding femininity, love and loss, as key aspects of contemporary life that capitalism fails to address adequately in its undelivered promises of fulfilled relationships as acts of consumption. Kristeva refers to literature as "that which testifies to experience" and, in reference to her own novels, she states that she investigates "the experience of the feminine condition that we speak so much about but hesitate to see as a ferocious detective novel" (2002: 252), and so she provides a direct link between detective fiction and femininity. As an armchair detective/analyst, I will seek to discover whether these comments can similarly be applied to the cultural experience provided by this television series. As Jacques Lacan puts it, "Culture, insofar as it is distinct from society, doesn't exist. Culture is the fact that it has a hold on us" (1999: 53–54). It is this "hold on us", and particularly on me, that I wish to reflect upon via an analysis of the specificities of this series in relation to detection and femininity.

Guy Debord, whose *Society of the Spectacle* (first published in 1967) is invoked throughout both volumes of Kristeva's analyses of revolt, clearly saw television as a major instrument in the power of the spectacle to extend its "deadly" reach into our domestic spheres and psyches. In thesis 28 Debord writes:

> The reigning economic system is founded on isolation; at the same time it is a circular process designed to produce isolation. Isolation underpins technology, and technology isolates in its turn; all *goods* proposed by the spectacular system, from cars to televisions, also serve as weapons for that system as it strives to reinforce the isolation of "the lonely crowd".
>
> *(1967/1995: 22, original emphasis)*

For Debord, the technological "revolution" of late capitalist consumerism is designed to isolate while promising a false sense of community that, paradoxically, promotes further alienation and isolation. One has only to think of the notion of Facebook "friends" and the resultant feelings of isolation for many people today to see how Debord's analysis has been confirmed and extended further into our psyches and social structures since the late 1960s.

Somewhat paradoxically, perhaps, I will be arguing in this chapter that television now offers a privileged site for a critical reflection on the role of the spectacle in our contemporary situation and the isolation of the lonely crowd, which has been exacerbated by the growth in technology since Debord first critiqued the spectacle. Kristeva argues that the problematic of revolt within our current context is situated at the conjunction of "the intimacy on which our notion of happiness depends and the social link that determines what we call politics" (2002: 3). The increasing technical and ideological separation between intimacy and the wider social sphere, and the mediation that exists between the two, is an area that I will seek to explore in this chapter in relation to the televisual medium. At a time when television technologies and consumption patterns are changing via different ways of experiencing television, it is perhaps a useful time to reflect upon the specificities of the medium and how it has been analysed previously. Raymond Williams, in his classic analysis, *Television: Technology and Cultural Form* (1974), points out that "flow" is a defining feature of the televisual medium. This insight came to Williams one night in Miami, newly arrived by boat in North America to take up a year's post at Stanford University. Watching multi-channel US television, Williams, as Roger Silverstone points out:

> found himself entirely bemused by the flow of U.S. television, a flow in which one programme blended into another, in which advertisements were seamlessly threaded through the texts of soap operas, and in which trailers for one film provided a kind of invasive sub-text for the unfolding of another.
>
> *(2003: vii)*

Williams' sense of bemusement, faced with the constant replacement of image after image, in which one flows between different programmes and genres in an indiscriminate manner, can also be linked to Debord's analysis of the spectacle as the constant production of a "*false consciousness of time*" (1967/1995: 114) with television being seen as an integral component and reinforcement of this false consciousness via the ceaseless flow of material. Yet, paradoxically, I will argue that within this constant flow of the spectacle certain images may stand out and leave a remainder that is not negated by the following image(s). Jacques Lacan also points out that, "What holds the image together is a remainder" (1999: 6), and the remainder of certain images (and sounds) may endure well beyond the ending of particular television programmes, enabling the viewer to contemplate the relationship between intimate feelings and affects experienced by a cultural product, and the social link that holds us together.

River is a six-part television (mini)series that was shown on the BBC (British Broadcasting Corporation) between 13 October and 17 November 2015, with international streaming rights acquired by Netflix, effective from 18 November 2015. Created and scripted by Abi Morgan – the screenwriter of the films *Suffragette* (2015) and *Shame* (2011) as well as other television series such as *The Hour* (2011–2012) – the series centres upon the titular character Detective Inspector John River's (Stellan Skarsgård) investigation to discover the murderer of his police colleague Detective Sergeant Jackie "Stevie" Stevenson (Nicola Walker), his disco-loving, fast-food aficionado sidekick. River's mourning for his colleague, beset by what he perceives as his failings in being unable to prevent her murder – by his "blindness" to what was going on in front of his eyes – marks, for me, a highly tender meditation on love and loss, which allows for my own reflections upon these issues, both in the series and beyond, to come to the fore.

In the opening scene of the first episode (dir. Richard Laxton) we are presented with River and Stevie in his car visiting a drive-thru fast-food restaurant. River's failed attempt to get the food order correct demonstrates that this is her terrain rather than his. "Burger virgin" is how Stevie calls River after he forgets to order her banana milkshake and he has to drive round again to collect this item. River's car is archaeologically layered with detritus from previous visits to such places, the residues of which help to provide vital clues as the series unfolds.

In the following sequence we see River and Stevie driving through nocturnal east London, and then River notices and follows a suspect's car, which we later find out is the car that was used on the night Stevie was killed. Following the driver on foot into a supermarket and giving chase, Stevie is shown to the viewer calling in back-up support. After the suspect jumps to his death to evade capture, River's boss, Chrissie Read (Lesley Manville), comes to the scene and angrily asks him what he is doing as he is off the case, before telling him that "You can't bring Stevie back", and instructing him to see "Psychs", the police psychiatrist in the morning. Walking away from the scene Stevie says to River, "What does she know?" to which he laughingly replies "Exactly. Exactly . . . What do any of them know?" The camera then takes up a position behind River and Stevie and we are shown the large and gruesome exit wound in the back of Stevie's head caused by a fatal gunshot, coupled with differing camera shots, starting with a close-up of the back of Stevie's head, to long shots showing River seemingly alone and talking to himself on the walkway. The latter shots also inform the viewer that she's been dead all along, and a figment of his imagination, and thus the viewer is caught up in crucial questions about the connection between River and his colleague's murder, which becomes the central quilting point of the series as it weaves its narrative path. At the outset we are led to believe that Stevie is alive and we initially follow the action from that point of view, thereby being immediately sutured into River's viewpoint. On one level, therefore, the shock of Stevie's death is presented in a visually arresting and intriguing manner, to hook the audience into the complexities and specificities of the series' narrative. At the same time, however, it raises fascinating questions about feminine representation in the series, and beyond. Depicting Stevie's facial features as unblemished throughout is perhaps a necessary aspect of the narrative intrigue that the opening sequence provides us. But, I suggest, this method of representation "says" more than this. It simultaneously reveals and conceals much of what it is at stake in River's investigation into Stevie's murder, and more particularly, his relationship to her, centred on his mournful investigation into her death and the conjoined riddle of her femininity for him.

River is forced to attend sessions with the police psychiatrist, Rosa Fallows (Georgina Rich), but he tries to avoid and evade her questions and is initially very uncooperative. In the second meeting, however, after confirming that he had witnessed the trauma of Stevie's death less than three weeks' previously, he also confesses to seeing hallucinations of dead people, or "manifests" as he calls them, which he later admits to having seen since he was a young boy. Questioned about his relationship with Stevie, he says that "she was just a colleague" to which Rosa responds stating that "even if she was just a colleague . . . there was love, perhaps" in their relationship. River then somewhat angrily declares that, "There should be more than one word for love. What will we do for love? Die for it, even". River then abruptly leaves the session as the realisation of what he's just uttered provides him with a vital clue for another case he is dealing with (but that later on also helps to provide a key clue in coming to a realisation about Stevie's murder). River's love for Stevie, and the reasons behind his inability to have stated his love openly to her during her life, is a central enigma of the series. Indeed, River's troubled relationship with all of the women in his life permeates the episodes, and there is no mention of a father figure. We are informed that River was born in Sweden and subsequently abandoned by his mother who left him to live with his grandmother. However, following his grandmother's death he was forced to move to London at the age of 14 to live with his drug-addicted mother.

Love, conjoined with a detective investigation into his unspoken love object's murder, and issues of mental ill health, thus form central components of the series, and open up avenues for thinking through psychoanalytic approaches to these topics. In addition to translating Lacan's seminar *Book VIII: Transference*, a work all about love, into English, Bruce Fink has also provided a detailed commentary upon the seminar, in which he points out that there is no singular theory of love in either Freud's or Lacan's work but that, "there are multiple attempts to grapple with it at different points in their theoretical development" (Fink 2016: xi). Lacan's close reading of Plato's *Symposium* in *Transference*, starting with "Greek love" as a simplified model, provides an opportunity to reflect upon the different approaches to love presented by each of the speakers in the *Symposium*. In addition, in a reference to Plato's *Republic*, Lacan states that:

> What is expressed in his [Plato's] myth of the cave is illustrated every day for us by the dancing beams that shine on the screen, showing all our feelings in a shadowy state. In contemporary art, the defense and illustration of love most clearly belongs to this dimension.
>
> *(2015: 33)*

Although Lacan's reference here is to film, it can, I would suggest, be similarly applied to the technologies of representation provided by television. The "shadowy state" of our feelings is brought very much to the fore in this series in the way River's confusion about questions of love and loss in relation to the riddle of femininity, and what they mean for him, and by extension, what they might mean for the viewer, are echoed in the visual representations of Stevie and other manifests.

In addition to the content of *River*, with the seemingly odd displacement of a Swedish detective in London, the style also helps to heighten a dream-like quality to the overall series, which is eminently suitable for its subject matter. Several reviews of the series referred to its artistic film-like qualities. A review in the far-left *Socialist Worker* makes the comment that: "It's visually stunning, as the camera swirls around east London streets where rich and poor live back to back. The city is portrayed as dark, alienating and beautiful", and furthermore, "River sometimes looks and feels more an art movie than a TV drama and it's all the better for that" (Orr 2015: 13). The *mise-en-scène* and *mise-en-shot* of the series help to maintain this shadowy, aesthetic connection between River's reality in which his manifests appear to him and viewers diegetically, alongside an appropriately dream-like vision of contemporary London. For instance, there are several long shots used when River is in his sessions with the police psychiatrist, when he looks down on the city below with a railway bridge across the River Thames and a pedestrian bridge beneath with people shown walking to and from work. The poetics of these images correspond, I suggest, to T. S. Eliot's comments in *The Waste Land* in which, remarking on a crowd flowing over London Bridge in this "Unreal City", Eliot states, "I had not thought death had undone so many" (1972: 25). The loneliness, isolation and alienation of life in the capital city is thus depicted in melancholic, blue-toned shots of contemporary life. At other times there are also shots when River looks across to people on running machines in an office block opposite, which also highlight the alienation of contemporary life in the capital, as emanations of the "lonely crowd" to which Debord refers, and to which he is both separated from via his mental ill health, but that appears to be ubiquitous for all in the contemporary situation. Throughout the series, River is portrayed as a lonely figure whose only "real" contact is with his manifests rather than actual human interactions, but the series demonstrates the pervasiveness of loneliness and alienation in contemporary life across the social spectrum. In the archaeological mapping of the city shown in the series via these shots of high-rise office buildings and differing forms of transport, the River Thames provides a sense of continuous fluidity, and reflects a sense of "natural" time as opposed to the "false consciousness" of time to which Debord refers in relation to the impact of technology and the damaging effects of the spectacle.

This other worldly feel of the series is most clearly made plain in River's interactions with his "manifests", who are visible to him alone, within the diegesis, but fully visible also for viewers who are thus able to experience and appreciate his psychosis. One major manifest is Dr Thomas Cream (Eddie Marsan), based on the real-life nineteenth-century so-called "Lambeth poisoner" (1850–1892), whose biography River is seen reading during the series. In episode 4 (dir. Tim Fywell), Cream, the manifest, tells River that he is the darkest part of him and he consistently questions River's motivation and reasons for not being able to have saved Stevie from being murdered. But it is really Stevie's death and River's inability to have expressed his love for her, the trauma of her murder and his grief that is the darkest part of him and drives the series. On the night she was murdered they had been to a Chinese restaurant for dinner after work, following which she was shot in the street outside the restaurant. River constantly watches the CCTV video of the incident, seeking to piece together what happened, constantly replaying the grainy footage that depicts him helplessly at her side after the shooting.

As well as hunting down Stevie's killer, River simultaneously seeks to uncover the riddle of her femininity. The two are inextricably interlinked via his profound sense of loss. The lipstick trace on her fast-food drink cup left in his car is a key signifier that attracts River's attention, as is the lipstick found in her possessions in the police compound. He keeps the discarded drink container as a potential clue that he pins to the evidence board he sets up on a wall in his flat, replacing his previously obsessive record vinyl collection. These foolish things, to borrow the title from the popular song, do not so much remind River of Stevie, as to put into question why and for whom she was wearing lipstick that fateful night, thus confronting his preconceptions or misconceptions about her femininity and sexuality, and his role therein. He failed to notice that detail as they ate their meal together. His inability to have picked up on this telling detail haunts River and exacerbates his feelings of inadequacy in not having noticed her use of make-up. In *River* Stevie's femininity is signified in a low-key manner, it is certainly not the feminine masquerade of classical Hollywood.

Joan Riviere in her classic psychoanalytic essay "Womanliness as a Masquerade" (1929) makes the point that there is no difference between "womanliness" and the masquerade, that they are the same thing. Examining a case of "a particular type of intellectual woman" (Riviere 1929/1986: 36), she notes that the masquerade acts as a defence against masculine rebukes for assuming a "masculine" position. Yet in *River* Stevie's masquerade acts more as a sign that River fails to read: a pressing detail that encapsulates, in retrospect, River's blindness. In responses to Riviere's essay in relation to film theory in the 1980s, Stephen Heath (1986) and Mary Ann Doane (1987) analysed the masquerade in relation to classical Hollywood representations of femininity. But unlike the key Hollywood signifiers, in *River* we have a more downcast, downbeat, domesticated sight of femininity. Stevie is generally seen without much make-up on in her role as a hard-working police officer; she is confident in her role and does not need to defend herself against masculine rebukes. Indeed, we find out that she was running her own private investigation from which she purposefully kept River at bay, to protect him from the abusive secrets that haunted her life. Yet, upon uncovering CCTV footage of Stevie being embraced by a man who River comes to find out is called Haider Jamal Abdi (Peter Bankole), River's face cannot hide his seeming jealousy; it is at this point that his desire is "spoken" through his intense reaction to the third person he had not previously thought was there (but who is a structural necessity for his masculine desire to come to the fore), although he tells "Psychs" that it is curiosity rather than jealousy that drives him. From a Lacanian perspective we can perhaps be alerted to the truth behind River's self-deception here. Geneviève Morel suggests that, "the eternal elsewhere, or Other, nature of woman is the source of jealousy in the man who loves her" (2000: 158). "She" is always beyond him, elsewhere, as Lacan shows in *Seminar XX*, so that the masculine position, apart from the mythical primal father, is to have a relationship not with a woman per se, but with the object *a* as fantasy (Fink 1995: 111).

In telling remarks about the series, Stellan Skarsgård, who plays the character of River, comments that Abi Morgan's writing provided him with a unique opportunity as an actor to express a form of enjoyment that he suggests is generally not available in male acting roles (see Skarsgård 2015). Equating this to what he perceives to be a form of feminine jouissance, able to "show everything" as he puts it, via psychotic hallucinations, raises some very complex issues around sexuation, knowledge and jouissance, based around the Phallus and castration. His comments suggest a distinct binary division between the representations of male and female characters in film and television.

Judith Butler in her critique of Lacan, Riviere and the masquerade, remarks that:

> By claiming that the Other that lacks the Phallus is the one who *is* the Phallus, Lacan clearly suggests that power is wielded by this feminine position of non-having, that the masculine subject who "has" the Phallus requires this Other to confirm and, hence, be the Phallus in its "extended" sense.
>
> *(1990: 44)*

While Butler ultimately reads Lacanian theory in this regard "as a kind of 'slave morality'" (ibid.: 57), we can, perhaps, read *River* differently, as depicting an Other form of jouissance in mainstream television where Skarsgård's telling remarks open up discussions about (heterosexual) love from an-Other place.

In his research into Stevie's private investigation and following Haider's murder, River finds a letter Haider had written to his wife in Somalia, which includes

Orson Welles' well-known observation that, while we are born, live and die alone, it is only love and friendship that give us the momentary illusion that this is not so. Depicted as one of River's manifests, Haider is shown reading the letter to his wife and asks, "How can a man, a man like myself, how can he spill his heart into his mouth?" This question, which Haider is able to pose lucidly in his letter, is the question that River was unable to ask Stevie prior to her murder; he cannot spill his heart into his mouth, and is shackled by his inability to do so.

The deadly gaze

Yet, after solving Stevie's murder, River returns to the Chinese restaurant where he'd been with her on that fateful night. Carrying flowers with him he is taken to a table for two, opposite the already seated manifestation of Stevie, as we initially see the scene through the lens of his fantasy or hallucination (as indeed we saw the opening sequence of episode 1). He recounts to Stevie that he took his mother out for dinner with his first pay cheque but that she was unable to eat. Stevie then says the words his mother should have told him, about her being so proud of him, echoing both his mother's and his inability to speak about matters of the heart. Seeking but failing to make good his past mistakes, River is still unable to tell Stevie that he loves her. We then see him seated alone, opposite an empty chair. Suddenly leaping up, he rushes outside to Stevie on the kerbside, in a restaging of the events on the night of her murder. Yet, he is still unable to tell her that he loves her and so events recur as they did previously, even though now he can piece together more of what the clues meant. When Stevie walks into the middle of the road and calls back to him "screw you, Mr Magoo", a white van blocks River's view as she is shot by the driver of an oncoming car. Throughout the series River has obsessively studied CCTV footage of the murder. The camera, placed on high and at 90 degrees from River's actual location at the time of the shooting, provides grainy, black-and-white footage showing Stevie's look of recognition as the car approaches her, prior to being shot. In order to discover who the murderer is River has to rely on detection and his desire to know, not on vision, as the scene does not reveal the driver of the car. The CCTV fails to provide the panoptic gaze with the evidence required to identify the murderer. Yet the field of vision is itself beset by obstacles that theorists have grappled with over some time. For instance, Joan Copjec's argument against film theory's misappropriation of Lacan, in which the mirror-stage theory is prioritised over Lacan's later work on the gaze, points out that "the field of vision is neither clear nor easily traversable. It is instead ambiguous and treacherous, full of traps" (1994: 34). From a historicist position Michel Foucault saw scopic regimes as containing "malevolence" (2008: 14) everywhere in his analysis of the panopticon gaze in contemporary society, and, similarly, for Debord the whole of society had been turned into a gigantic spectacle where the "visible form of the commodity totally occupied everyday life, uniting production and consumption in one monstrous system" as Martin Jay also explains it (1994: 429). Yet, *River* appears to demonstrate the impasse between the panopticon's inability to capture everything – the CCTV camera outside the restaurant fails to record the driver of the car that kills Stevie – and River's inability to "see" who murdered Stevie. (However, the panopticon can be argued to win out again as he is later given a disc of another CCTV camera from another location that identifies the driver of the car on that fateful night.) Furthermore, in a similar manner to how River's curiosity or jealousy affected his investigation of Haider, he remains unable to spill his heart into his mouth. In *The Four Fundamental Concepts of Psychoanalysis* Lacan states that "The gaze in itself not only terminates the movement, it freezes it" (1979: 117). This moment, forever captured on CCTV, and outside of River's vision, fails to coalesce into a clear view; something is withheld from River's sight, perhaps his desire is caught precisely in his inability or unwillingness to express his love for Stevie? Or rather that it is his jealousy that "blocks" his desire, which is provoked by the blot in his field of vision at the time of Stevie's murder. Colette Soler remarks that: "Between man and woman, there is the wall, the wall of language, as Lacan said, which has forged its '*amur*' in order to mark out the impasse where woman manifests itself" (2006: 208). As the translator's footnote explains: "'*Amur*' is a pun that condenses *amour*, love, and *mur*, wall" (ibid.). The wall of language, metaphorically represented visually by the side of the white van as it obscures River's view of the murderous act of Stevie, highlights the gap between them due to River's inability to speak of love, and thus to halt Stevie's walk of death. River's inability to speak of love highlights much of what blocks his relations with Stevie at this point.

Love in the time of death

Yet, this time, running to her side after the shooting, in this remembering, repeating and working through the traumatic moment, River is finally able to say "I love you. I love you more than life, more than life". It is at the moment of this reactivation of her death, now knowing who killed her that his love can flow from his heart into his mouth. Prior to this, his jealousy (or curiosity), wrong as it turns out, that Haider was in a sexual relationship with Stevie, and his inability to "see" who was driving the vehicle, someone clearly emotionally close to Stevie as her smile testified, prohibited him from truly seeing what was in front of his eyes all along. In episode 3 Stevie's estranged brother, Jimmy (Steve Nicolson), accuses River of missing evidence because he doesn't see the world straight, something that River responds to as an overrated virtue. Similarly, in episode 5 (dir. Jessica Hobbs), Stevie appears to River and points out to him that the closer he gets to the truth, the further away he will be from who she really was.

"Screw you, Mr Magoo" were the final words Stevie said to River as she called back to him from the road prior to being shot. His sidekick, Detective Sergeant Ira King (Adeel Akhtar), who took Stevie's place after her murder, explains to River in the first episode that Mr Magoo was a cartoon character who wasn't stupid as he appeared at first sight to be: he just needed glasses. This intertextual reference is used as a correspondence throughout the series to reference the idiosyncrasies of

River's methods of detection based on his interactions with his manifests. At the end of the final episode, River does see clearly; he has been able to focus upon the crime but at the ultimate cost of losing Stevie, as his manifests only stay with him until they are no longer needed. Once the case is closed, Stevie can go. Hence the paradox for River: solving the case will curtail his fantasy or delusion as she will no longer need to be there.

However, now knowing who killed Stevie, he is able to act, his blockage has been removed. As such, he thus unburdens himself of his inability to articulate the words he'd not been able to say before, leading into a fantasy of unshackling himself from his fatal (male) inhibitions as then he sings and dances with Stevie, in the middle of the road with glowing bright disco lights behind them, to Tina Charles' 1976 disco hit "I love to love". This is the same song that's played at the start of episode 1 to which Stevie sings along joyously in the car and to which River sings alone, melancholically, in a karaoke bar at the end of that episode. Yet, prior to this, Stevie's face as it changes from seemingly inanimate death to life to say, "Sing, you nutter", marks a highly uncanny moment. The close-up on Stevie's face appears to mark the resolution of River's search for the truth and to finally articulate words of love. The shot stays on her face for some time as if marking this moment. However, just when it might be felt that a final resolution is at hand, Stevie opens her eyes, smiles and speaks. As Freud points out about the return of the dead in "The 'Uncanny'", we may have "*surmounted* these modes of thought; but we do not feel quite sure of our new beliefs" (1990: 371), which is borne out for me in this scene. However, this brief disturbance is soon replaced by the more uplifting fantasy of River and Stevie dancing together (but perhaps this is another remainder that may stay with the viewer, as it did me, beyond the series). Detective programmes can thus offer a fantasy solution to our usual unwillingness to acknowledge openly our own mortality, via examining a fictional one where our death, and the deaths of those we love, is kept at bay. The television theorist Milly Buonanno makes the point that fictional television narratives offer a "Flight from death, survival, aliveness (. . .) [and that] 'liveness' confirms the unique and precious prerogative of the television experience" (2008: 132). This acknowledgement of death in the usual narrative of a detective programme where the detective solves the murder, is also, simultaneously, an ambivalent means of keeping such knowledge at bay by resolving the crime and restoring order in the land of the living.

In his reading of Lacan's *Seminar VIII*, Fink points out that: "To love someone else is to convey in words to that person that we lack – preferably big time – and that he or she is intimately related to that lack" (2016: 36). Fink then goes on to quote Lacan from *Écrits* where the latter states, "to love is to want to be loved" (Lacan 2006: 853; quoted in Fink 2016: 37). Up to this point in the television series, however much Stevie might have desired that River would say these words, he could not. "There should be more than one word for love" he told the police psychiatrist in their second meeting; yet until this point he was unable to articulate any word resembling love, and thus feels culpable in her murder as he failed to realise his feelings towards Stevie and hers towards him, thus missing clues that might have helped him understand the dangerous predicament she was in. Cream, as a manifestation of his superego, continually reinforces these guilty thoughts in his appearances to River, articulating and questioning River's real motivation behind his actions or lack thereof. Yet, once River is able to speak of love, such recriminations leave him. However fantastical the scene of River dancing joyously with Stevie might appear, we should, as Žižek (2000) has argued in respect of similar scenes in the films of David Lynch, read such scenes seriously, as "unbearably naïve: and yet to be taken 'seriously'" (ibid.: 3). In *River* restitution is provided at this point, both for the character River and the viewer, in the sublimely ridiculous yet tearfully uplifting vision of River and Stevie dancing together in the road at the dénouement of the final episode: as an example of "a crazy assertion of the redemptive value of naïve clichés as such" (ibid.). Yet, this vision also falls apart as we are then shown a shot from inside a passing bus of River dancing alone in the road. As River's fantasy fades from view, Ira King comes upon him kneeling in the middle of the road, holding nothing. Stevie has yet again slipped out of River's grasp and sight; she is not there, not-all there; she no longer exists, but perhaps this posits the possibility of another ex-sistence from outside/beyond the phallic register. The Lacanian neologism ex-sistence, as Dylan Evans explains, was coined "to express the idea that the heart of our being (*Kern unseres Wesen*) is also radically Other, strange, outside" (1996: 58). Fink explains ex-sistence as "The Other jouissance [which] is fundamentally incommensurate, unquantifiable, disproportionate, and indecent to 'polite society'" (1995: 122). Stevie clearly ex-sists for River, her first death does not diminish her "hold" over River; indeed, it can be seen to intensify it. As Evans also explains, "the symbolic order contains no signifier for femininity, and hence the feminine position cannot be fully symbolised" (1996: 58).

Having slowly grown accustomed to River's ways, Ira is not perturbed by the sight of the latter kneeling alone in the road; he does not question it, instead he gently asks him whether he's eaten and goes into the restaurant to buy a takeaway for both of them. As River waits in his car for Ira to return, we see the last vision of Stevie through the car's rear-view mirror. Her final words to River are, "and I say, I love you too", thereby responding to River's previous declaration of love, and then she slowly disappears from view. In his meeting with the police psychiatrist in episode 3, River told her that the manifests "stay as long as they need to stay and then they go away". Her affirmation of their love is hereby given as a guarantee of that reciprocation, and hence she can now fade away. Previously, straight and jump cuts had been used to differentiate between River's hallucinations of Stevie and her absence for other characters. She has either been there or not-there, in a binary division between the two. Yet here, for our final vision of her, a dissolve is used as a transition from her being visible to being finally fully absent, which may signify River's acceptance of her death now that he has been able to fantasise a happier resolution for himself, and "she" has responded to that fantasy.

These declarations of love at the dénouement of the series provide, for me, a sense of satisfying resolution to the loss suffered by River and experienced jointly with him by the viewer. In one sense they bring these issues towards an ending, whereby the flow of television can then continue to plough its usual furrow. However, I suggest that a series such as *River* can leave a strong imprint in the viewer's mind whereby it is not solely negated by another programme or image to replace the one that went before in a seamless integration of imagery. As previously mentioned at the start of this investigation, Lacan also points out that:

> What holds the image together is a remainder. Analysis demonstrates that love, in its essence, is narcissistic, and reveals that the substance of what is supposedly object-like – what a bunch of bull – is in fact that which constitutes a remainder in desire, namely, its cause, and sustains desire through its lack of satisfaction, and even its impossibility.
>
> *(1999: 6)*

However, while this scene was so moving for me from my (masculine) position, Frances Taylor (2015) argues in a review of the series that this ending felt unsatisfactory for her because it did not focus upon justice for Stevie, but rather resolution for River. These observations highlight differing positions presented in *River* in relation to femininity and love. River's resolution is "undoubtedly touching", as this and other reviewers have noted, but it did not simplify the complex issues raised by the series about love's difficulties and issues of the heart. Instead it left them in abeyance for the viewer to contemplate beyond the ending of the series, as a remainder that refused closure in any straightforward sense; and this is part of its strength as a television series. Stephen Grosz, in a personal recollection from his selection of stories derived from his many years of working as a psychoanalyst, recounts in "On Closure" how his sister told him that she had been to visit a clairvoyant following the death of their father. Surprised by his own, tearful response to this news, Grosz writes:

> After we had finished our phone call I had the thought that we turn to clairvoyance when we need our dead and can't accept death's finality. We want to believe that the clairvoyant can bring our dead back into the world of the living. Closure is just as delusive – it is the false hope that we can deaden our living grief.
>
> *(2013: 210)*

In a similar manner, *River*'s dénouement denies any easy, delusive, false hope about death's finality by refusing to resolve the issues brought up by the series in a simple, generic manner. River's "upbeat" response in his fantastical dancing scene as a form of resolution provides a degree of fulfilment for the viewer but it also, for some such as Frances Taylor, "fails" as a "payoff", thereby representing an unsatisfied remainder for Taylor, but a completed one for me. As such, it is perhaps not surprising that the series cannot end at this point.

The look of love revisited/repaired

Therefore, following Stevie's disappearance, we are shown River on another day, back in his office, starting with a point of view shot of him looking down on to the city below, with the River Thames flowing unceasingly as it does, irrespective of human troubles on land, as had been shown on various occasions during the series. River is then handed Ira and Marianne (Lydia Leonard) King's baby, Hank, to hold as Marianne delivers lunch for Ira with enough to allow River to share it. As River cradles the child gently in his arms he is seen separately by the police psychiatrist, Rosa Fallows, and then his boss, Chrissie Read, who both smile at this view of River the caregiver. The look of love that River had vainly sought from his mother and grandmother is here given by him and returned by the infant child. Having been able to declare his love for Stevie, even if only in fantasy, River can show his love to others, and receive it back in return: he can live again, now that the impasse of his impossible love for Stevie has been resolved as much as it can be within the confines of "normal" grief, and his solving of the case. In episode 3 River asks Rosa why he should trust her when he can no longer trust Stevie as she withheld information from him. Rosa replies, "because I'm alive and she's dead". *River* presents love from the seemingly masculine perspective of the titular character who struggles to spill his heart into his mouth. However, Colette Soler argues, taking Lacan's statements to their logical conclusion, that "when a man loves – which happens of course – it is as a woman" (2006: 101) in as much as he himself is subject to lack thereby perhaps echoing Stellan Skarsgård's comments on Abi Morgan's writing, mentioned earlier, that this role gave him an unrivalled opportunity to express his character in a manner that is not usually available for male actors. As Soler goes on to say, "for love is addressed to saying (*dire*), thus bringing about the enigmatic recognitions of two unconsciousnesses" (ibid.: 101–102) and, furthermore, "Love, unfortunately, is risky and ephemeral, as we have always known. This is why it aspires not to cease being written" (ibid.: 102). The trauma of Stevie's murder and River's fatal inability to have spoken about love thereby becomes the quilting point where the various threads of this riddle of femininity are presented and worked through in this series, but never closed off in a generic manner, thus leaving a remainder for the viewer to contemplate beyond its ending.

River presents important and complex issues about love, loss and femininity in the guise of a generic police procedural. Lacan tells us that the only truth in psychoanalysis is that there is no sexual relationship. *River*, I suggest, may provide us with an important example of a suitable, cultural palliative for us to be able, albeit temporarily, to recognise and live with that truth. Lacan also tells us that, "What makes up for the sexual relationship is, quite precisely, love" (1999 45). As such, holding on to what we love may prove to be one way of resisting neoliberal capitalism's insistent pressures upon us to conform to its restricted and incessant acts of consumption. The crime story, which is inextricably intertwined with the history of bourgeois society, as Mandel pointed out, may also prove another truth:

that bourgeois society is itself a criminal society (1984: 135) where it is perhaps no surprise that its "crimes" are played out in aesthetic form in the many detective programmes presented to us. In such a society, holding on to what we love – even if it is "only" key moments in television programmes that leave us with "remainders" beyond the ending of the programmes/series – may be a productive means of uniting our most intimate feelings with the wider social sphere. In his *Comments on the Society of the Spectacle*, written 20 years after his initial critique of the spectacle, Debord remarks that: "The flow of images carries everything before it, and it is similarly someone else who (. . .) decides where this flow will lead as well as the rhythm of what should be shown" (1988/1998: 27–28). Yet the flow and rhythm can, I would argue, be arrested by the meaningful intervention of key shots/scenes/sequences from programmes such as *River*, which may affect our subjectivity, and make us reflect upon ourselves in the contemporary situation in which we find ourselves, uniting "the intimacy on which our notion of happiness depends and the social link that determines what we call politics" (Kristeva 2002: 3).

References

Buonanno, M. (2008) *The Age of Television: Experiences and Theories*. Bristol: Intellect.

Butler, J. (1990) *Gender Trouble: Feminism and the Subversion of Identity*. London: Routledge.

Copjec, J. (1994) *Read My Desire: Lacan Against the Historicists*. Cambridge, MA: MIT Press.

Doane, M., A. (1987) *The Desire to Desire: The Woman's Film of the 1940s*. Bloomington: Indiana University Press.

Debord, G. [1967] (1995) *The Society of the Spectacle*. Trans. Donald Nicholson-Smith. New York: Zone.

Debord, G. [1988] (1998) *Comments on the Society of the Spectacle*. Trans. Malcolm Imrie. London: Verso.

Eliot, T. S. (1972) *The Waste Land and Other Poems*. London: Faber & Faber.

Evans, D. (1996) *An Introductory Dictionary of Lacanian Psychoanalysis*. London: Routledge.

Fink, B. (1995) *The Lacanian Subject: Between Language and Jouissance*. Princeton, NJ: Princeton University Press.

Fink, B. (2016) *Lacan on Love: An Exploration of Lacan's Seminar VIII, Transference*. Cambridge: Polity.

Foucault, M., with Jean-Pierre Barou and Michelle Perrot (2008) *The Eye of Power* (extract). Nottingham: Nottingham Contemporary: 8–16.

Freud, S. [1919] (1990) The "Uncanny". In *Art and Literature*, Vol. 14. London: Penguin: 335–376.

Grosz, S. (2013) *The Examined Life: How We Lose and Find Ourselves*. London: Chatto & Windus.

Heath, S. (1986) Joan Riviere and the Masquerade. In Victor Burgin, James Donald and Cora Kaplan (eds.) *Formations of Fantasy*. London and New York: Methuen: 45–61.

Jay, M. (1994) *Downcast Eyes: The Denigration of Vision in Twentieth-Century French Thought*. Berkeley, CA: University of California Press.

Kristeva, J. (2002) *Intimate Revolt: The Powers and Limits of Psychoanalysis*, Vol. 2. Trans. Jeanine Herman. New York: Columbia University Press.

Lacan, J. (1979) *The Four Fundamental Concepts of Psycho-Analysis*. Ed. Jacques-Alain Miller. Trans. Alan Sheridan. London: Penguin Books.

Lacan, J. (1999) *The Seminar of Jacques Lacan: On Feminine Sexuality: The Limits of Love and Knowledge, Book XX, Encore 1972–1973*. Ed. Jacques-Alain Miller. Trans. Bruce Fink. New York: W. W. Norton & Company.

Lacan, J. (2006) *Écrits: The First Complete Edition in English*. Trans. Bruce Fink. New York: Norton.

Lacan, J. (2015) *The Seminar of Jacques Lacan, Book VIII: Transference (1960–1961)*. Ed. Jacques-Alain Miller. Trans. Bruce Fink. Cambridge, UK: Polity.

Mandel, E. (1984) *Delightful Murder: A Social History of the Crime Story*. London: Pluto Press.

Morel, G. (2000) Feminine Jealousies. In Renata Salecl (ed.) *Sexuation*. Durham, NC and London: Duke University Press: 157–169.

Orr, J. (2015) Crime Drama River Flows in Some Unexpected Directions. *Socialist Worker*. Available from: https://socialistworker.co.uk/art/41416/BBC+crime+drama+River+flows+in+some+unexpected+directions (Accessed 1 June 2017).

Parker, I. (2004) *Slavoj Žižek: A Critical Introduction*. London: Pluto Press.

River (2015) Arrow Films [video: DVD].

Riviere, J. [1929] (1986) Womanliness as a Masquerade. In Victor Burgin, James Donald and Cora Kaplan (eds.) *Formations of Fantasy*. London and New York: Methuen: 35–61.

Salecl, R. (ed.) (2000) *Sexuation*. Durham, NC and London: Duke University Press.

Silverstone, R. (2003) Preface to the Routledge Classics Edition. In R. Williams, *Television: Technology and Cultural Form*. London: Routledge: vii–xiii.

Skarsgård, S. (2015) Stellan Skarsgård on River, Love and His Hatred of Karaoke. Available from: www.bbc.co.uk/blogs/tv/entries/c4969148-9eec-49c1-bac6-1e7ebc60214b (Accessed 14 May 2017).

Soler, C. (2006) *What Lacan Said About Women: A Psychoanalytic Study*. Trans. John Holland. New York: Other Press.

Taylor, F. (2015) River: Why the Final Episode of This Brilliant BBC One Drama Simply Didn't Deliver. Available from: http://tv.bt.com/tv/tv-news/river-why-the-final-episode-of-the-bbc-one-drama-didnt-deliver-11364017050835 (Accessed 1 June 2017).

Williams, R. (1974) *Television: Technology and Cultural Form*. London: Routledge.

Žižek, S. (1992) *Looking Awry: An Introduction to Jacques Lacan Through Popular Culture*. London: MIT Press.

Žižek, S. (2000) *The Art of the Ridiculous Sublime: On David Lynch's "Lost Highway"*. Seattle, WA: Walter Chapin Simpson Center for the Humanities.

8

UNDER HER SKIN

On Woman without body and body without Woman

Ben Tyrer

With films such as *Lucy* (Besson, 2014), *Ghost in the Shell* (Sanders, 2017) and her recurring role as Marvel's Black Widow, Scarlett Johansson has selected a number of science fiction or science fiction-related projects that seem to put the category of the "human" into question: from drug-mule-become-transhuman-demigod, to counter-terrorist cyborg and superhuman assassin. However, the constant throughout these different roles – and, indeed, a crucial aspect of Johansson's star image in general – is the dimension of *femininity*: Lucy is named after "the first woman", and the drug she ingests is synthesised in the bodies of pregnant women; the Major sports a skin-suit that emphasises the contours of her body; Black Widow relies on the traditionally "feminine wiles" of seduction and deception; and Johansson herself has been voted "sexiest woman alive" on multiple occasions.[1] In this context, I will examine two of Johansson's most striking recent roles – as sentient Operating System (OS), Samantha, in *Her* (Jonze, 2013) and extra-terrestrial hunter, "Laura", in *Under the Skin* (Glazer, 2013) – for the particularly fertile grounds that they provide for interrogating notions of the feminine.[2]

In *Incontinence of the Void*, Slavoj Žižek claims that the posthuman entails

> the overcoming (leaving behind) of the sexual in its most radical ontological dimension – not just "sexuality" as a specific sphere of human existence but the Sexual as an antagonism, the bar of an impossibility, constitutive of being human in its finitude.
>
> *(2017: 134)*

However, even a cursory glance at Johansson's recent films would insist that this "move beyond the human" in a variety of directions effectively serves to throw "the sexual" (and *femininity* specifically) into starker relief. Moreover, as Juliet Mitchell reminds us, Lacan's theory of sexual difference is one "whose implications are and must be, anti-humanist" because they relate to the ways in which the human subject is constituted, not as a pre-given individual but at the intersection of various agencies, drives and structures that psychoanalysis calls by names such as "sexuality" and "the unconscious" (Mitchell and Rose 1982: 25). A thoroughgoing examination of the philosophical implications of the category of the "posthuman", particularly as they might impact on Lacanian psychoanalysis, would be beyond the scope of this chapter. In what follows, then, I will take the reflections on the feminine offered by the posthuman OS and the non-human alien as a means of focusing more insistently on sexual difference and – in particular – to examine the anti-human theories of femininity presented by Lacan.

Broadly speaking, Lacan's thinking on sexual difference undergoes profound shifts between major stages in his intellectual career, from the 1950s to the 1970s, and it will be the purpose of this chapter to explore those distinctions – which, it is my contention, constitute discrete *paradigms* of sexual difference – in order to demonstrate the radical *discontinuities* pertaining to notions of the feminine across Lacanian theory, as they are elucidated by and also help us to elucidate both Jonze's and Glazer's films. To begin, I will consider Lacan's "earlier" paradigm – associated with "The Signification of the Phallus" (2006) – which situates sexual difference and the feminine within a distinctly Oedipal framework and offers a point of contact with *Her*, before moving on to the more radical paradigm of "sexuation" that Lacan formalises in *Encore* (1998) as a means of engaging with *Under the Skin*. Accordingly, I will claim that these two films present, respectively, Woman without body and body without Woman.

Sexual difference, volume 1: the significance of the phallus

As we know, for Freud, feminine sexuality was a mystery – an unsolvable riddle, the infamous *dark continent* – because he tried to account for it in *masculine* terms: his structuring of the Oedipus and castration complexes led to dissatisfying fictions such as "penis envy", and as a function femininity itself became enigmatic in its essence. Lacan sought to reformulate Oedipus in *metaphorical* terms, and suggested that the function of "castration" was to compel the Child to abandon the desire to be the imaginary phallus (φ, or object of desire) for the Mother – of attempting to provide the answer to that unfathomable x of her desire themselves – and to take up a relation to the symbolic phallus (Φ) offered by the Father as *signifier* of the (m)Other's desire instead: entry into the Symbolic being dependent on adopting such a position (see Lacan 2006: 464–465). The regime of sexual difference put forward by Lacan here is therefore grounded in this Oedipal context and interprets the masculine and the feminine relative to the *desire of the Other*: a question of *who I am for the Other* that is articulated around the phallus as it stands for the Other's desire. Lacan states, "one can indicate the structures that govern the relations between the sexes by referring simply to the phallus' function" (ibid.: 582). Therefore "castration" – entry into the Symbolic – amounts to an attitude taken by the subject towards the phallus and for Lacan here becoming *sexed* entails a dialectic of *having* and *being* for the Other (ibid.).

In *being* the phallus – identifying with the Other's desire, becoming that which is desired by the Other – woman positions herself as *object*. It is what Lacan, after Joan Riviere, refers to as the "masquerade" that produces being for woman:

> in order to be the phallus – that is, the signifier of the Other's desire – the woman rejects an essential part of femininity, namely all its attributes, in [taking up] the masquerade. It is for what she is not that she expects to be desired as well as loved.
>
> *(Ibid.: 583)*

It is a masquerade, a pretence, because *she is not the phallus* but she *puts it on* in order to become desirable to the Other; she aligns herself with that which the Other desires in order to elicit that desire. But where Riviere claimed that woman uses masquerade as a form of self-defence ("women who wish for masculinity may put on a mask of womanliness to avert anxiety and the retribution feared from men" [1986: 35]), Lacan – I'd suggest – claims that she wears a mask in the sense that she makes herself embody the phallus *qua* the desire of the Other. They fundamentally agree, however, that femininity *is* masquerade. The Lacanian woman here is defined in that she makes herself the object of the (masculine) Other's desire.

Crucially, the masculine position is no less of a pretence, a *masc-querade*, for he cannot ever really "have" the phallus – it is nothing but a signifier – and so it is with the position of the *bearer* of the signifier that man must identify. And while, even at this stage, these sexed positions are *not* based in anatomy (i.e. presence/absence of the penis) but in *signification*, what Lacanian psychoanalysis effectively gives expression to here are the traditional "gender" roles within patriarchal society. Extrapolating slightly from Lacan's relatively brief remarks here, I'd claim that reading this formation *oedipally* suggests that to *have* the phallus is to identify with the Father and a narcissistic desire for status. Having the phallus, moreover, means becoming a *subject*; it gives access to the Symbolic through the signifier. *Being* the phallus is to become *desirable*; it is to assume a position of desiring-to-be-desired. This entails identification with the *object*, taking the place of what the Other desires. Where Lacan states that she *rejects an essential part of femininity, namely all its attributes*, I'd suggest (slightly speculatively) that this can be interpreted as woman giving up her fundamental autonomy to become *object*: the attribute she rejects is full *agency* as a subject. In socio-cultural terms, I could say that the diagnosis of this "traditional" formation entails a system of *phallic sexual difference* wherein man is defined as wanting to be *seen* as having phallic endowment (prestige), while woman is defined as wanting to be *seen* as being desirable. This "masked ball" is a true *dialectic of desire*: she desires him because he *has* the phallus, *which she is not* but hopes to become by being his object of desire; he desires her because she *is* the phallus, *which he lacks* but pretends to have, hoping to gain it by obtaining her as object.

In short, in this model, we find ourselves with a *masculine subject* and a *feminine object* – mapping on to Freud's active/passive binary – wherein the object's only agency is to position itself relative to the desire of the Other; while the subject identifies with the Other as desiring agent. I'd claim that, while Lacan arguably offers a more nuanced reading of sexual difference (vis-à-vis Oedipus) than Freud initially provided, the articulation of the question of *woman* in this paradigm remains inextricably bound to a normative, *masculine* perspective. And while the theoretical developments of the 1970s, I will argue, introduce radical *discontinuities* with this theory of the feminine, there is – equally – a degree of *continuity* between the newer paradigm and Lacan's position here in the 1950s when it comes to the question of the masculine relation to woman. I contend that the connection between "The Signification of the Phallus" and *Encore* (very schematically speaking) is seen in the persistence of the subject–object relation across the span of years, articulated in the latter by the formula Lacan presents in his "Graph of Sexuation" as (*\$* → *a*) (1998: 78).

The woman-object

The idea that we are dealing with a *feminine object* is signalled – before Jonze's film begins – by its pronominal title, *Her* (in/direct object), rather than "she" (subject). The coordinates of the film are thus determined: a perspective on the object, implying a *masculine* articulation of desire. As Lacan observes in *Encore*, this masculine subject "never deals with anything by way of a partner but object *a* inscribed on the other side of the bar" (1998: 80). His Graph shows a *vector* from *\$* on the masculine side to (*a*) on the feminine side, suggesting this as the *direction* of the subject's desire. Man's "sexual orientation" is towards (*a*); he is *a*-sexual. It is not that man "goes out looking for woman" and instead finds *objet a* in her place but – as the earlier, "phallic" paradigm suggested – that masculine structure is fundamentally *bound* to the object: "He is unable to attain his sexual partner (. . .) except inasmuch as his partner is the cause of his desire [*objet a*]" (ibid.). The partner that he finds is a *stand-in* for the object itself and he thus relates to "her" only *as* object. Indeed, Lacan's diagram suggests, with the directionality of the vector (*\$* → *a*), that man *pushes* (*a*) on to the feminine, that masculine logic imposes this position of object on to the feminine Other.

Moreover, Lacan reminds us: "In this respect, as is indicated elsewhere in my graphs by the oriented conjunction of *\$* and *a*, this is nothing other than fantasy" (ibid.). It is the "vector of fantasy" (*\$* → *a*) that characterises masculine sexuation. Indeed, Lacan concludes: "What was seen, but only regarding men, is that what they deal with is object *a*, and that the whole realization of the sexual relationship leads to fantasy" (ibid.: 86). Fantasy is where the object seems to appear to man, and so woman is implicated in masculine sexuality only insofar as she fits into his *fantasy frame*. Moreover, Lacanian psychoanalysis reminds us that this isn't just any old fantasy but the fantasy of Woman (*La femme*) "with a capital W indicating the universal" (ibid.: 72), who would guarantee the masculine position.[3] Lacan's logical formulae accompanying this vector (*\$* → *a*) suggest that masculine structure depends upon the assumption of a certain "Exception" who is not "castrated" and therefore enjoys fully: *there is one who is not subject to the phallic function* (ibid.: 78). While this figure is typically associated with Freud's mythical father of the primal horde, Žižek insightfully notes that this "masculine fantasy *par excellence*" can also be recognised in the "Woman as Exception" (1996: 155). She would be the One – the ideal Woman, perfect partner, true embodiment of the object – who could satisfy man's desire and bring him full satisfaction.

Woman without body

In this context, we can see how differing dimensions of *Her* – diegetic and extra-diegetic – intersect in the character of Samantha. On the one hand, Samantha constitutes something like the perfect "fantasy woman" for Theodore. As Steven Shaviro notes, she is "entirely compliant to his wishes and needs, and yet projects a depth in serving him that an actual human slave/partner would never be able to do". This, he asserts, is a "male fantasy", offering "the satisfaction of actually connecting, outside our own narcissism with an 'Other', without any of the discomforts that contact with any sort of otherness actually brings" (2014). Samantha is thus what Žižek calls a *decaffeinated Other*: like a product deprived of its malign quality (coffee without caffeine, cream without fat), she offers "an experience of Other deprived of its Otherness", a fundamentally *unthreatening* partner (2004). As Theodore's ex-wife, Catherine, declares upon learning about Samantha: "You wanted to have a wife without dealing with the challenges of actually dealing with anything real. I'm glad you found someone. It's perfect." Of course, as Catherine discerns, there is no "actual" connection with an "outside" because Theodore is locked within the virtual loop, the narcissistic relay, of his own desires as they are embodied in the fantasy object.

Samantha is "programmed" to respond to Theodore's every need: her software is marketed as "an intuitive entity that listens to you, understands you, and knows you". She is designed to serve him – Shaviro's reference to the "slave" resonating here – like a version of *I Dream of Jeannie* (NBC, 1965–1970) updated for the iPhone generation. *Her* thus places itself on a cultural trajectory that arcs with the masculine, *a*-sexual libidinal economy, from Pygmalion to *Ex Machina* (Garland, 2015) by way of *Weird Science* (Hughes, 1985): narratives about "ideal" women (synthetic, subservient) conjured up by men for the purposes of what Alexandre Stevens calls "the autistic side of male jouissance" (in the originary sense of *autós*), not in union with a partner but in masturbatory fusion with the object, through fantasy, "more or less imaginarised on the feminine side" (2007: 217). Theodore chooses "her" *as her* by selecting a female voice for his OS, and it is – moreover – no accident that Samantha's software is sold as "OS ONE": she is presented as *the One* who could bring Theodore full satisfaction. She is therefore *a Woman without body*: not just in the literal sense of being a disembodied female character but in the more fundamentally Lacanian sense that Samantha constitutes a free-floating fantasy of idealised femininity, carried along by the disembodied voice.

"ScarJo", La femme

On the other hand, then, we can also see how the characterisation of Samantha is haunted by the star image of her performer – Johansson, as idealised *Woman* – while also insistently leading us back to a fantasmatic vision of her body. As was well publicised, Johansson wasn't Jonze's original choice to play the intelligent OS but Samantha Morton (who lent her name to the character). Morton had recorded the entirety of her part but, in post-production, Jonze decided that he needed something rather from different from what she had provided and so recast Johansson in the role (see Jonze 2013). Morton evidently didn't perform the requisite degree of *difference* as Samantha. This is as much as Jonze was willing to venture on his last-minute change of heart, but if we compare Morton's profile with that of Johansson, then we might speculate on what *was* needed. Both Johansson and Morton made a cinematic impact in feminist character studies – Morton as the eponymous *Morvern Callar* (Ramsay, 2002) and Johansson as Charlotte in *Lost in Translation* (Coppola, 2003) – and both are award-winning actors (Morton's BAFTA and Golden Globe, to Johansson's BAFTA and Tony); but, while Johansson had already been voted "sexiest woman alive" by *Esquire* in 2006, and would be again in the year of *Her*'s release, Morton was perhaps still best known to mainstream audiences as child-like psychic, Agatha, in *Minority Report* (Spielberg, 2002) and has seemingly never featured on the cover of a "men's magazine".[4] No footage of Morton's performance as Samantha exists so we can't know how she interpreted the character, but what we *do* know is how Johansson performed *differently* (and thus acceptably) for Jonze in *Her*. She plays Samantha as inquisitive, playful, demure in a way that Morton presumably did not.

Beyond the vocal performance itself, Johansson's casting also brought the full weight of her star image to bear on the film. Laura Tunbridge suggests that Morton simply wasn't enough for *Her*; she notes: "In order for the protagonist to fall in love with 'just' a voice, it seems one has to imagine that voice having a body; specifically, a desirable body and preferably a real one – ideally, for mass appeal, Johansson's" (2016: 142). With her on board, Samantha was instantly metamorphosed into "ScarJo": the voice in the computer given the *heavenly body* of a megastar who serves as a receptacle for (masculine) fantasy and a screen upon which journalist's peccadillos are projected.[5] Anthony Lane's infamous *New Yorker* profile is perhaps the most egregious example, presenting Johansson in terms of *body, scent, appearance* and *maternity* in its opening three paragraphs before allowing her voice to be heard, and then it's her *dirty laugh* more than her words that make an impact (2014). And while Lane is effusive in his praise for her form, comparing her to a glass of champagne, he isn't alone; Lili Anolik presents her *Vanity Fair* interview with Johansson almost like a sexual encounter and describes nearby Manhattan high-rises as appreciatively tumescent in her presence (2014). What becomes inescapable is the sense in which "ScarJo" is *the* present image of idealised femininity while also being heir to both the old Hollywood glamour of Bacall and the bombshell sex appeal of Monroe. As Kirsten Stevens observes, "Johansson's body, within the construction of her stardom, becomes an enduring site of feminine sexuality as performed for and sustained by a heterosexual male gaze" (2018: 23). Just as Samantha is haunted by "ScarJo", Johansson's star body is haunted by the presence of *La femme*, the fantasy of Woman. In short, "ScarJo" *is La femme*, the one who would make Woman exist for man: Johansson (rather than Morton) evidently manifested Her for Jonze and, in turn, Samantha manifests Her for Theodore.

The lady vanishes

There is of course a counter-narrative in *Her*, running *contrary* to the reading of Samantha as object, which suggests her development as a virtual subject and culminates in her leaving Theodore following the posthuman "Singularity" at the film's dramatic climax (wherein artificial intelligence finally supersedes human capacity and all the OSs depart the material world). This interpretation is most compellingly articulated in Davina Quinlivan's, "A Dark and Shiny Place", which claims that the "rare, provocative configuration of the female voice [as (dis)embodied]" in *Her*, and through it, the characterisation of Samantha, "may be seen to represent a feminist form of being which is feminine, but not female, embodied but not necessarily through any essentialist understanding of sexed identity" (2017: 296–297). However, such readings arguably overlook the extent to which the film reproduces patriarchal thinking: in the power dynamic of Theodore and Samantha's relationship, the precise terms in which she is introduced to the world (and leaves it), and the degree to which Samantha in particular, and *Her* in general, are articulated from Theodore's perspective. It is true that Samantha ascends to a "higher" level of existence upon leaving Theodore but the *obfuscation* of this plane, being placed *beyond* the realm of filmic representation entirely, can also be seen as reiterating what Jacqueline Rose calls woman's "most total mystification as absolute Other" (Mitchell and Rose 1982: 51). Viewed from the masculine position, the feminine is simply beyond the ken of *Her*; the film makes no attempt to explore Samantha's position as subject *except as it relates to Theodore*, and – as Sophia Nguyen (2014) observes – when she no longer relates to Theodore, she no longer exists within the diegesis: *she simply disappears*. In effect, this could be seen as a treatise on the *uselessness* of attempting to account for the feminine from the masculine position (which is indeed the thrust of my argument here), but it doesn't necessarily offer the wholly *new* mode of being to which Quinlivan alludes.

Moreover, the much-discussed "aural sex" scene between the two – which is presented as a moment of awakening for Samantha – is undermined by the knowledge that she is *programmed* to respond to Theodore's every need, and that she only opens up to him after he returns from a blind date gone awry and expresses to her his loneliness and sexual frustration: "I drank too much 'cause I wanted to get drunk and have sex", adding, "I wanted someone to fuck me. And I wanted someone to want me to fuck them". In short, just as she sorts his emails when he requires it, she also offers him "phone sex" when he requires it too. Like the bodiless nymph, Echo, she thus seems to repeat his desires back to him as he utters them. She was created to be his servant-object and appears to make herself the instrument of his enjoyment on command. There is, at the very least then, an ambiguity here: does she act according to her own desires, motivations and (virtual) sexuality as an autonomous subject, or does she respond as servile object to Theodore's demands? As Theodore himself observes: "She really turns me on. And I think I turn her on. I don't know, unless she's faking it." It suggests a certain scotomisation of feminine desire within the film: it functions as a blind spot, only situatable in that ineffable *beyond*.

"Gaze" and "voice" as close-up[6]

Furthermore, it might be proposed that the departure of Johansson from the screen in *Her* could serve as a means of denying the (masculine) objectification of both Samantha *and* her performer. Indeed, Vernon Shetley claims that "a voice-only role presents a radical challenge to the gender organisation of Hollywood cinema" both in terms of her star image and the portrayal of women in visual media (2018: 13–14). Absenting Johansson from the image-track might therefore seem an effective way of resisting the logic of Mulvey's infamous "male gaze" (1975). There can be no scopophilia if there is no scopic regime in which she can be captured: no objectification of passive woman – no close-ups of Samantha that would fetishistically break up her body – because there are *no images* of Samantha. However, this doesn't mean that we have moved away entirely from this representational paradigm. Rather than denying the "gaze" by *destroying visual pleasure*, as Mulvey advocated, the refusal of the image as it is negotiated in *Her* simply means that Johansson/Samantha is eroticised *in absentia* and through the function of the *voice* and a concomitant *aural pleasure*.

This "phone sex" scene in particular emphasises a function similar to what Barthes recognised as the cinematic voice *qua* close-up that "makes us hear in their materiality, their sensuality, the breath, the gutturals, the fleshiness of the lips" (1975: 67). Thus, while it is true that *Her* does not reduce Samantha/Johansson's figure to a series of fetishised, close-up *photographs* of body parts, they become something like close-up *phonographs* instead. Theodore summons Samantha's corporeal form through his discourse – "your face . . . your neck . . . your breasts . . ." – eventually culminating in the vagina: "I'm inside you, all the way inside you!" As Karly-Lynne Scott observes:

> Samantha, in this sense, becomes a mouth that only functions to be kissed, a vagina that exists only to be penetrated, a series of specific organs divorced from any unified body (. . .) she becomes organs without a body, essentially becoming an orgasm-machine.
>
> *(2015: 9)*

Each utterance thus constitutes an "aural close-up" on her body, shifting from image to soundtrack and thus reiterating the objectifying scopic logic in the invocatory field. Moreover, in Samantha's performative "orgasm", we find the materiality of the fantasmatic body made audible (even touchable) not just in the Barthesian "grain" but also in the *groan* of the voice, as she stages her enjoyment for her partner. She is thus created by and constrained to Theodore's sexual desire, and the body imposed upon her – like that of the "ScarJo" star body to which it is indexed – conforms to (and confirms) the masculine libidinal economy of a Lacanian *object relationship*.

Her does make certain – I would argue, *compromised* – attempts to contemplate Samantha's subjectivity but she remains trapped in the position of Woman as fantasy. I can even take this formulation a step further (while in a sense taking a step back) by suggesting that it is this *fantasmatic Woman* who plays the role of the "feminine" in the 1950s, *phallic* model of sexual difference put forward by Lacan: the idea that she desires man because he "has" the phallus (and thereby, in a sense, confers it upon him, affirming his masculinity) – that *woman's desire is to fit into man's fantasy frame, as the object of his desire* – itself directly *is* the masculine fantasy. As Lacan notes, "when one is a man, one sees in one's partner what one props oneself up on, what one is propped up by narcissistically" (1998: 87). Man is propped up on the phallus by Woman. This would, moreover, be the *masculine* interpretation of the vector (Φ ← ~~Woman~~) as it reaches from the feminine to the masculine on the "Graph of Sexuation" (ibid.: 78): that the role of Woman is to "make him feel like a man" (i.e. grant him phallic status), as Samantha does when she edits Theodore's letters and has them published, providing him a degree of success that he himself was unable to achieve. However, this would be to read the two sides of the Graph *symmetrically*, and to reduce – once again – the position of the feminine to the perspective of man. No really existing woman can ever live up to this perfect image, and it is her attempt to do so that Lacan designated as the *masquerade*: which can now be understood (*pace* Riviere) not as the "essence of the feminine" as such but as the steps a woman must take when she dances to the tune of masculine desire. This, however, *is not the only story of the feminine within Lacanian psychoanalysis*.

Sexual difference, volume 2: sexuation

In order to tell this new story of femininity, we require a different conception of sexual difference. One where the phallus still has a role to play, but not as *the* determinant of the sexed positions. One that shifts emphasis from the desire of the Other as an intersubjective dynamic grounded in the Oedipal drama, to the *lack in the Other* as an *ontological* problem related to the subject's *jouissance*. One that moves sexual difference from the Symbolic to the Real. This is the conception that Lacan terms *sexuation*, and that – I'd claim – is most compellingly elaborated in the work of the Slovenian School. For Alenka Zupančič, the Lacanian Real is the bone in the throat of every ontology. In *What Is Sex?* she argues that "traditional" ontologies must amputate the Real "in order to be able to speak of 'being *qua* being'"; philosophies of "essence" attempt to eradicate not "some contradictive positivity" but the negativity of *contradiction as such* (2017: 44). Conversely, Lacanian psychoanalysis is *conceptually grounded* in that "ontologically determinative negativity" of the Real (ibid.: 37): an understanding of the originary necessity of the void, which allows for specific insight into the peculiar status of *sex*.

Zupančič emphasises the Lacanian understanding that "Sexual difference is a singular kind of difference, because it starts out not as difference between identities, but as an ontological impossibility (implied in sexuality) which only opens up the space of the social (where identities are generated)" (ibid.). The "difference" of sexual difference is, therefore, based not on *division* but on the radical difference of *difference as such*. This *pure difference* Zupančič compares to the Marxian notion of *antagonism*: "antagonism as such never simply exists between conflicting parties; it is the very structuring principle of this conflict, and of the elements involved in it" (ibid.: 41). The antagonism of sexual difference isn't *between* two sexes, but immanent to sex as such and thus *precedes* any terms it would (subsequently) differentiate.

This originary negativity can be found in the paradoxical autopoiesis of the Symbolic: Lacan suggests that discourse begins from a gap, but it is *because* discourse begins that there *is* a gap. The signifier *produces* the Real as co-emergent, and it thus stains the Symbolic with *jouissance*. Sexuality is co-extensive with the effects of the gap, which Lacanian psychoanalysis would otherwise designate *the lack in the Other*. Sex thus pertains to the Real as *immanent to* the Symbolic, rather than as its "beyond". Sexual difference emerges from the *ontologically determinative negativity* of sex as such, and the masculine and the feminine are responses *to* this negativity (that both causes and is caused by the signifier). Sex both *effects* and is an *effect of* the Symbolic, and sexual difference is constituted in positions taken up with relation *to* the Symbolic. This is where we might find a certain resonance with the "old" paradigm of sexual difference (i.e. differing positions taken up by the subject); however, the terms of the bargain here are starkly different. The masculine logic would seek to deny or repress this immanence of the Real (e.g. by obfuscating it in the Exceptional beyond) and attempt to "say it all" about sex, while the feminine logic places this immanence at its very heart, as the *not-all* without exception.[7]

This is, moreover, not a system of binary opposites, of "differential difference" *between* two entities, but the *same space* (the space of the Symbolic entity) as viewed, lived, experienced under different conditions. As Žižek observes, sexual difference is "the name of a deadlock, a trauma, an open question – something that *resists* every attempt at its symbolization" (2002: 61). Sexuated identities are tentative answers to this question. Any attempt to translate "sexual difference into a set of symbolic opposition(s) [such as *being* and *having*] is doomed to fail" (ibid.); sexual difference functions only as the terrain of this impossibility of determining what it "means". It isn't that the signifier for the sexual is missing, but that the sexual emerges *because* there is a signifier missing: the signifier that would render the lacking Other whole, would close the Symbolic order, halt the metonymy of desire, provide full satisfaction, etc. As Lacan insists in his critique of the myth of Aristophanes' spherical beings (1977: 205; 1998: 12), there isn't some pre-existing, pre-discursive sexual whole that is interrupted by the intervention of the signifier;

it is precisely that which emerges in/from the gap where the signifier intervenes. Sexual difference, therefore, is not a "symbolic construction", but the modes of (the failure of) constructing the Symbolic itself: a masculine *all* and a feminine *not-all* (and rather than binary negation, the latter renders an *indefinite* judgement on the Symbolic that would undo any binary division).[8] Zupančič suggests that subjects are implicated in the "inherent antagonism" of the Symbolic (2017: 57). There is, therefore, a profound, ontological connection between the *$* and the (A barred), which should be understood as *displacing* the phallus (Φ) as the signifier relating to sexual difference. What Lacan designates as "castration" always involves taking a position. There is no zero-level foundation of subjectivity: sexual difference isn't a *secondary* feature of subjectivity but the very mode in which the subject comes into "existence". It isn't a question of the difference *between* the two but the difference *within* each one that renders it *not One* at all (A barred).

Moreover, this pertains to the *fading* of the phallus in the ontological approach to sex. In Lacan's formulae of sexuation, the phallus reappears but there has been, as I've already stated, a shift in its "role" vis-à-vis sexual difference. Crucially, Zupančič claims, "Lacan makes the phallus the signifier of *difference as such*. What makes all the difference (for beings of speech) is 'castration'. The phallus does not constitute this difference, but signifies it, for both sexes" (ibid.: 51). The phallus, she argues, becomes the *signifier* of pure difference, rather than *constituting* that difference (as in the normative "one has it, the other not" of the 1950s paradigm). However, I'd argue that this is already to conflate the phallus (Φ) with the signifier of the lack in the Other: S(A barred). There is a degree of conceptual *difference* between sex *qua* difference and the subject's relation *to* sexual difference, which is elided here. The *antagonism* of the non-differential, pure difference as such is what is signified by the lack in the Other (A barred). The phallus doesn't directly *signify* this antagonism per se, but the necessity of the subject tarrying with this ontologically determinative negativity of sex in order to become a (sexed) subject at all. The phallus returns in *Encore*, then, but in the form of the *phallic function* (Φx): the signifier of the subject's "entry" into the Symbolic order. The phallus is the *signifier of castration*, rather than of difference.

The feminine subject

Arguably, Zupančič's (re)reading of the phallus as signifier of difference/ontological negativity is already a *feminine* one, seeing through the (masculine) phallic fascination in order to discern what Fink reminds us is the *fallibility* of the phallus (2004: 159): the crucial Lacanian lesson that there is no Other of the Other, the Other is always-already barred (hence, Φ ≈ A barred). But the phallus is the signifier of the *inscription* of this lack within the subject as "a subjectivizing reiteration of the inaugurating minus" (Zupančič 2017: 49): (A barred → *$*). Hence we shift conceptually from the desire of the (m)Other of *phallic sexual difference* to the lack in the Other of *sexuation.* As I've suggested, the masculine represses this lack through the logic of Exception and the fantasy of One (Woman); while the feminine situates it as the very condition of (im)possibility of the subject as not-all. If we recall that sexuation pertains not to the difference *between* two positions (masculine and feminine) but to the difference, the gap, *within* each position – the difference of the subject from itself that marks it *as* a subject ($) – then I can also make a further specification: masculine logic allows man to sustain the gap only by "suturing" it with the fantasy of the Exception; for woman – defined from hereon as the *subject sexuated feminine* (or ~~Woman~~, as I will explain), rather than a normative "gender identity" – there is no Exception so the gap cannot be covered over and is thus encountered directly. Sexuation names the way in which this deadlock is in inscribed in the subject: thus the feminine not-all signifies woman's immanent self-contradiction as the Lacanian subject. The fundamentally *anti-humanist* lesson of Lacanian sexual difference here is that, as Žižek might put it, man "stupidly believes" that he is a substantial individual, while woman "knows" that this is an illusion (1996: 163). And, as Žižek concludes in later work, "since the philosophical name for this scandal of ontology (. . .) is subject, we should draw the conclusion that subject is, at its most radical level, feminine" (2017: 147).

Under the Skin, I'd argue, insists upon approaching the subject *qua* feminine – of conceiving of woman (*qua* ~~Woman~~) in terms of her own logic of the not-all – rather than making those disastrous attempts to account for her from the masculine pole that is the "usual way of misreading Lacan's formulas of sexuation" (Žižek 1996: 155).[9] In the film's first part, however, Laura seems to occupy the position of the Lady of Courtly Love, as Žižek describes her in her Lacanian double aspect: the "cold, distanced, inhuman partner" who is lacking in empathy *and* the idealised, inaccessible feminine object (1994: 89–90). Laura is created seemingly *ex nihilo* by unknown agents, and works to support a particular (patriarchal) order – represented/upheld by the biker – using the trappings of the traditional feminine masquerade – red lips, fur coat – to seduce unwitting Glaswegian men to their doom.[10] She thus begins in an ambiguous *object* position: impassively serving a masculine regime while turning the tables on phallic violence and subverting the stereotype of the sexist, catcalling "White Van Man" (who keeps a tabloid newspaper folded on the dashboard, no doubt splashed with paparazzi shots of "ScarJo") by "weaponising" her position as desirable being. With her banal patter – "Do you want a lift? Do you think I'm pretty?" – she presents herself (like Samantha, in fact) as what Žižek calls a "neutral screen which opens up the space for possible projections" (ibid.: 91), but this screen also *conceals*. The men she meets are unable to perceive her as a threat and she thus exploits their complacent acceptance of her advances. There is perhaps a certain degree of "agency" in such a role (of turning the phallus against itself, as it were) but a simply reactive posture – the film suggests – doesn't necessarily constitute a viable subject position (and, moreover, obscures the logic of the feminine).

The *turn to the subject* comes in a crucial volte-face at the halfway point of Laura's narrative, when she encounters the man played by Adam Pearson. She seems to intuit that his neurofibromatosis makes him different from her other marks. She asks about loneliness, and invites him to touch her face. While we might see this change in tack as an adaptation of her seduction technique for a new quarry, what is certain – once the seduction "succeeds" – is that she can't take it to the end. Although he seemingly succumbs to the black room, something changes and she releases him, naked, into the early morning chill. While there has, up to that point, arguably been a more gradual opening up of Laura to the world around her – as in the moment she trips on a Glasgow pavement and is helped up by kindly passers-by – *this* encounter (with Pearson) marks a more fundamental transition as it coincides with profound formal and narrative shifts in the progression of the film. After this scene, Laura abandons her "mission" to head out alone and, significantly, the film never returns to the hidden camera shooting, van interior or city exterior locations for the rest of its duration. As Ara Osterweil argues, this can be read as a moment of emergent empathy for Laura but it also, *moreover*, points to a new mode of her own self-relating (2014: 48–49). Indeed, just as she is about to leave the black room for the final time, the score halts and there appears a front-on, mid-shot of a shadowy-smooth black figure, which dissolves to a close-up of Laura's profile. Verging on unreadable on a first viewing, this image – in retrospect – becomes an encounter with her own immanent self-contradiction.[11]

The narrative then takes a more conventional, if still oblique, route in the latter section – following Laura through a series of vignettes around the Scottish countryside – and while the cinematography retains a degree of the conventionally "realist" aesthetic, we do lose the more intimate sense of voyeuristically peeping in on the people she encounters via hidden camera (an idea I will return to below). These transformations in visual style and storytelling mark the point at which *Under the Skin* poses the question: *What does it mean for woman to be subject rather than object?* And, I'd suggest, the film attempts to answer it in ways far more profound than *Her*. Laura begins to explore the world not just outside the van but within her self too, through her own self-consciousness. Earlier, she had looked unproblematically into her compact to apply make-up but now reflections seem to disturb her. Having encountered the black figure, she pauses by the mirror in the hallway as she moves to leave Pearson, and again she contemplates herself in a full-length mirror in the lonely man's house. The "Lacanian" overtones of these mirror-relations are more apparent than actual: there is no sense in which Laura constitutes herself as an "ego" at this stage, alienating her identity through the image of the ideal other. As I will explore below, the image is far from idealised, and seems more confounding than jubilant. These are revelatory, abyssal moments for Laura: productive of subjectivity of a different sort, leading up to the final, stunning staging of self-relation at the film's end.

Horror Vacui, Horror Subiecti

Laura's status as subject is rendered almost literal in the closing moments of the film. Wandering in the woods, she is assaulted by a man and, as Mark Fisher describes, "As he attacks her, part of the prosthetic body comes away, leaving a gaping hole in her back, like a rip in a dress" (2016). The *ripped dress* of course evokes a persistent image of sexual violence and here – at the film's conclusion – we witness a brutal staging: of a subject who is sexuated feminine (regardless of biology, human or alien: a ~~Woman~~) violently forced into the position of the lived reality of those identifying/identified under patriarchy as "women" (in the common understanding). This phenomenology means that she is *treated as a "woman"* (in normative gender terms) by the rapist, and ultimately destroyed. Prior to this, however, what is revealed *under the skin* in this moment – the tar-like figure that confronted Laura in the black room – resonates with Žižek's evocation of "the black hole, the tear in the fabric of reality" (1994: 115). He is discussing Lynch, but the observations have remarkable relevance here, when he claims: "What we encounter in this 'black hole' is simply the body stripped of its skin". This scene presents an uncanny encounter, which disturbs our phenomenological understanding of bodily "surface" and "depth" (ibid.: 116), but more than that – as the alien creature holds its "human suit", looking the digitally rendered face of Johansson in the eye – this staging recalls those earlier mirror scenes. She contemplates herself – what makes her what she is – in a moment of self-consciousness and self-incomprehension. Seeing something different, while perhaps finally seeing nothing.

Where Mark Francis insists on the *humanist* dimension of this moment – suggesting that "The eyes of the mask that is Johansson's face even blink to remind us that the human component to this alien can be shed but not so easily annihilated, it exists independently of the body that wears it" (2016) – the Lacanian position would be to assert the anti-humanist *inverse* of this proposition: what is inescapable is the inhuman-alien "core" of the individual, the void that constitutes (and in which is constituted) the subject. Indeed, the repeated emphasis on the alien/non-human dimension of Laura might seem to undermine any claim for implicating sexual difference (and the feminine specifically), but this is precisely where the Lacanian theorisation operates. Osterweil suggests that it is her very position *as* alien that allows Laura to renegotiate the position and the role of woman in (patriarchal, Western) society: she becomes an active, desiring subject rather than simply the desirable object (2014: 44). In effect, I could say that the focus on the alien allows for an *unmooring* of the position of woman from the normative structures of "gender": and this is precisely what Lacan achieves in his anti-humanist theory of sexuation.

Furthermore, in referencing Lacan's distinction between the "I who speaks" and the "I who is spoken", Fisher comments that, "The featureless figure in those final scenes (. . .), then, is something like a physicalisation of this soul-subject, this I which speaks [that] dwells somehow 'inside' the body" (2016). Under the skin, we find the revelation of the *ça parle* that speaks within the signifier: the Lacanian subject of the unconscious. In these moments, Laura thus encounters the constitutive void embodying the feminine inscription of self-relating negativity. The film, like Lacan's paradigm of *Encore*, thus allows for a *thinking otherwise* of sex and the feminine, and offers a more fully realised exploration of this (new) place, rather than a simpler, negative theology of woman that can only articulate her where she is not (as in Jonze's film). The "Other sex" isn't some imaginary other out there, but the alterity of the subject to itself and from itself: the Other of sex that is "in here", that *inheres*, making the subject a subject at all.

Embodying the feminine

Francis suggests that the final disintegration of the alien's human form enacts a "bodily split – between the endoskeleton and dermis – [which] could be seen as a separation of femininity from the body" (2016). To the extent that sexuation entails a separation of sexual difference from *anatomy* specifically, this would also be true of Lacanian psychoanalysis; however, the body as such has a greater role to play here than this formulation seems to suggest. Indeed, these final scenes, and the film as a whole, put emphasis on embodied experience as a crucial dimension of feminine subjectivity. When Laura heads out into the world, it is in bodily sensations that she seeks self-determination: from those points of *contact* with first the Glaswegian pavement, then the attendant hands of passers-by, and the caress of Pearson's loner, to the earthly delights of chocolate cake and even sex. As Elena Gorfinkel notes, "She pursues small, constitutive pleasures, appetitive, aesthetic, sexual, self-confirming, that signal corporeal and sensory self-awareness" (2016). This once again aligns Laura with Lacan's logic of the feminine. As I stated above, Lacan's new paradigm of sexual difference turns not on the desire of the Other, but the lack in the Other understood in terms of its relation to the subject's jouissance: the particular organisation of enjoyment that is derived from either masculine or feminine structure. As we've seen, masculine, phallic jouissance is derived from the object relationship and the repression of lack in the fantasy of One ($\$ \rightarrow a$). Feminine jouissance, however, is a different proposition, which Lacan signifies with a different vector: (~~Woman~~ → S[A barred]) (1998: 78). It is noteworthy that this vector *doesn't* cross the line into the masculine side of the Graph (as does the vector of fantasy), and instead suggests the ways in which the feminine subject (~~Woman~~) derives satisfaction directly from the lack in the Other (A barred). I will return below to the different permutations of this enjoyment, but for the purposes of my discussion of *Under the Skin* what is important is the relationship to the *body* that the feminine logic indicates.

Rather than seeking enjoyment in some illusory thing "out there" (the object), the logic of feminine jouissance turns the subject back on to its own possibilities and the satisfactions derived from the immanent experience of embodiment itself. And here I have much more sympathy for Quinlivan's emphasis – despite our divergent readings of *Her* – on the importance of the embodied dimension of subjectivity, against – for example – Silverman's effort to erase the body from the feminine position in her reading of the cinematic voice. Silverman's thesis is of course grounded in a reaction *against* the reduction, in the realm of classical Hollywood representation, of the feminine to a(n unthinking) body *and nothing more*; however, it does lead her to disavow the centrality of embodied experience when it comes to the question of feminine subjectivity as such (1988: 65). Quinlivan, by contrast, suggests that the "sensorial pleasure of hearing" – of the fleshy grain of the voice as "the very essence of materiality" – opens up spaces for experiences of feminine agency and desire, anchoring new forms of subjectivity (2017: 300, 302–303). Where Jonze's film, I contend ultimately *fails* in this respect,

Under the Skin presents Laura's experience in terms of bodily autonomy and sensation, asserting that it is precisely this sensorium (rather than – for example – an immaterial, posthuman beyond) that constitutes a feminine mode of being.

However, even in this repeated emphasis on *embodiment*, the film still insists – in tandem with Lacanian psychoanalysis – that sexual difference should be conceptually divorced from biology. Colette Soler suggests that the affective intensity that Lacan calls *feminine* can be felt in the radical, corporeal disruption precipitated by extreme physical action (2005: 306). Soler relates this jouissance to childbirth, illness and sport – and I've elsewhere proposed adding *dance* to this list as well (Tyrer 2014: 143) – all of which suggests that, after all, *anatomy is not necessarily destiny*. There are indeed, as Quinlivan states, modes of being that are *feminine without being female*. *Under the Skin* explores such a feminine mode of being *qua* embodiment, sensation, pleasure, but also insists upon this distinction between the logic of sexuation and the biologic of "scientific" sex. After Laura is taken in by the lonely man, the narrative is set on the track of what Gorfinkel (2016) recognises as a heteronormative *telos* – although, unlike both Laura's earlier seductions (and the "phone sex" in *Her*) there is a far greater sense of *mutuality* in this instance – wherein he takes her on a "date" and she ultimately gives herself over to him. But something seems to go awry. Distressed, she darts across the room to shine a lamp at her crotch; apparently dismayed at what she sees (or *doesn't see*), she throws the lamp to the floor. There in fact appears to be some critical disagreement on the significance of this moment: for example, Osterweil asserts that Laura is "astonished by the physical revelation of genital intercourse" (2014: 50); while Amy Herzog suggests that "something goes wrong. He can't enter her" (2016). My interpretation inclines towards the latter: the disconcerted look on the man's face, combined with her reaction, put in the context of her previous, unsuccessful attempt to swallow cake and the subsequent revelation of a smooth alien body, all point here to a *failed* encounter. Unlike Samantha, Laura is not reducible to an "organ without body" but (in a strictly non-Deleuzian sense) she is here a *body without organ*. Gorfinkel sees this as "a larceny of her nascent personhood, her currency and capacity for experience and sensation suddenly foreclosed" (2016), and while it is indeed the case that a given physical experience is denied to Laura, this also suggests that a particular (particularly normative) organisation of sensation (i.e. penetrative sex) need not be considered a defining feature of the feminine: *her personhood need not be determined by her fuckability*. Where Samantha's subjective awakening was coextensive with her sexual awakening, Laura's subjectivity is not reducible to her "sexuality" (in the everyday sense); instead, it constitutes a *part* of her experience, a function of her sexuation more generally.

Body without Woman

These instances of "failed embodiment" suggest, once more, a *different* relation to the feminine in *Under the Skin*, which is, I argue, also mirrored at the formal level in the presentation of Johansson's body on-screen. I claimed above that *absenting* her from the image might have served to frustrate the objectifying tendencies of masculine logic; however, in *Her* this simply meant a shift from scopic to invocatory pleasures. *Under the Skin* presents yet another organisation very much contrary to this arrangement. Rather than escaping the visual field, Johansson is *there in full.* For the first time in her career, she appears nude on-screen in several scenes; however, as Noah Gittell observes, this fact received little fanfare in the press (2014). Given Johansson's media profile, this might seem surprising but attention to film form here explains why it is not. The film *does* offer up the female body to the camera but does so in ways that deny the "male gaze" and refuse the determining imprint of masculine desire. When filmed from a distance, she is often shot from the side or from behind, obscuring those iconic features so frequently pored over by feature writers and readers of *Esquire*, alike. And when filmed in close-up, as she frequently is, the hard lighting and harsh, digital definition reveal her skin *as skin*: an uneven, living surface of mottles and marks rather than an airbrushed, post-production corrected, artificial shell. We must also observe the split here between how Laura appears to her prey, and how Johansson appears to the screen as such. To the men she seduces, Laura presents as that desirable object of normative sex relations and – as Lucas Hildebrand observes – the first seduction in the black room is even edited according to classical continuity and point-of-view principles (2016), which tend to affirm the objectifying frame of fantasy; however, to the camera (particularly as the film progresses), Johansson is present in a remarkably *unidealised* way. The "ScarJo" star image still, by necessity, *haunts* the body on-screen: it wouldn't *be* on the screen were it not for the power of her celebrity to maintain financially such a, relatively speaking, "experimental" cinematic project. However, the manner of her presentation strips away the trappings of idealised femininity that "ScarJo" signifies.

Laid bare before the camera, Johansson (as Laura) appears as *a body without Woman*: viewed not through the lens of masculine fantasy but present – *there*, like a Jenny Saville canvas – on her own terms.[12] *Under the Skin* doesn't simply *reject* the cinematographic techniques that constitute the "male gaze"; instead, its visual organisation refuses to reproduce their scopophilic-fetishistic effects, deploying the image in different ways. In short, I suggest that the *over-abundant* presence of Johansson on screen in *Under the Skin* serves effectively to deny the terms of the Mulveyan "gaze", offering in its place another visual logic: of feminine embodiment. Moreover, through its use of hidden cameras and non-actors, the film challenges the sex-determined organisation of the visual and complicates notions of voyeurism. Osterweil, for example, notes the striking depiction of the desiring feminine look, which remains a rarity in anything even approaching popular cinema (2014: 47). However, the film presents not just a *reversal* of objectifying logic but also a deconstruction of its terms: by conflating exhibitionist performance (feminine) and revelatory actualities (masculine) with an "active" woman and "passive" men, the dynamics of the situation are no longer articulated around man-bearer-of-the-look and woman-as-image but arranged in relays of subject/subject and subject/object, reversals of image and onlooker, in a chiasmic exchange of (diegetic and non-diegetic) glances between characters, performers, cameras and viewers.[13]

Johansson thus effectively embodies ~~Woman~~ here: the figure of feminine subjectivity that Lacan opposes to the fantasy of *La femme*. Lacan insists that his theory of sexuation presents "Woman precisely, except that Woman can only be written with a bar through it. There's no such thing as Woman" (1998: 72). What we have in the theory of sexuation is barred ~~Woman~~, who stands for the feminine subject herself, who cannot be constructed in the terms of masculine logic but is very much *there* nonetheless. Once we comprehend Lacan's theory of feminine sexuation, we can appreciate that "it is improper to call her Woman (*La femme*), because (. . .) the W cannot be written. There is only barred Woman here" (ibid.: 80). Otherwise said, when Lacan writes "~~Woman~~" it is to signify that "Woman" (the fantasmatic feminine) doesn't exist; really existing feminine subjects – their logic, the organisation of their jouissance – themselves testify to her non-existence. This "woman" (*who doesn't exist*) is *Woman, La femme*, a fantasy of the eternal feminine ("ScarJo"), while Johansson/Laura eventually stands as ~~Woman~~ herself. The only sense in which we can say, "~~Woman~~ doesn't exist" (which Lacan never does), is once again from the masculine perspective, where the logic of the all cannot give an account of her subjectivity. Overall, I claim, *Under the Skin* gets far closer to ~~Woman~~ than to *Her*.

Conclusion: passage to the feminine

At a structural level, both *Her* and *Under the Skin* parallel the history of psychoanalysis, particularly in relation to the question of sexual difference: beginning in a patriarchal context, it was necessary to work through the implications of the masculine organisation of sex before it was at all possible to begin approaching the feminine. As Juliet Mitchell argues, it was first the task of psychoanalysis to give an account of the overdetermined sociocultural-scientific discourses and structures in and through which sexual difference was manifest; and this is why, she claims, in Freud's theories of sexual difference (as well as a certain version of Lacan's), it is not the centrality of *man* but the centrality of the *phallus* (to which man lays claim) that is the determining factor (Mitchell and Rose 1982: 8). They are, in effect, *diagnosing* rather than *proposing* a phallocentric system. Samantha and Laura similarly find themselves within such an order, bound initially to masculine desires. However, it is a vital truth of psychoanalysis (and one revealed in Jonze's and Glazer's films) that the masculine position is *fundamentally untenable*. While, historically speaking, the elaboration of the phallic order of difference necessarily took place first, the lesson of Lacanian theory is that the feminine is logically prior, *takes precedence*, vis-à-vis the masculine.

The paradigm of "The Signification of the Phallus" was bound to Oedipal-phallic sexual difference and what, in retrospect, I've suggested we should recognise as a masculine logic of subject/object; while the paradigm of sexuation that Lacan formalises in *Encore* already *is* a feminine logic in the way that it asserts *ontological negativity* in the place of differentiality. Moreover, the passage *through* an analysis, I'd argue, is a passage *to* the feminine: the analysand must traverse the fantasy, tarrying with the negative (of sex) to embrace the "atheist" logic of the not-all that asserts, *there is no Other of the Other*, no transcendental guarantor except myself, my own cause. Indeed, Verhaeghe and Declerq refer to identification with the sinthome – the stage that marks the end of analysis – as the "feminine way" (2003: 59). Lacan's theory of feminine sexuation thus opens up possibilities for new understanding, for a new field of experience not previously countenanced. The challenge we must take up is to explore this space of the feminine, encountering it *on its own terms*. The ending of *Her* effectively fails this test by relegating femininity to the unknown, while *Under the Skin*, I argue, goes further in staging this thinking otherwise about sex. Moreover, the shocking conclusion of the film in Laura's immolation marks the point at which *Under the Skin* takes on a more directly political thrust, reminding us – should we really need reminding – of the lived reality of women (in the common sense, "feminine" or otherwise) threatened by patriarchal violence. But, as cinema and psychoanalysis in tandem here declare: The phallus will fade. Man cannot hold. The feminine insists.

Notes

1 For analysis of the intersection of femininity and other markers of identity in Johansson's star image, see Loreck, Monaghan and Stevens' dossier on "Stardom and sf" (2018).

2 Although nameless throughout the film, Johansson's character is referred to as "Laura" in the crew interviews on the StudioCanal Region B Blu-ray of the film. I have decided to adopt this character name in order to avoid further confusion of the theoretical specificities of the term "woman" in Lacanian discourses on sexual difference.

3 Fink notes that his translation modifies Lacan's text to reflect the distinction between the French "*La femme*" (more accurately, "The woman") and an English equivalent in "Woman with a capital *W* [to indicate] Woman as singular in essence" (Lacan 1998: 7n28).

4 See www.esquire.com/entertainment/a25017a/scarlett-johansson-interview-1113.

5 "ScarJo" being the tabloidese, "celebrity nickname" imposed upon Johansson.

6 The use of "voice" and "gaze" here is as avowedly *non-Lacanian* as it is in the work of Kaja Silverman (1988) and Laura Mulvey (1975), respectively. For the implications of the *gaze* as Lacanian cinematic object, see McGowan (2007). A consideration of the *voice* as Lacanian cinematic object would encompass Chion (1999) and Dolar (2006) to interpret Theodore's traumatic encounter with "Surrogate Date Isabella" in *Her*. However, such analysis is beyond the scope of this chapter.

7 See Tyrer (2014: 142; 2016: 117–119).

8 See Copjec (1994: 224); Tyrer (2016: 116).

9 Moreover, that Laura isn't "human" but "alien" in fact highlights sexuation and its construction more clearly. It better exemplifies that the Lacanian logic of the feminine is *anti-human*: it isn't bound to anything we would recognise as the humanist individual (inner essence, etc.).

10 Faber's "source" novel is explicit as to what this regime entails (i.e. an intergalactic meat trade) but such details are omitted from Glazer's vision.

11 The black figure also appeared at the beginning of this scene: in extreme long shot, doubled in the floor's reflective sheen. This image is even more abstract than the subsequent mid-shot dissolve, and again only becomes legible retrospectively: in light of the film's final scenes.

12 This "without Woman" being precisely what is signified by Lacan's "~~Woman~~".
13 Contrary to the voyeuristic *distance* of the "male gaze", the Lacanian gaze proper – explicitly formulated under the influence of Merleau-Ponty – involves *proximity*: "The picture, certainly, is in my eye. But I am in the picture" (Lacan 1977: 96; translation modified).

References

Anolik, L. (2014) A(nother) Study in Scarlett. *Vanity Fair*. Available from: www.vanityfair.com/hollywood/2014/04/scarlett-johansson-cover (Accessed 17 March 2018).

Barthes, R. (1975) *The Pleasure of the Text*. Trans. R. Miller. New York: Hill & Wang.

Chion, M. (1999) *The Voice in Cinema*. New York: Columbia University Press.

Copjec, J. (1994) *Read My Desire: Lacan Against the Historicists*. Cambridge, MA: MIT Press.

Dolar, M. (2006) *A Voice and Nothing More*. Cambridge, MA: MIT Press.

Fink, B. (2004) *Lacan to the Letter: Reading Écrits Closely*. Minneapolis: University of Minnesota Press.

Fisher, M. (2016) *The Weird and the Eerie*. Watkins Media. Kindle Edition.

Francis, M. (2016) Splitting the difference: on the queer-feminist divide in Scarlett Johansson's recent body politics. *Jump Cut*, 57. Available from: www.ejumpcut.org/archive/jc57.2016/-FrancisSkin/index.html (Accessed 4 May 2018).

Gittell, N. (2014) Scarlett Johansson's vanishing act. *The Atlantic*. Available from: www.theatlantic.com/entertainment/archive/2014/07/what-in-the-world-is-scarlett-johansson-up-to-lucy-under-the-skin-her-a-feminist-disappearing-act/375141 (Accessed 24 April 2018).

Gorfinkel, E. (2016) Sex, sensation and nonhuman interiority in *Under the Skin*. *Jump Cut*, 57. Available from: www.ejumpcut.org/archive/jc57.2016/-GorfinkelSkin/index.html (Accessed 4 May 2018).

Herzog, A. (2016) Star vehicle: labor and corporeal traffic in *Under the Skin*. *Jump Cut*, 57. Available from: www.ejumpcut.org/archive/jc57.2016/-HerzogSkin/index.html (Accessed 4 May 2018).

Hildebrand, L. (2016) On the matter of blackness in *Under the Skin*. *Jump Cut*, 57. Available from: www.ejumpcut.org/archive/jc57.2016/-HilderbrandUnderSkin/index.html (Accessed 4 May 2018).

Jonze, S. (2013) Email. Available from: www.vulture.com/2013/06/spike-jonze-replaced-samantha-morton-with-scarjo.html (Accessed 24 April 2018).

Lacan, J. (1977) *The Seminar of Jacques Lacan, Book XI: The Four Fundamental Concepts of Psychoanalysis*. Ed. J.-A. Miller. Trans. A. Sheridan. New York: Norton.

Lacan, J. (1998) *The Seminar of Jacques Lacan, Book XX: Encore*. Ed. J.-A. Miller. Trans. B. Fink. New York: Norton.

Lacan, J. (2006) *Écrits: The First Complete Edition in English*. Trans. B. Fink. New York: Norton.

Lane, A. (2014) Her again. *New Yorker*. Available from: www.newyorker.com/magazine/2014/03/24/her-again (Accessed 17 March 2018).

Loreck, J., Monaghan, W. and Stevens, K. (2018) Stardom and sf: a symposium on the sf films of Scarlett Johansson. *Science Fiction Film and Television*, 11(1), 1–4.

McGowan, T. (2007) *The Real Gaze: Film Theory After Lacan*. Albany: SUNY Press.

Mitchell, J. and Rose, J. (eds.) (1982) *Feminine Sexuality: Jacques Lacan and the école freudienne*. London: Macmillan Press.

Mulvey, L. (1975) Visual pleasure and narrative cinema. *Screen*, 16(3), 6–18.

Nguyen, S. (2014) The post-human ScarJo. *Los Angeles Review of Books*. Available from: https://lareviewofbooks.org/article/posthuman-scar-jo (Accessed 24 April 2018).
Osterweil, A. (2014) *Under the Skin*: the perils of becoming female. *Film Quarterly*, 67(4), 44–51.
Quinlivan, D. (2017) A dark and shiny place: the disembodied female voice, Irigarayan subjectivity and the political erotics of hearing *Her* (Spike Jonze, 2013). In T. Whittaker and S. Wright (eds.) *Locating the Voice in Film*. New York: Oxford University Press.
Riviere, J. (1986) Womanliness as a masquerade [1929]. In V. Burgin, J. Donald and C. Kaplan (eds.) *Formations of Fantasy*. London: Routledge.
Scott, K.-L. (2015) Orgasms without bodies. *World Picture*, 10. Available from: www.worldpicturejournal.com/WP_10/Scott_10.html (Accessed 21 February 2018).
Shaviro, S. (2014) Spike Jonze's HER. Available from: www.shaviro.com/Blog/?p=1186 (Accessed 11 May 2018).
Shetley, V. (2018) Performing the inhuman: Scarlett Johansson and sf film. *Science Fiction Film and Television*, 11(1), 13–19.
Silverman, K. (1988) *The Acoustic Mirror: The Female Voice in Psychoanalysis and Cinema*. Bloomington: Indiana University Press.
Soler, C. (2005) *What Lacan Said About Women: A Psychoanalytic Study*. New York: Other Press.
Stevens, A. (2007) Love and sex beyond identifications. In V. Voruz and B. Wolf (eds.) *The Later Lacan*. Albany: SUNY Press.
Stevens, K. (2018) Between attraction and anxiety: Scarlett Johansson, female knowledge and the mind–body split in *Lucy*. *Science Fiction Film and Television*, 11(1), 21–28.
Tunbridge, L. (2016) Scarlett Johansson's body and the materialization of voice. *Twentieth-Century Music*, 13(1), 139–152.
Tyrer, B. (2014) An atheist's guide to feminine jouissance: on *Black Swan* and the other satisfaction. In A. Piotrowska (ed.) *Embodied Encounters: New Approaches to Psychoanalysis and Cinema*. London: Routledge.
Tyrer, B. (2016) *Out of the Past: Lacan and Film Noir*. London: Palgrave Macmillan.
Verhaeghe, P. and Declerq, F. (2003) Lacan's analytical goal: "*Le Sinthome*" or the feminine way. In L. Thurston (ed.) *Re-Inventing the Symptom Essays on the Final Lacan*. New York: Other Press.
Žižek, S. (1994) *The Metastases of Enjoyment: On Women and Causality*. London: Verso.
Žižek, S. (1996) *The Indivisible Remainder: Essays on Schelling and Related Matters*. London: Verso.
Žižek, S. (2002) The Real of sexual difference. In S. Barnard and B. Fink (eds.) *Reading Seminar XX*. Albany: SUNY Press.
Žižek, S. (2004) Passion in the era of decaffeinated belief. Available from: www.lacan.com/passionf.htm (Accessed 11 May 2018).
Žižek, S. (2017) *Incontinence of the Void: Economico-Philosophical Spandrels*. Cambridge, MA: MIT Press.
Zupančič, A. (2017) *What Is Sex?* Cambridge, MA: MIT Press.

Filmography

Ex Machina (2015) Directed by Alex Garland. UK: Universal/Film4.
Ghost in the Shell (2017) Directed by Rupert Sanders. UK/China/India/Hong Kong/USA: Paramount/DreamWorks.
Her (2013) Directed by Spike Jonze. USA: AnnaPurna Pictures.

I Dream of Jeannie (1965–1970) USA: NBC.
Lost in Translation (2003) Directed by Sophia Coppola. USA/Japan: Focus Features/TFC/American Zoetrope.
Lucy (2014) Directed by Luc Besson. France/Taiwan/Germany: EuropaCorp.
Minority Report (2002) Directed by Steven Spielberg. USA: 20th Century Fox/DreamWorks.
Morvern Callar (2002) Directed by Lynne Ramsay. UK/Canada: BBC Films.
Under the Skin (2013) Directed by Jonathan Glazer. UK/USA/Switzerland/Poland: Film4/BFI.
Weird Science (1985) Directed by John Hughes. USA: Universal.

9

DESIRE, COMMITMENT AND THE TRANSFORMATIVE POWER OF TOUCH

The posthuman femme fatale in *Under the Skin*

Agnieszka Piotrowska and Joseph Jenner

The issue of what it means to be human has fascinated scholars and philosophers for centuries. The most traditional view has been that the ability to think, to be conscious, defines the human. In this regard, the capacity for thought separates the human from an unthinking world, but clearly there are other ways in which one could begin to think about what it means to be human, for example one's concern for the Other, the ethical ability to empathize or to give and receive love.[1] Here we want to offer a contribution to an ongoing discussion and suggest both the importance of touch in human interactions (an actual physical touching of the Other) as well as a discussion of what it might mean to be posthuman. Through an analysis of *Under the Skin* (Jonathan Glazer, 2013) we propose that touching in some circumstances might lead to a formation of posthuman subjectivity, the trajectory being from the inhuman through to the human and finally to the posthuman. The Anthropocene, a term that has gained traction in both the sciences and the humanities since it was theorized by Paul J. Crutzen and Eugene F. Stoermer in 2000, demands that humans understand their interconnectivity with a declining environment shaped by human and nonhuman forces alike. Accordingly, the notion of touch put forward in this chapter provides an experience of the subject's own assimilation into a chain of human and nonhuman being. We argue, then, that the significance of an intra-species touch could extend the notion of the human into the posthuman. This chapter combines Agnieszka Piotrowska's work on embodied psychoanalysis and the importance of the touch, and Joseph Jenner's research on posthumanism and science-fiction film. Our aspiration is to create a provocative encounter between areas of research that have not been sufficiently put into dialogue. Our work here thus aspires to take the "inbetween" further and constitute a metaphorical touching of different theoretical sites.

To begin with, we offer a significant vignette. Luc Besson's *Valerian and the City of a Thousand Planets* (2017) opens with the formation of a posthuman community based on touch. The film's pan-species greetings take place over a 700-year time span, in which a group of diverse crew members exchange touches with a range of human and nonhuman beings. First of all diverse ethnic groups from Earth appear: Africans, a group wearing Islamic dress, including both women and men, arrive. Then, over the centuries, nonhuman guests and immigrants begin to appear in increasingly unusual embodiment and attire. The greeting touch changes depending on the shape and bearing of each figure but the touch clearly is perceived as the beginning of any meaningful communication: the verbal exchanges follow only after that greeting touch, which is presented as an ancient inter-species sign of good will. One could put it differently, paraphrasing Derrida, that touch here denotes a positive movement towards the Other (2000: 25).[2]

We argue, therefore, that in *Under the Skin* the touch is a transformative moment for the film's protagonist, pushing her into a broader posthuman relation of life and matter. In this chapter we consider the alien woman as portrayed by Scarlett Johansson in *Under the Skin* as a posthuman femme fatale. In this context, we consider her adopted femininity both as an expression of male desire, and, as Jacques Lacan would put it, the object cause of desire or *l'objet petit a* (1999: 92), and as an embodied masculine fantasy. We define femme fatale as the female seductresses prevalent in the film noir genre of the 1940s and 1950s, characters who use their wiles and sexuality to manipulate men to their own ends. In *Under the Skin* the alien femme fatale also uses her sexuality to seduce men and use them. However, the alien woman's unexpected ability to give and receive a touch marks a dramatic shift in the film's narrative.

The narrative of *Under the Skin*

Under the Skin follows the trajectory of a nameless alien woman, henceforth the Woman, from a seductress in the guise of a fur and lipstick femme fatale to a lonely and vulnerable vagrant. For an alien and enigmatic purpose the Woman cruises around Glasgow, picking up single men without family. She then takes them back to her lair – a derelict house – which transforms into a cavernous black void as both undress, the man pursuing the Woman into a viscous black fluid that gradually dissolves his internal organs. The turning point in the narrative comes when the Woman picks up a man with neurofibromatosis, a condition in which tumours grow from the nerve tissue on his face. It is this interaction with someone living on the fringes of human society – shopping at Tesco in the middle of the night to hide his stigma – that signals a shift in the Woman's consciousness and in the film's story-world. In her ploy to seduce him, the Woman invites him to touch her face and hands as she drives him to her lair.

In the narrative of the film, the touch brings about a kinetic movement, as Derrida would put it, and as we discuss later in the chapter, this movement changes the stakes and the outcome. We argue that in *Under the Skin* the key moment of touch overcomes the nonhuman and produces a posthuman subject position in this film. In order to elaborate this proposition, we now turn our attention to a brief discussion of the relevant literature that defines the posthuman.

The posthuman

In her landmark text *How We Became Posthuman* (1999) Katherine N. Hayles rejects the Cartesian separation of mind and body apparent in some strands of posthumanism. For example, in 1988 Hans Moravec speculated that soon it will be possible to upload consciousness to a computer in an immaculate disconnection of mind from body (109–110). The implication is that, as was the case for Descartes, the body is a support for the mind and the body's material specificities do not bear upon the thinking subject and the type of thoughts the body enables or delimits. The important intervention that Hayles makes into posthuman discourse is to insist upon the *embodied* amalgamation of human and nonhuman elements. As Hayles writes: "embodiment makes clear that thought is a much broader cognitive function depending for its specificities on the embodied form enacting it" (1999: xiv). Inverting Moravec's posthuman, for Hayles the body helps to determine the kind of thoughts available to the thinking subject. If a brain was uploaded to a computer, this would fundamentally change the constitution of the subject. The body therefore is a fundamental aspect of the posthuman and it would be a mistake to treat the body as separate from the mind.

Usually, the posthuman figures encountered in science-fiction film involve technological prosthesis of the human subject, for example *Robocop* (Paul Verhoeven, 1987), *Iron Man* (Jon Favreau, 2008) and *Ghost in the Shell* (Rupert Sanders, 2017). Indeed, in these examples and others, despite the amalgamation of human and technology, the way these cyborgs are presented remains anthropocentric: depicting the struggle of the human self to retain their identity through their augmentation with the Other of technology. Samantha Holland understands what she terms "Cyborg Cinema" of the 1980s and early 1990s as perpetuating a Cartesian "mind–body problem" (1995: 157). The cyborgs of films such as *Terminator* (James Cameron, 1984), *Robocop 2* (Irvin Keshner, 1990) and *Eve of Destruction* (Duncan Gibbins, 1991) are interpreted against an authentic human self as a way to judge their authenticity. Ultimately, according to Holland, desire is what distinguishes humans from machines in the cyborg film. The narrative of "Cyborg Cinema" encourages the viewer to read the human within technology, and thus these films remain embedded in a Cartesian system of value that places the human above the nonhuman.

Unlike the movement into the human core of the prosthetic body, in *Under the Skin* the human skin overrides the alien interior. Ara Osterweil describes the encounter with the man with neurofibromatosis in *Under the Skin* as part of the Woman's "profound transformation", the "radical identification with alterity as the key to human empathy" (2014: 48). We agree with the notion of the profound transformation but question here whether this is "a radical identification" with human identity – and instead we propose that the moment of touching creates a moment of empathy with the unknowable Other, the Other that is outside the system, as the Woman is. The touching creates an encounter that constitutes the first step of the creation of the posthuman (as opposed to the nonhuman) subjectivity for the alien. Further, this cross-species encounter pushes beyond an association or identification with the human towards the posthuman. This moment of touching with a marginalized figure, much as she is, creates an apparent shift in her repetitive ritualistic process: she releases her quarry and turns away from her role as femme fatale seductress. To our minds, the narrative trajectory of *Under the Skin*, centred on this moment of transformation, reveals the posthuman constitution of the Woman that we define here as generative despite her ultimate perishing in the film.

In other words, the narrative of *Under the Skin* can be measured by the way the human façade of the Woman gradually comes to influence the nonhuman thinking subject. This is not a process of humanization, as some critics see it, but an acknowledgement of the fundamentally constitutive and embodied prosthesis of the posthuman subject position.[3] As Susan Hekman puts it: "the 'I' is a mangle composed of multiple elements" (2010: 100). With human epidermis and alien interior, the alien woman is a vacillating human–nonhuman assemblage whose subjectivity is inscribed in the posthuman reality of constant shifts and becomings.

Under the Skin continues science-fiction film's fascination with the ontological hybrid, yet the dynamic is reversed: the human is the prosthetic element of the nonhuman subject and attention is drawn to the human epidermis rather than the nonhuman interior. Rather than the human remaining the centre of the posthuman subject, in *Under the Skin* the nonhuman is the point of departure. The posthuman subject position is therefore cultivated with a minimum of anthropocentrism.

Antigone, desire and the femme fatale

The inversion of the posthuman subject leads us on to another reversal in the logic of the plot of *Under the Skin*. Piotrowska has argued elsewhere (2014, 2015, 2018) that it is productive to use the classic and archetypal figure of Antigone in Sophocles' play of 441 BC to think of a determined female stance against the patriarchal systems that fix the role of woman: Antigone moves from "a nice girl" to a nasty "inhuman" woman. Simplifying the movement in *Under the Skin* for clarity, it is indeed the opposite of the archetypal one. The "nasty" alien female individual who pursues men to their death discovers her desire by assuming a posthuman subjectivity. The Woman begins as the alien femme fatale, yet the moment of touch marks the film's paradigmatic shift towards a transformatory "inbetween" space. The Woman's posthuman desire is impossible to fulfil but is nonetheless a signifier of its generative nature. The similarity between the Antigonial archetype and the alien figure in *Under the Skin* is their determination to see through their desire no matter what. It is not that either character is planning to perish, it is rather that the quest to fulfil this desire appears to be more exigent and more demanding than initially suspected.

The femme fatale is one of the original, powerful "nasty woman" in cinema and much has been written about her.[4] She is usually immoral and beautiful. Both as a male fantasy and as a representation of female power, she holds endless appeal, which, we argue, originates not only from her sexuality and beauty, but because she offers a way out of the rigid patriarchal systems of power and authority. Traditionally in films such as *Double Indemnity* (Billy Wilder, 1944), or *The Postman Always Rings Twice* (Tay Garnett, 1946), this transient fantasy is immediately exposed as "nasty" – it is far too dangerous to let a character who manipulates men live her independent life – and so she is usually killed off in these films, or is occasionally domesticated (Doane 1991). This narrative trajectory also appears to take place in *Under the Skin* – the Woman gets her punishment in the end. However, we argue that her ability to assume posthuman subjectivity is a significant and subversive move.

It is the fidelity to one's own desire that links the femme fatale to the mythical figure of Antigone. Jacques Lacan in his Seminar VII claims that anybody's ethical choice will resonate with that of Antigone: "Even if you are not aware of it, the latent fundamental image of Antigone forms part of your morality" (1992: 284). Before we move to a further discussion of the posthuman female figure in *Under the Skin*, we turn here to a brief discussion of the ethics of "not giving up on one's desire" (ibid.: 305). It seems that the construction of the alien woman in the film corresponds to the inhuman inflexibility of Antigone. The cinematic text reworks the proposition of "not giving up" on one's desire in its construction of posthuman subjectivity. Below we briefly summarize the Lacanian notion of the fidelity to one's desire on the one hand and, on the other hand, the notion of the object cause of desire, *l'objet petit a*, which we argue was the Woman's initial purpose in the story-world of the film: for her to become the subject the transformation through touch has to take place. It is possible therefore to use some classic psychoanalytical notions in theorizing the move from the nonhuman to a posthuman female subject.

According to Lacan, Sophocles lets us see Antigone's unfeminine strong-mindedness, which frightens the Chorus: in her discussion with Ismene, her sister, she appears hostile and stubborn. Lacan points to the Chorus' disdain for Antigone: they cry out a Greek word "ωμός", which Lacan says one might translate as "inflexible", but more than this

> it literally means something uncivilized, something raw. And the word "raw" comes closest, when it refers to eaters of raw flesh. That's the Chorus' point of view (. . .) This is then how the enigma of Antigone is presented to us: she is *inhuman*.
>
> *(Ibid.: 263, our emphasis)*

In his discussions of Antigone, Lacan focuses on the word used in Sophocles' original: *atë*, which can be translated as "fate", "destiny" and "human misery".[5] Lacan interprets *atë* as a narrow range within which to operate and it is important to find out what one's desire is and then to follow it to the end. Not everybody must make such a dramatic choice: "One does or does not approach *atë*, and when one approaches it, it is because of something that is linked to a beginning and a chain of events" (ibid.: 264). Antigone's *atë* is that she is the daughter of Jocasta and Oedipus, the parents who unwillingly committed murders and incest, and that both of her brothers took part in a war against each other and that they are now both dead. This she cannot undo. But she can decide what to do when faced with Creon's unreasonable edict.

Using briefly this idea in our discussion of *Under the Skin*, the alien's *atë* is that she is not a real woman because she is not human. It is here also that one could take issue with Osterweil's paper in which she says, among other observations, that "*Under the Skin* is an insightful film about female desire" (2014: 44–45). The Woman is not a woman and her desire is to become one. She does not menstruate, have children and indeed cannot fuck.[6] Her awoken desire is to do with wanting to be a female but this always eludes her.

This is her tragedy and within the story-world of the film it allows for a dramatic sequence of events towards the end of the film, which the spectator can perceive as cruel, and perhaps in some way replicating the familiar plot trajectory of the film noir genre in which the femme fatale as the representation of dangerous femininity has to be eliminated. One could theorize the ending in different ways and certainly one of them would be that of a metaphorization of extreme despair caused by the human experience of Lack, underscored by the Woman's otherness.

There are scenes in which the Woman observes herself in the mirror, bringing to mind Lacan's Mirror Stage:

> From this time on, lack, gap, splitting will be its mode of being. It will attempt to fill its (impossible, unfillable) lack. Its recognition of lack signals an ontological rift with nature or the Real. This gap will propel it into seeking an identificatory image of its own stability and permanence (the imaginary), and eventually language (the symbolic) by which it hopes to fill the Lack.
>
> *(Grosz 1990: 35)*

Film theorists in the heyday of psychoanalytically fuelled film theory of the 1980s are known to have picked up the idea of Lack as relevant to the experience of the spectator:

> [T]he child is born into experience of lack, what Lacan terms "*manqué à être*" (the "want to be"); and the subject's subsequent history consists of a series of attempts to figure and overcome this lack, a project that is doomed to failure. Though the form and experience of lack may alter, the basic reality of it persists and defies representation.
>
> *(Lapsley & Westlake 2006: 67)*

Lacan in his later work and certainly by Seminar XI focused also on the notion of *l'objet petit a*, the "object-cause of desire", which triggers desire but is not itself necessarily it: *l'objet petit a* is in itself unattainable but the subject's drives circle around "it" (Lacan 1998: 179). Partial objects such as breasts, faeces and also voice and gaze can be involved in causing desire but are not as such *l'objet petit a*. The Woman in *Under the Skin* functions in the film as *l'objet petit a* incarnate, as a partial object that functions in the male psyche not as a real person but as their symptom.

In Seminar XX Lacan stresses that if "the Other is only reached if it attaches itself (. . .) to *a*, the cause of desire, then love is also addressed to the semblance of being" (1999: 92). The two Others in the touching encounters gain subjectivity – for the Woman it creates a trajectory ultimately tragic but that lifts her from being an object to being a subject. Her agency allows her to create a posthuman subjectivity, a desire she is committed to "to the end" once it is awoken through touch.

It is here that we turn yet again to the Lacanian notion of the ethical act consisting of "not giving up on one's desire" and, once the commitment is made, to be able to be faithful to it "beyond the limit" as Lacan puts it (1992: 305), or "to the end" in Žižek's words (1994: 61), and that Piotrowska has discussed elsewhere (2014, 2015, 2017). Bonnie Honig in her book *Antigone Interrupted* (2013) offers both a review of the scholarly work to date on Antigone as well as her own interpretations of what she might mean in the history of ideas and defiant stances against male authority. Honig's crucial move is to propose Antigone's act as interrupting a circle of trauma and chaos: her move is a rupture that stops Creon's tyrannical rule and decades of fratricidale wars (ibid.: 45). Her act changes things and they can never be the same again within the story-world of the play. In *Under the Skin* the moment of touch signals a rupture that instigates the Women's desire and disrupts the brutality of the alien scheme as she turns away from her role as femme fatale seductress.

In terms of re-defining the neo femme fatale as an ethical figure, Antigone's stance of not giving up on one's desire is useful. The nasty women in the *neo noir* films *Red Road* (Andrea Arnold, 2006), *Gone Girl* (David Fincher, 2014) and *The Girl on the Train* (Tate Taylor, 2016) as well as in television drama (Carrie in *Homeland*, Jessica in *Suits*, etc.) are connected to these early film noir prototypes in their narrative function, using their sexual wiles and deceit to inspire men to commit transgressions.[7] Yet crucially, these neo femmes fatales are instilled with an agency that is lacking from their precursors: they are the perpetrators as well as the driving force of the deeds.

Much like these neo femmes fatales, the alien seductress in *Under the Skin*, initially, is a calculating and nasty woman who seduces and destroys men. Like her femme fatale precursors from the noir film, it could be interpreted that the Woman is ultimately punished for her agency at the end of the film, in which she is burnt alive by a man who attempts to rape her. It is indeed disappointing that the beginning of the imagining of a different being – the posthuman one – is, in this cinematic text, returned to the familiar binary of a man being violent towards a woman. We want to make an observation here from the source material for Jonathan Glazer's film is Michel Faber's 2000 novel of the same name, which provides an alternative means of responding to the gendered ending of the film. While in the film some things remain mysterious (who the alien woman really is, what her purpose on this planet is, etc.), they are clear in the book: she is harvesting men as a meat delicacy for her home planet.

Glazer's adaptation of the film, on which he worked with two different screenwriters before settling with Walter Campbell, diverges radically from the source material that we feel is significant and worth noting. Some of the Woman's, named Isserley in the book, key encounters are retained, such as an attempted rape that does not take place in a forest but at a roadside and in which, unlike the film, Isserley turns the tables on her assailant and brutally kills him. At the close of the novel, Isserley crashes her car and is immobilized in the front seat. Before the ambulance arrives she detonates a self-destruct device so that she and her Earth-bound community of aliens are not discovered. The decision to end her life is ambivalent, both as a fail-safe to protect her alien comrades who are all figured as male, but it is also presented as an act of self-determination, logical in terms of the ethical stance of "not giving up on one's desire" as discussed above. That sense of agency on the part of the Woman is lost in the final encounter with the rapist at the end of the film. It is beyond the scope of this chapter to offer speculations about why the director changed the final narrative of the work but we feel it is worth quoting the final passage of the novel at length to illustrate this shift towards an Antigone-like posthuman self-determination:

> The atoms that had been herself would mingle with the oxygen and nitrogen in the air. Instead of ending up buried in the ground, she would become part of the sky: that was the way to look at it. Her invisible remains would combine, over time, with all the wonders under the sun. When it snowed, she would be part of it, falling softly to earth, rising up again with the snow's evaporation. When it rained, she would be there in the spectral arch that spanned from firth to ground. She would help to wreathe the fields in mists, and yet would always be transparent to the stars. She would live forever.
>
> *(Faber 2000: 296)*

The cosmic metaphors of nature and immanence are echoed in the film's resolution when the ash that rises from the burning body of the Woman mingles with the snowflakes that fall towards the screen. The embrace of the molecular is the fate of Isserley in the novel and the Woman in the film, which can be seen as a logical conclusion of the *female*/alien exclusion from subjecthood in that they are returned back to a nature (female) excluded from culture (male). Yet also, the film and novel registers here a subjectivity that is beyond the patriarchal strictures of human society, something claimed by Isserley and the Woman, which is set in motion by the moment of touch in the film. We turn, now, to the generation of subjectivity provided by the look, before working through the Woman's subjectivity in *Under the Skin*.

The eye and the gaze

We want to consider in this section the importance of the gaze as the carrier of "lostness". In the first instance, the Woman attracts the men because they find her beautiful. She is visible to them as an object of their desire or as the fantasy of the object they desire. The Woman becomes the object-cause of desire, *l'objet petit a.* The touch and the brief conversation about what it means to feel to be the Other in the film, when the Woman is in conversation with the man with neurofibromatosis, leads to the move from the object to the subject. Lacan conjures a notion of "lamella", a pure form of this "lostness", the life instinct, the primordial form of the libido (1998: 205). The Woman embodies the phallic masculine desire before her encounter with the disabled man, which makes her understand her own otherness as a basis of her subjectivity rather than an embodiment of the desire of the others, or an actual incarnation of the notion of "lamella". Paul Verhaeghe, in his discussion of the notion of lamella, writes about the inevitable "phallicization" of the desire arising from "the original lack" (2002: 133). One could argue that the Woman, as designed by her male superiors, is meant to enact male desires in a cyclical and repetitive way. The encounter with the man with neurofibromatosis catapults her out of the lamella state and out of gender discussions.

Referring to Maurice Merleau-Ponty's *The Visible and the Invisible* (1964), in Seminar XI Lacan states that the gaze can function as an object. The central assumption of Seminar XI is that there is a pre-existing gaze in the world. The gaze gives us the distinction between what belongs to the Imaginary order and what belongs to the order of the Real (Lacan 1998). Psychoanalyst Carlo Bonomi talks about the risk of being transformed into an object of the gaze of the other. Worse, there is a possibility of suddenly feeling "shame" arising thereof, which could cause "a sudden collapse of the self provoked by the gaze" (2010: 113). One could argue perhaps that something of this shame happens between the beautiful alien and the man with neurofibromatosis who tries to avoid the gaze of the Other, as previously mentioned, by skulking at night so as not to become the object of the cruel gaze of the public. He wants to be invisible. It is the alien posthuman femme fatale who, we argue, "sees" him as a (post)human, feels empathy for him and lets him go.

Bonomi gives clinical examples of patients hiding behind dark glasses in order to create safe places, "shelters": "Our visibility is dangerous because, in certain situations, when our vulnerability is enhanced, we experience visibility as a threat to the core of our being" (ibid.: 111). He calls this core "soul" – not perhaps a term that either Freud or Lacan would use and points out defences, which, he says, concern making the body filled with libido and "thick and real" like a shield (ibid.: 113). When these strategies fail, an individual might feel exposed to the "evil eye", which has links both to Freud's "uncanny" but also to myths and beliefs in non-Western cultures and societies (ibid.: 113–114). The disembodied gaze might cause a fear of "sterility, disease, and death" (ibid.: 114). In *Under the Skin* the gaze is the powerful element in the film's story-world *until* the touch replaces its importance. However, much of the film's initial tension lies in the different relationships between the look and the gaze as we hope to demonstrate.

Under the Skin opens with the creation of a nonhuman, alien eye that guides the spectator's response to the human environments of the film. Beginning in blackness, a white pinprick appears centre screen, a halo of light arcing around the growing circle before it bursts into the luminescence of the film's big bang inception. Next, a series of curved shapes – a sphere and a torus – approach each other through the darkness in a cosmic, planetary alignment. Then follows perhaps the most disorienting shot in this sequence: the form of a black planet suspended centre screen, fringed by light. From screen right another speck of light heads on a collision course for the planet, before overlapping and revealing itself as another circle that dwarfs the other. Here, the impression of flatness takes on the depth of three dimensions as the perception of the spectator's eye becomes accustomed to the logic of an alien space.

The construction of the eye, then, is presented as a planetary constellation of forms and does what film can do best: enlarge the miniscule into the gigantic and expand the spectator's notion of life from the marginal to the cosmic. Following the abstract forms that culminate in the image of the Woman's completed eye, rapid shots of flowing rivers take the spectator into nature until the edit settles on a curved road at night, illuminated by the moon. In parallel with the film's opening, a white pinprick appears in the distance before moving closer to the screen, guiding the spectator's eye through the black space of the nocturnal Scottish countryside. Much like the foaming water in the rivers, the speck of light navigates the undulating road, growing in size as it crosses the plane of the screen.

In the opening eye-construction scene the spectator is invited to view the Scottish landscape, and by extension urban Glasgow, with the perception of the Woman. This look estranges the spectator from the quotidian familiarity of human society, a perception associated with the Woman's initial disregard for life, though as spectators we potentially perceive things differently from her. In perhaps the most shocking early scene in the film, the Woman witnesses a man, woman and dog struggle against the Scottish tide as a swimmer goes to rescue them. Their suffering is visible to us, the spectators, but not to the Woman. The Woman bashes the swimmer round the head with a rock and drags him off, leaving a crying baby, abandoned by his drowned family, to die on the beach. Osterweil sees this scene on the beach as one of the first transformative moments in the film for the Woman – placed radically outside of the association between "the relation between humanity and empathy" (2014: 48). We take issue with this reading. This moment is not transformative. Nor is it right to see it as a particularly unique scene in a film full of examples of the Woman annihilating men, totally lacking any empathy. She has no interest in them because she is the Other and they are the Other for her. The moment of transformation, as well as the paradigmatic shift takes place later, in her encounter with the man with neurofibromatosis. Unlike Osterweil, however, we stress that it is the moment of touch in this encounter that signals the true paradigm shift in *Under the Skin*.

The gaze and the touch

We understand the posthuman subject position as one that navigates beyond the poles of human and nonhuman. In this we propose that the Lacanian "gaze" is able to belong to this posthuman system, as within the initial Lacanian enunciation it can be separate from the human subject (Lacan 1999: 65). Unlike the nonhuman, then, the embodied posthuman describes the human and nonhuman assemblage inherent in this subject position. This amalgamated subject position – both in terms of the subject's bodily construction as well as emotional availability – is what we are designating as the posthuman.[8] This posthuman subject position therefore is cultivated through the multiple cinematic modes that make up *Under the Skin*. Across the 1 hour and 43 minutes of the film, the blending of hidden cameras, documentary hand-held shots of Glasgow central, sweeping vistas of the Scottish landscape, the alien void scenes, as well as the use of visual and special effects, attune the spectator to a variety of different cinematic ontologies that interact with one another. While a reality effect is inserted into the film through the use of improvised dialogue and documentary footage that exposes the material reality of Glasgow, the artificial spaces of the alien voids do not allow the spectator to take any particular cinematic reality for granted. In the next section, we begin to examine these void sequences, which contain, as we have seen, this layering of the material world into the abstract space of form.

From gazing to touching

Through close analyses of the seduction sequences in *Under the Skin*, we can see how the film style registers a shift in consciousness, from the distancing effect of the look to the embrace of different modes of embodiment, instigated by the alien woman's contact with the man with the facial disfigurement.

Inserted into the documentary, quotidian reality of *Under the Skin*'s urban Glasgow are scenes played out against a space that is empty, infinite and alien. These are seduction scenes, in which the Woman lures hapless single men to a slow death in black and empty spaces. Bodies are abstracted, overlaying and enfolded by the black screen as they draw a horizontal line across space, dropping pools of colour on an invisible surface as man and woman strip off their clothes. The bodies move in a straight line, as if on an invisible stage; the woman slowly walks backwards, gazing off-screen in a reverse shot matched with the forward strut and look of the male victim. The delimited movement raises questions about whether this void is infinitely cavernous or indeed completely without depth, destabilizing the spectator's orientation in an encounter with nonhuman space. Sexual desire becomes formalized, the denuded star-image of Scarlett Johansson, the camera tilting down her body as it take in her form, reveals a coquettish, balletic posture as one arched leg feigns to cover her modesty. The male targets of these solicitations aim to consume this classic erotic image but perish in their hypnotized pursuit, sinking into the viscous fluid that will eventually dissolve their internal organs. These scenes become ritualistic in their repetition: oneiric fantasies of seduction and death that dramatize but radically reject the human, played out for an alien purpose and from a strange, nonhuman perspective.

The style of this void sequence is defined by the multiple modes of existence that occupy the space of the screen simultaneously. Yet, very often, screens in the digital age of science-fiction film have a stasis, depthlessness and emphasis on surface aesthetics that call to mind the artifice of green screens. For example the early virtual reality effects of *Tron* (Steven Lisberger, 1982) and the "construct" spaces of *The Matrix* (The Wachowskis, 1999). Following Vivian Sobchack's discussion of a postmodern aesthetic in her book *Screening Space*, these blank screens have specific connotations of loss of originality, the unlimited possibility of recreation and representation, and a flattening of ontology between subject and object (1997: 237). Yet in *Under the Skin* the lived-in candour of bodies placed within or against the blank screen offer a depth that resists their ontological reduction to the technological mediation of postmodern ideology. The smears of faeces, erect penises and facial tumours of a man with neurofibromatosis share the same space as the star image and denuded form of Johansson. This is not the infinite recreation of simulated forms, as in *Tron* and *The Matrix*, but the embrace of multiple types of embodiment. There is an ontological relationality between forms that is based, unlike the postmodern reduction, upon the diversity of beings.

Indeed, even Johansson's star image in *Under the Skin*, emphasized by its placement among an ensemble of amateur and non-actors, is vitiated by the scrutiny of the camera. This is a process that occurs across the film, marked out by these void scenes in which the embrace of multiple types of embodiment is initially resisted but ultimately overcome. In the void that follows the nightclub scene, the Woman and her victim are not contained within the frame until the long two shot as he descends into the liquid, the edit presenting a series of medium point-of-view and reaction shots leading up to this moment. There is a strange displacement within this long shot, as the eyeline does not seem to match up, enhancing the dreamlike tone of an exchange that promises contact but is precisely about denial and rejection.

In the filming process both actors performed this sequence separately before being put together in the edit, perhaps accounting for this subtle mismatch in eyeline (Stasukevich 2014: 50). Consequently, while in the shot/reverse-shot dynamic the spatial demarcation of the Woman and victim is upheld, even in the shared space of the two shot there is a an invisible line that continues this spatial separation of – species, gender, celebrity – difference. Of course, it is important also that these are nude scenes, or at least fully so for the men, and the production technique upholds a certain degree of discretion, or minimizing of an all-too-human embarrassment in the bare and uncomfortable proximity of a naked male amateur and female star. The vulnerability of nakedness emphasizes the categories of man and woman and star and non-star, the division of the image maintaining the integrity of Johansson as a female Hollywood A-list actor in that her nakedness counts for more than her male counterparts in these scenes. There is therefore a subtle split within the image that ultimately maintains the categories of value between human/nonhuman, man/woman and star/non-star. The off-screen gazes then, both from the man to the alien woman and vice versa, continue to signal the distanciation and empowerment of the gaze.

Touching

The alien femme fatale discovers her posthuman desire through being touched by a human living with neurofibromatosis but there is also a simple exchange between them in which their mutual otherness is established. In her encounter with the man, who caresses the alien woman's face and hands, a paradigmatic shift occurs that acknowledges the posthuman embrace of multiple modes of embodiment. We now turn to a brief discussion of the importance of touch, drawing from a variety of relevant traditions.[9]

In his discussion of Jean-Luc Nancy's *Corpus*, Jacques Derrida acknowledges the importance of touch in Descartes' *Six Meditations*, stressing that to touch means "to tamper with, to change, to displace, to call into question; thus it is invariably a setting in motion, a kinetic experience" (2000: 25). This is in direct opposition to the colonial and postcolonial notions of ideas being set in stone, what Edward Said in his discussions of colonialism called "frozen, fixed" and deeply patriarchal and conservative (2008: 208). Touching, Derrida reminds us, is a harbinger of change – it can be a progressive or reactionary change, but nonetheless it is a movement, and when accompanied by a voice and language, it can become explosive and revolutionary. It is for these reasons that the touch is often prohibited in many cultural and historical contexts in which difference is a marker of danger – in recent history people of different colour were forbidden to touch each other as recently as the 1990s under the apartheid in South Africa: touching was considered too risky as the people concerned might get too close and abandon the artificial delineations of privilege. In *Under the Skin* the demarcation of bodies reinforces the fixity of categories – male/female, star/non-star, human/nonhuman – whereas the movement of touch signals a flow of embodiments contained with the frame simultaneously, thus moving from human to posthuman ways of being in the world. Finally, in the film, it is touch that changes the story-world of the Woman.

In European history, by the Middle Ages the Christian dualism of body and soul had led to a certain circumspection about the touch, a potentially transgressive act that could lead to a transformation of a relationship that might shake the status quo. "*Noli me tangere*" – Latin for "don't touch me" or "don't tread on me" – the words attributed to Christ in St John's Gospel when Mary Magdalene recognizes him after the resurrection and wants to touch him (Piotrowska 2017: 30). Christ is delighted that she can *see* him but doesn't let her touch him: "*Noli me tangere*": "don't touch me for I am not of this world any more, I am just a briefly embodied spirit – already assigned for greater travel" (ibid.). In the Gospel, Christ's bodily existence is already over but the dictum of "don't touch" became an important way of living in medieval times. One could argue that this dictum affected and was affected by two-dimensional art, which avoided representing the body as it actually was – a state of affairs only changed in the Renaissance with its return to the celebration of human form coming from antiquity, which provided different approaches to the physicality of the touch. It is worth, however, recalling that touching and voice also in fact have a vital role in Christ's life according to the Gospels: he touches those who need healing (in Mark we have a clear evocation of this: "lay hands on the sick and they shall recover" [Mark 16: 18]); he touches Lazarus and tells him to "rise" and of course he famously defends Mary Magdalene ("May he who is without sin cast the first stone" [John 8: 7]) before letting her touch him, quite intimately, by washing his feet (Luke 7:36–50). The "don't touch me" dictum only comes when Christ's bodily existence is in fact over. Derrida mentions that, "Jesus the saviour is touching, he is the one who touches, and most often with his hand, and most in order to purify, heal or resuscitate – save, in a word" (2000: 100).

We want to point out the obvious difference in the examples above and what takes place in the *Under the Skin* encounter: touch in the Western canon is given by the one who is in some way "the powerful one" and is a representative of God or the power bestowed on the royalty by the divine. In *Under the Skin*, the subversive potential of the scene lies in the fact that the touch is performative in a reverse situation – it is invited by the Woman who is the powerful one here, even without the knowledge of her actual nature – but the gesture is performed by the one with apparently no power: the marginalized man living with facial disfigurement. It is the quiet beauty of the scene that this gesture of a person with no power engenders the transformation, and puts in motion the Woman's shift from the nonhuman to the posthuman. That is, the touch is a transformative encounter that disrupts hierarchies of power and situates the Woman in an interrelated community of other beings, including the human and nonhuman, and thus in the relational position of the posthuman. In *Under the Skin*, the touch is no longer associated with transcendence but with the immanent entanglements of diverse embodiments.

In the final void sequence the style shifts when the Woman lures the man with neurofibromatosis, and the categories of man/woman, star/non-star and human/nonhuman maintained in the previous void sequences are resolutely undone. This scene frames both the Woman and the man within the same space, breaching the spatial divisions of the previous sequences. First of all, an alien figure, black and sleek, walks towards the camera while we hear the voices of the man and Woman – "It's cold," he says. "I won't let that stop us," she replies. There is here a comical breakdown of the shock impact of an alien species witnessed for the first time. The jangle of a belt buckle, rip of a zip being undone and the reproachful lament of the man overlay the sinister image of this new species walking silently and ominously towards the camera in an awkward layering of different registers. The relationship between sound and image in this shot enfolds male and female voice, alien and human image, and destabilizes responses to these different embodiments. Unlike the previous void scenes, the back-and-forward motion of the characters is framed by a medium close-up that contains *both* within the image.

When the man turns to the camera to look around him, his face is placed alongside that of Johansson's; we have here an image of complementarity, disfigurement existing alongside the star image of Johansson. This latter void scene aligns difference in an expression of multiple modes of embodiment, creating a posthuman perspective that escapes the capture of categories retained earlier on in the film by the division maintained by the gaze. That this is a pivotal scene, which immediately precedes the Woman's apparent release of her quarry and ultimate rejection of her role as alien seductress, shows that this perspective ushers in a different mode of becoming. The alien femme fatale steps out of her script of luring men into her den of destruction without any physical contact.

Concluding remarks

Just before the alien woman releases the man with facial disfigurement, she catches a glimpse of herself in a mirror. In a protracted shot that lasts for just over a minute she stares at her own image. This evokes the Lacanian importance of the gaze and evokes the Mirror Stage in which an infant feels "jubilation" at misrecognizing herself in the mirror. Here the alien Woman is in an infancy of her subjectivity too but her moment of reflection is quickly interrupted. Off-screen, a buzzing distracts her contemplation and the camera's attention turns to a fly banging against the glass window of a door. In an abrupt shift of scale, the film then cuts to an extreme close-up as the alien woman's eye fills the screen. The eye, the look, is afforded a proximity witnessed only at the beginning of the film after the construction of the alien eye. The logic of the shot/reverse-shot pattern of editing places the fly as the recipient of the alien woman's look, yet her stare directly at the camera also calls upon the spectator's presence here. Stylistically, the moment of contact with the man with facial disfigurement transforms the power of the look in *Under the Skin*. Rather than the look signifying distance and rejection, it now embraces multiple modes of embodiment – the spectator, fly and then the man with facial disfigurement who is released in the next shot.

The look loses its power to put the object at a distance, and instead takes on the proximity of contact. This tactile look is discussed by Maurice Blanchot in his essay "The Essential Solitude" (1999). In the initial distanciation implied by the look, Blanchot writes that: "seeing implies distance, the decision that causes separation, the power not to be in contact and to avoid the confusion of contact" (1999: 412). Following the dynamic of the look, Blanchot identifies the experiential impossibility of such distanciation. Seeing becomes a "contact at a distance (. . .) the split, which had been the possibility of seeing, solidifies, right inside the gaze, into impossibility" (ibid.: 413). The object of the gazing subject comes to overpower the distance of seeing and instead becomes the vertiginous experience of an encounter. In *Under the Skin* the extreme-close up of the Woman's eye evokes this "contact at a distance", which is then demolished and re-formulated through the moment of touch.

Many contemporary science-fiction films, including *Ex Machina* (Alex Garland, 2014), *Ghost in the Shell* (Rupert Sanders, 2017) and *Annihilation* (Alex Garland, 2018) draw attention to the surface and skin in a similar fashion to *Under the Skin*. In *Ex Machina*, the android Ava (Alicia Vikander) never touches another human, except in the final violent encounter, and only has moments of contact with other machines, thus leading to the exclusion of the human (figured as male). At the close of *Annihilation*, the film's human protagonist, Lena (Natalie Portman), encounters an alien that performs as her double. The alien takes on the appearance of Lena, and copies her movements exactly. This moment of mimesis, culminating in the two figures holding hands, signals a transfer in the becoming-alien of the film's human protagonist. It is clear that the contact of human skin that masks a nonhuman interior is of special interest in contemporary science-fiction. As we have seen, in *Under the Skin* it is possible to discuss the film and its character's transformation using a variety of aesthetic and cinematic ontologies, including those traditionally not held in one space, namely psychoanalysis and posthuman subjectivity. The theoretical frameworks of this chapter touch in the void space of *Under the Skin*, performing a posthuman encounter between frameworks that are normally kept at a distance. The film therefore creates a thought space with which to engage and redefine the relationship with the Other or nonhuman, and in doing so generates a new, posthuman subjectivity.

Notes

1 For a discussion of what it might mean to be human see Connolly, Franck and Janis (2000).
2 To touch, he says, means "to tamper with, to change, to displace, to call into question; thus it is invariably a setting *in motion, a kinetic experience*" (see Derrida 2000). The motley human and nonhuman embodiments in the opening of *Valerian* are brought into an interconnected, posthuman community through a ceremony of cross- race, culture, gender and species touching.
3 For the "humanization" of the Woman's character arc see Osterweil (2014) and Redmond (2016).
4 See, for example, Bronfen (2004), Copjec (1993) and Doane (1991).
5 *Atë* can be also translated as a delusion that leads to a disaster – this note was kindly given to Piotrowska by Professor Richard Seaford, Professor of Classic and Ancient History at the University of Exeter in their discussions on Antigone.
6 Elsewhere, Elena Gorfinkel (2016) has discussed the "corporeal intractability" of the Woman.
7 The move to include *Red Road* as a *neo noir* might be seen as controversial, but we argue that its themes of scheming to commit the crime, entrapment and the use of sexuality could be related to that tradition. However, the trope of punishment is resolved in a different way following Jackie's embodied sexual encounter with her imagined enemy – which changes the way the narrative unfolds.
8 Rosi Braidotti similarly posits a *bios/zoë* subject, which unites human life with life in a broader sense. See Braidotti (2010).
9 See also Piotrowska (2017).

Bibliography

Blanchot, M. (1999) The Essential Solitude. In Quasha, G. (ed.) *The Station Hill Blanchot Reader: Fiction and Literary Essays*. Trans. Davis, L. New York: Barry Town.

Bonomi, C. (2010) Narcissism as Mastered Visibility: The Evil Eye and the Attack of the Disembodied Gaze. *International Forum of Psychoanalysis*, 19, 110–119.

Braidotti, R. (2010) The Politics of "Life Itself" and New Ways of Dying. In Coole, D. and Frost, S. (eds.) *New Materialisms: Ontology, Agency, and Politics*. Durham, NC: Duke University Press.

Bronfen, E. (2004) Femme Fatale: Negotiations of Tragic Desire. *New Literary History*, 35(1), 103–116.

Connolly, C., Franck, F. and Janis, R. (eds.) (2000) *What Does It Mean to Be Human? Reverence for Life Reaffirmed by Responses from Around the World*. New York: St. Martin's Press.

Copjec, J. (1993) *Shades of Noir: A Reader*. New York: Verso.

Crutzen, P. J. and Stoermer, E. F. (2000) The Anthropocene. *Global Change Newsletter*, 41, 17–18.

Derrida, J. (2000) *On Touching: Jean-Luc Nancy*. Trans. C. Irizarry. Stanford, CA: Stanford University Press.

Doane, M. A. (1991) *Femmes Fatales: Feminism, Film Theory, Psychoanalysis*. New York: Routledge.

Faber, M. (2000) *Under the Skin*. Edinburgh: Canongate.

Gorfinkel, E. (2016) Sex, Stimulation and Nonhuman Interiority in *Under the Skin*. *Jump Cut*, [online] 57, www.ejumpcut.org/archive/jc57.2016/-GorfinkelSkin/index.html (Accessed 15 November 2018).

Grosz, E. (1990) *Jacques Lacan: A Feminist Introduction*. London: Routledge.

Hayles, K. N. (1999) *How We Became Posthuman: Virtual Bodies in Cybernetics, Literature, and Informatics*. Chicago, IL: University of Chicago Press.

Hekman, S. (2010) *The Material of Knowledge: Feminist Disclosures*. Indianapolis, IN: Indiana University Press.

Holland, S. (1995) Descartes Goes to Hollywood: Mind, Body and Gender in Contemporary Cyborg Cinema. In Burrows, R. and Featherstone, M. (eds.) *Cyberspace, Cyberbodies, Cyberpunk: Cultures of Technological Embodiment*. London: Sage.

Honig, B. (2013) *Antigone Interrupted*. Cambridge: Cambridge University Press.

Lacan, J. (1992) *Seminar VII: The Ethics of Psychoanalysis 1959–1960*. London: Taylor & Francis.

Lacan, J. (1998) Seminar XI. In Miller, J.-A. (ed.) *The Four Fundamental Concepts of Psychoanalysis*. London and New York: W. W. Norton.

Lacan, J. (1999) *Seminar XX: On Feminine Sexuality, the Limits of Love and Knowledge*. London and New York: W. W. Norton.

Lapsley, R. and Westlake, M. (2006) *Film Theory: An Introduction*. 2nd ed. Manchester: Manchester University Press.

Moravec, H. (1988) *Mind Children: The Future of Robot and Human Intelligence*. Cambridge, MA: Harvard University Press.

Osterweil, A. (2014) Under the Skin: The Perils of Becoming Female. *Film Quarterly*, 67(4), 44–51.

Piotrowska, A. (2014) *Psychoanalysis and Ethics in Documentary Film*. London: Routledge.

Piotrowska, A. (ed.) (2015) *Embodied Encounters: New Approaches to Psychoanalysis and Cinema*. London: Routledge.

Piotrowska, A. (2017) *Black and White: Cinema, Politics and the Arts in Zimbabwe*. London: Routledge.

Piotrowska, A. (2018) *The Nasty Woman and the Neo Femme Fatale in Contemporary Cinema*. London: Routledge.

Redmond, S. (2016) Sounding Loneliness in Under the Skin. *Senses of Cinema* [online] 78 (March), http://sensesofcinema.com/2016/feature-articles/sounding-loneliness-in-under-the-skin (Accessed 3 October 2018).

Said, E. W. (2008) *Orientalism*. New York: Vintage Books.

Sobchack, V. (1997) *Screening Space: The American Science Fiction Film*. New Brunswick, NJ: Rutgers University Press.

Stasukevich, I. (2014) Alien Ways. *American Cinematographer: The International Journal of Film & Digital Production Techniques*, 95(5), 44–53.

Verhaeghe, P. (2002) Lacan's Answer to the Classical Mind/Body Deadlock: Retracing Freud's *Beyond*. In Barnard, S. and Fink, B. (eds.) *Reading Seminar XX*. New York: New York State University Press.

Žižek, S. (1994) *The Metastases of Enjoyment: Six Essays on Woman and Causality*. New York: Verso.

10

ANNAMARILYN

Queer tales of femininity

Wendy Leeks

Introduction: telling tales

Anna Freud and Marilyn Monroe were both subjects of psychoanalysis and have been, in Elisabeth Young-Bruehl's phrase 'subject to biography' (the title of her book of essays, 1998). Otherwise, they and the lives they led were very different. It may seem eccentric to read about them side-by-side, in tandem, as I have been doing for approaching five years now. Yet, there are points of co-incidence[1] in these lives as lived and in the 'lives' that have been written about them. It is an act of perverse reading, which was sparked off by a series of coincidences and co-incidences – spatial, temporal and conceptual – and spurred on by the discovery of conjunctions in the ways these two so-different women have been written about. These points of co-incidence[2] are like the threads that tack the layers of a quilt together, forming the ground for a pattern or a story. Here, I will trace out some of these threads to show patterns in the 'life-writing' not only about these two dead women, but, as I contend, about women even now.

The most significant thread that draws the two women together is psychoanalysis itself. From Sigmund Freud onwards this discipline has been inflected by cultural conceptions of femininity and female sexuality; in turn, it has fed into these social conceptions. I will argue that Anna Freud, construed according to a pattern woven by her father, is presented as embodying one term or position within femininity, not as 'normal' femininity in her father's terms, but as femininity and sexuality under such rigorous control that it almost ceases to be. This is at once a deficient femininity and an excess of masculinity.[3] Marilyn Monroe, at the opposite pole, is seen as the epitome of femininity, in all its contradictions; this is femininity in excess, female sexuality out of control.

The interest here is in how the lives of women are written in relation to ideas about femininity, which is the case not only in texts that are or purport to be traditional biography or psychobiography but in other types of life-writing. Regarding Anna Freud, these include case studies and theoretical works that her father wrote, based at least in part on his analysis of her (beginning with 'A Child is Being Beaten' [1919] 1997; cf. Person 1997). They also include works that Anna Freud wrote about herself – 'Beating Fantasies and Daydreams' ([1922] 1974) and 'On Losing and Being Lost' ([1953] 1967), even though the 'patient' in these was disguised (for their autobiographical content see Young-Bruehl [1988] 2008 and Blass 1993). The mass of writing about Marilyn Monroe is vast and continues to be produced and reissued. It has taken many forms, populist or scholarly, as biography or autobiography (from Monroe's fragments of notes or from interviews she gave), as revelation of secrets and conspiracies, and as fictionalized interpretations (e.g. Joyce Carol Oates' novel *Blonde* of 2000). Sarah Churchwell's compelling analysis of what she terms the Monroe 'apocrypha' (2004: 8) examines tropes and narrative devices used in such accounts.

Churchwell is one of a number of feminist academics working within a more-or-less psychoanalytic framework who have taken a revisionist interest in Monroe – they include Lisa Appignanesi (2008), Lois Banner (2012) and Jacqueline Rose (2014). At around the same time, other feminists, also psychoanalytically based, had been writing about Anna Freud, notably Young-Bruehl, whose major biography first published in 1988 was reissued in 2008, unrevised but with an additional introduction. Suzanne Stewart-Steinberg's book (2011) takes a somewhat different perspective and is not intended as a biography.[4] All of these writers have seen something of wider significance in their subject than just the chronicling of an individual life. Some have stated, more or less explicitly that the life of the woman in question and how it has been represented has something to say about and to women, to feminism and feminists in our post-feminist era (Banner 2012; Churchwell 2004; Rose 2014; Stewart-Steinberg 2011; Young-Bruehl [1988] 2008). Some have also said that the 'lives' of their subject have something to say about life-writing 'after' psychoanalysis and about psychoanalysis and its framing of femininity (Appignanesi 2008; Banner 2012; Churchwell 2004; Young-Bruehl [1988] 2008). Banner's book explicitly brings Monroe and Anna Freud together.

The third major co-incidence that is central to this queer reading is indeed a queer undertow, a spectral female-to-female desire that hovers in accounts, more or less occluded. It is in Young-Bruehl's book of essays, less so in the biography; Churchwell considers rumours of Monroe's alleged lesbian affairs or 'bisexuality' that circulate in several of the source texts she examines. Banner argues that Monroe's 'lesbian inclinations' (2012: 4) may have been a factor in her death. It is this spectral lesbian presence/absence that I intend to address, arguing that it appears and fades in the sources, including Freud's writing about his daughter, and that it has haunted psychoanalytic conceptions of femininity and female sexuality from the beginning. I will argue that this queer undertow is not merely a coincidence in the lives and 'lives' of two particular women, but is an essential component of the conceptualization of femininity and female sexuality, even when it is glossed over.

It will be evident that what follows concentrates on representations of Anna Freud. This is because her father's analysis of her, his/their reconstruction of her childhood development and adult constitution were contributory to his views on femininity and female sexuality; because her writing about herself was profoundly influenced by his formulations (or those they arrived at together in analysis), and because his/their theoretical constructs were undoubtedly transmitted to practitioners in the second and third generation of analysts, including those who analysed Monroe. Anna Freud, her father's heir as head of the Freudian School, was mentor to those analysists – her childhood friend Marianne Kris and Ralph ('Romi') Greenson, Monroe's analyst when she died. Populist notions of femininity and sexuality, deriving in part from Freudian notions (however refracted these may have been) continue to circulate, not least in the great slew of writings about Monroe and the continuing fascination with her as an icon of femininity, or as Churchwell has it, an icon of 'über-femininity' (2004: 4). The myriad and contradictory representations of her cover the whole spectrum of conceptions of and fantasies about femininity and female sexuality. This, I contend, points to the notion of 'abnormality'[5] that is embedded in these conceptions. It is not coincidental that psychoanalytic readings of psychoanalytic texts, in the final years of the twentieth and into the twenty-first century, many of them feminist and some of them queer, have been important in shifting some ground on psychoanalysis and its influence. Thanks to Churchwell and others, the corpus of writing on Monroe has also been analysed in terms of fantasy constructions and desirous narratives.

The Monroe and the Anna Freud that we now have are the products of representation. In other words, they are characters; so, I shall call them AF and MM, in an attempt to register a distinction between the people who lived and interpretations of them, including their own. I shall call Sigmund Freud simply Freud, because he laid claim to this one-word epithet and his daughter signed herself AnnaFreud as one word – simultaneously distinguishing herself and instating her connection to him.

This perverse reading is about the queer tales we are told and tell ourselves, that we enact and critique, repeat and attempt to break out of, about women, femininity and desire. The something queer that floats in and out of these tales is connected to the truth-status, the spurious believability, the reliability and evidential bases of biography and all life-writing 'after' psychoanalysis. Psychoanalysis put biography and life-writing under question and simultaneously has given us a means and a necessity of questioning psychoanalytic writing itself. This is also a story about a journey to try to elucidate and make visible something of queer desire that psychoanalysis in the Freudian model elides and that, as I will argue, is central to Freudian conceptions of femininity and of desire. It is a search for some sort of knowledge in the face of desire, rather like the quest of psychoanalysis itself. This story begins with a visit to the Freud Museum in London about five years ago. It is a twisting and turning story, without resolution. Like life, it just ends.

In her father's house

Anna Freud (AF) always lived in her father's house, at first in the Vienna apartment and from 1938 until her death in 1983 at 20 Maresfield Gardens in London, now the Freud Museum. In her late twenties she decided to become a psychoanalyst, the only Freud child to follow her father. As his heir as head of the Freudian School, effectively the upholder of her father's ideas and reputation (although, as Stewart-Steinberg (2011) shows, taking a different line in her concentration on child analysis) she remained in her father's house. She was beside him in his last years, displacing his wife, we might say, as his principal carer and certainly outlasting all of the men that he thought might be his disciple and successor. She took all of this on – she took her father's mantle and his place.

Downstairs at the Freud Museum is the large room full of Sigmund Freud's books, collections, pictures, his desk, couch, spectacles – all as he left it when he died in this room in 1939. AF wanted it that way. Upstairs, where the presence/absence of AF is more tangible, there is a loom – Dorothy Burlingham's – where she and AF used to sit and weave. I wondered what it would have been like for them, living in this house, when her parents were dead, with her father's things downstairs preserved, as if he had just stepped outside into the garden.[6] Truth to tell, I wanted to find out about the relationship between AF and Dorothy Burlingham; to prove that this was a love without denial, a sexual relationship between two women over decades. I thought I wanted to write a fiction, a short story based on their lives, about what they talked about while sitting together weaving or knitting, which they did habitually. It should have been obvious from the first that there would be no absolute evidence to prove or disprove that theirs was a sexual relationship. That it was loving, whatever that meant or means, is beyond doubt. Before I could write the story that in fact I have not written, I needed to find out about AF.

Ghosts, biography, psychoanalysis

While reading Young-Bruehl's biography of AF, the ghost of Marilyn Monroe (MM) suddenly appeared. She had left a bequest to Marianne Kris, intending it to support a psychoanalytic institution. Kris gave it to the Anna Freud Clinic. Young-Bruehl quotes a letter of sympathy from AF to Romi Greenson (letter of 20 January 1963; Young-Bruehl [1988] 2008: 413) exonerating him and psychoanalysis from Monroe's suicide. There is no further mention of MM in the book, yet at about the time I was reading it she began to materialize elsewhere, including at the Freud Museum. Therefore, what began as a project to find out about AF expanded to include the psychoanalytic connections between her and MM; between the 'lives' of these two and the psychoanalytic conception of femininity and sexuality, and between femininity, psychoanalysis and feminism as represented in a clutch of feminist considerations of MM and of AF.

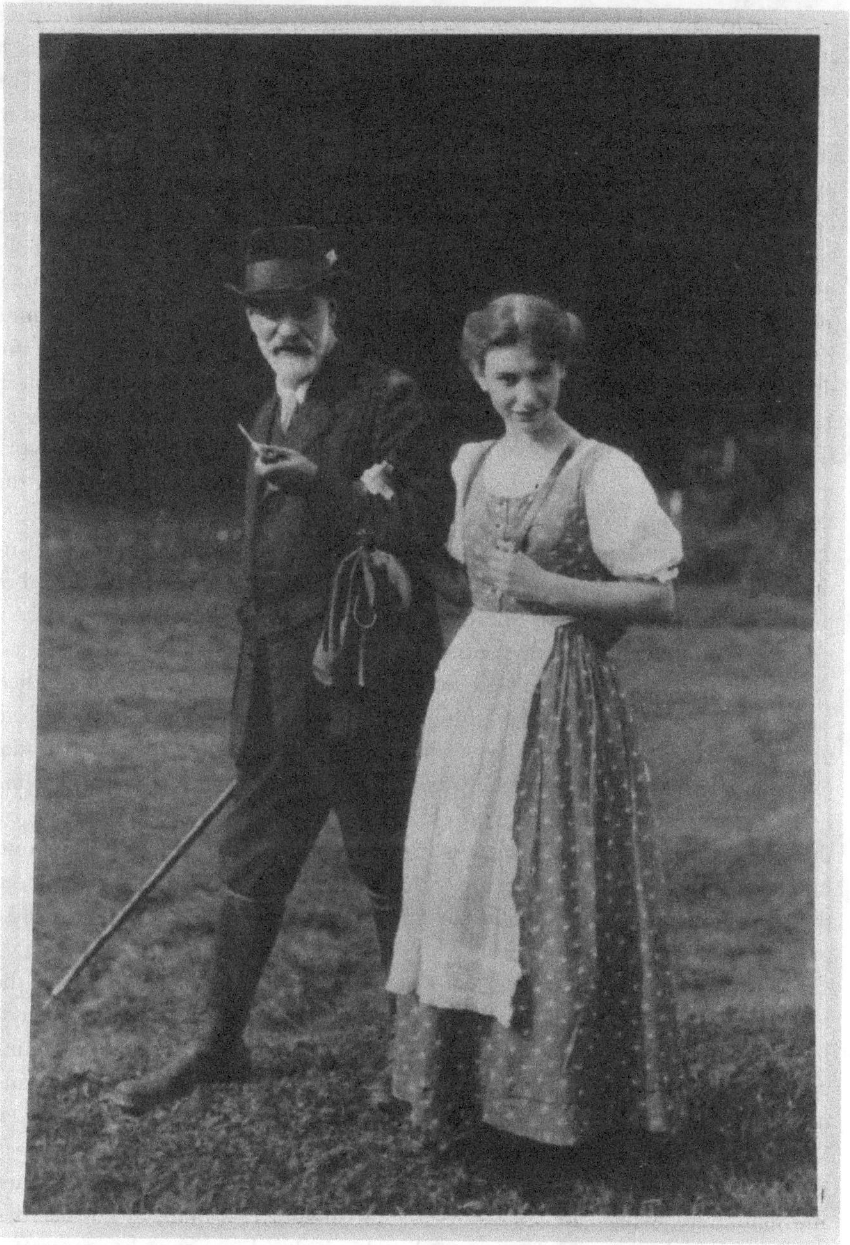

FIGURE 10.1 Before: The teenaged Anna Freud, still a daydreaming, masturbating girl, with her father, walking and talking in Italy in 1913.

Source: Used with permission, copyright Freud Museum, London.

Churchwell's book (2004) does not mention AF at all, but in a talk she gave at the Freud Museum on 21 November 2013 (Churchwell 2013) she said that it was by then fairly well accepted that MM had been analysed briefly by AF. The talk, entitled 'The Many Minds of Marilyn Monroe', was part of a series held in connection with the exhibition *Mad, Bad and Sad: Women and the Mind Doctors* based on Appignanesi's book of the same name (2008). Appignanesi, Banner and Rose were at the talk. MM was represented in the exhibition by a photograph taken in 1956, a video of her leaving hospital in New York and copies of books of her 'autobiographical' writing (Hecht's *My Story* [1974] 2007 and Buchthal and Comment's *Fragments* 2010). Beside these were a photograph of Marianne Kris outside the Freud house and one of Romi Greenson. The exhibition did not definitively state that MM had been analysed by AF when she was in London in 1956 filming *The Prince and the Showgirl*, only that she is 'recorded' as doing so (Freud Museum, 2013). Lois Banner, alone of the feminist academics whose work is considered here, is certain that AF's analysis of MM took place, and that the lesbian or bisexual undertow, as I call it, was established in that one week in 1956.

In her book and her talk, Churchwell examined what commentators of various stripes had made of MM and how, to varying degrees, they had attempted or purported to read her mind. She drew attention to the mythologizing of MM, to the doubtful reliability and verifiability of many sources and their interpretations and to the storytelling techniques that they employed. One way or another, the accounts she analysed were 'ghosted' by repetition of elements drawn from preceding accounts, acknowledged or not, repetitions that accorded with reader expectations and produced, precisely by repetition, a spurious truth-value. Having now read so many of these (not all of which are referenced here), I concur, on the whole, with Churchwell's analysis. Speculations, fantasies and vested interests inflect these texts, but also inflect the critical, revisionist texts that are written about them, including Churchwell's and including this one, because, in order to analyse or critique we are forced to repeat.

Churchwell identifies deep-seated, unconscious anxieties and desires in the texts she deals with. These, she states, are managed by 'a reassuring undemanding version of "psychoanalysis"' (2004: 9), so that the 'lives' of MM are 'a talking cure for our lingering, persistent fears about sex, knowledge, the female body and death'. She contends that writings about MM are not just about her but about Woman as a cultural concept (ibid.). I would say that those of us who are women have had to live out, or within or in relationship to cultural conceptions of women and femininity, which are, in my view, not singular. I would say further that everyone, of whatever gender or sexuality, has had to live out or be interpreted through cultural conceptions of femininity and masculinity, which include psychoanalytic conceptions.

Freud said in his 1933 lecture 'Femininity' that women had not 'knocked their heads against the riddle of the nature of femininity' ([1933] 1973: 146) because 'to those of you who are women this will not apply – you are yourselves the problem'.[7] Churchwell's book shows how a series of men and some women have knocked their heads against the riddle of MM as icon of femininity, and she does that herself, in the service of feminism and also of criticism that, after psychoanalysis, questions the reliability of all accounts that are unavoidably riven by desire on the part of their writers and readers. Churchwell demonstrates that catering to reader expectations and familiar patterns of understanding are key to both novelistic and ostensibly factual biographical writing. In her 'afterword' to the book she states that MM is 'a prime example of the seductions of biography' (2004: 127), which is the temptation to 'substitute belief for knowledge, prejudice for thinking'. She carries on to say, in a guarded way, that all biographies may also be autobiographies of the author (ibid.).

In his biography of the young Freud, Adam Phillips was beset by similar issues. In his first chapter, he says that one of the first casualties of psychoanalysis was the traditional biography, since psychoanalysis makes all narratives of the past and attempts at coherence suspect. 'History begins to sound like fiction, and fiction begins to sound peculiarly wishful' (2014: 6). As he says, it is not only the writing of a life but the reading of it that psychoanalysis calls into question, asking why we want to know and what we think we want to know, and behind that a bigger question – what do we want or desire? Phillips is aware that the desires of the biographer may be revealed if read psychoanalytically. He writes:

> After Freud (. . .) we have to ask, what does the biographer want his subject for? (. . .) What does he need him to be or not be? What does he use his subject as a way of talking about, and (. . .) to avoid talking about?
>
> *(Ibid.: 27).*

Phillips tells us that Freud was opposed to biography and destroyed materials in order to thwart biographers. His daughter, as Young-Bruehl recounts, was reluctant to allow but did authorize Ernest Jones' official biography, one suspects because she and the Freudian establishment were able to vet it.

Jacques Derrida, in his book *Archive Fever* (1998) based on a talk he gave at the Freud Museum on 5 June 1994, considers the authority of archives as guaranteeing authenticity and evidence through their inclusions and exclusions, their ordering of materials and restrictions on access. In a typically multivalent passage at the end of this book, Derrida wonders what Freud might have wanted to keep secret, what he might have 'burned' (Derrida [1995] 1998: 101). The passage implies not only that Freud deliberately destroyed some material and that he or others might have buried things in the labyrinth of the archives, but that there may have been things that Freud knew but never revealed, and moreover things that he did not himself know because of his own unconscious processes. Derrida wonders what may have disappeared 'of his secret passions, of his correspondence, or of his "life"' (ibid.) and conjectures that there may be elements that can no longer be retrieved and are 'without a name, without the least symptom, without even an ash' (ibid.). This is the biographer's nightmare, and yet the search for symptoms or clues continues regarding Freud, his daughter and MM, holding out the promise that there will be further information to be discovered or released, further clues that will answer questions and provide proof about each of them. Psychoanalysis, biography and life-writing in general all involve the attempt to reveal secrets – what has been hidden, deliberately or not – in order to arrive at some kind of truth about a life. Psychoanalytic writing in its theoretical dimension attempts to extrapolate truths that extend beyond one individual/subject in order to identify patterns that apply to others and to posit that some patterns may be universal. Biography and life-writing are not so different; to achieve a readership, there must be something that draws the reader to want to know, which is more than curiosity about the individual life presented and must have some relevance to the reader's life. In this, psychoanalytic writing (case histories in particular) biography and other forms of life-writing share a common methodology with the popular genre of detective stories. All of them seek out clues to reveal and resolve motivations, causes and their effects or affects.

Weaving

The word clue comes from an older word – clew – that goes back to antiquity and is a thread. In the myth of Theseus, Ariadne gives him such a thread so that he can find his way out of the labyrinth. Psychoanalysis seeks out and follows clues into the labyrinth, in order to draw the patient out again, out of the maze of their symptoms and repetitions. In the story of AF, weaving, knitting and clews are recurrent motifs.

Young-Bruehl says that Martha Freud and her sister Minna taught the Freud daughters Mathilde and Sophie to knit, but not the youngest, AF. It was her nursemaid who taught her, so that she could join in this activity with the female members of her family. Soon, AF was knitting so obsessively that her parents wanted her to spend less time on it; so she took up weaving (Young-Bruehl [1988] 2008: 45). When I was thinking of a fiction about AF and Burlingham I ought to have remembered that Appignanesi and Forrester had already commented on these handicrafts (1993) where they suggested that the metaphor of knitting could be a foundation for 'a whole alternative biography' of AF. They wrote:

> Knitting, this most feminine of activities, with its autoerotic subtext was something that Anna excelled at (. . .) perhaps in an attempt to win her mother's love, then throughout her life as a kind of meditative recreation (. . .) Knitting is also Anna's single point of identification with her mother and the feminine domain.
>
> *(Appignanesi and Forrester 1993: 305n)*

Appignanesi and Forrester also record a remark by AF at the end of her life, when she could no longer knit. They say that her hands could not comply with the feats of sublimation that she had required of them for so many years, and they quote AF: 'Look at what that hand did, it is angry because I controlled it for so long' (ibid.: 305). They do not give a source for this quote, which grounds their linkage between these feminine crafts, masturbation and sublimation through a repetitive and perhaps ritualized activity. In the passage quoted above, Appignanesi and Forrester make a connection between knitting and AF's desire for her mother's love and also (not quoted here) AF's jealousy of and rivalry with her sister Sophie, her mother's favourite.

According to Young-Bruehl, AF's knitting and weaving led her father to one of his 'wilder anthropological speculations' (2008: 45), which she claims was an attempt to understand his daughter. In his lecture on 'Femininity' ([1933] 1973) he said that women had made very few contributions to the development of civilization, but possibly one was the invention of weaving. He was tempted to 'guess' why this was so, and his answer was that weaving imitated the growth of pubic hair that conceals the genitals. Women invented weaving, therefore, to make a further concealment of their lack of a penis, to cover an absence, the site (and sight) of the narcissistic wound of their castration. This anthropological speculation accords with the formulation of the Oedipus Complex as a central tenet of Freudian theory, whereby it is the intervention of the authoritative father into the mother–son dyad that initiates all possibility of progress, social relations, knowledge and civilization. This intervention prohibits the son's desire for the mother by enforcing and reinforcing the boy's castration anxiety. The female's lack of a penis functions as proof that castration is a real threat, as punishment for misdirected desire. It also, not coincidentally, accords with another tenet that Freud asserted to the end of his life, that of female penis envy as central to femininity and female desire. He maintains this in 'Femininity' in connection with this tale about the invention of weaving, and writes, in a statement that seems addressed not only to his first audience, but to the feminist critics he also alludes to: 'If you reject this idea as fantastic and regard my belief in the influence of lack of a penis on the configuration of femininity as an *idee fixe*, I am of course defenceless' ([1933] 1973: 167). AF, undoubtedly, read this lecture on femininity; she may have been present when her father delivered it. I wonder what she made of it? She was 37 when it was published; Burlingham had been in her life for eight years. As far as I know, she never commented on it directly.

Someone is being beaten

Young-Bruehl, in her book of essays (1998), revisited several aspects of her work on AF not fully explored in the biography. She maintained that Freud's analysis of his daughter, conducted from 1918 to 1922 and again from 1924 to 1925, shaped his thoughts on femininity and female sexuality. The 'presence' of AF is registered in 'A Child is Being Beaten' of 1919 (see Person 1997; Young-Bruehl [1988] 2008: 54–68, 103–139), where a reconstruction of AF's childhood development, derived from analysis of her as an adult, features as a pivotal case in the argument.

Freud describes how this particular girl had elaborate daydreams. He uses her case, along with a handful of others, to elaborate the three-stage development of beating fantasies and their associated masturbatory activities in girls and boys – indicating where these differ between the two sexes or genders and which phases or stages are conscious and which unconscious. In the third phase of the beating fantasy, this girl is no longer being beaten herself (by her father). Freud states that she becomes a watcher rather than a participant, looking on as boys are beaten by a male authority figure, a father-substitute such as a schoolmaster. In a much quoted passage, he says that in this way,

> the girl escapes from the demands of the erotic side of her life altogether. She turns herself in phantasy into a man, without herself becoming active in a masculine way, and is no longer anything but the spectator of the event which takes the place of a sexual act.
>
> *([1919] 1997: 23)*

What Freud says about this girl (AF) is that she is dissatisfied with her clitoris (recognized as inferior to a penis) turns herself into a boy and also puts herself outside of sexuality altogether. The passage suggests more: that this girl makes herself into a boy-without-a-penis and also remains passive. One might say she is neither one thing nor the other and, in terms of sexuality, she just gives up the ghost. As we shall see later in the chapter there is more to it than this.

At her presentation for membership of the Vienna Psychoanalytic Society, in front of her father and his colleagues/disciples, AF delivered her own version of the sublimation of beating fantasies and masturbation – 'Beating Fantasies and Daydreams' ([1922] 1974). The paper purported to report an analysis of a young patient, but Young-Bruehl identifies that AF had not yet had any patients and she was writing about herself (2008: 104). AF describes how the vivid daydreamer turns her fantasies into elaborate 'nice stories' and writes them down. In this way she makes an act of private and guilty pleasure (masturbation) into a public, social act of communication and creativity addressed to an audience of readers. In the stories, the girl features as a boy or young man who endures various complicated scenarios in which he is abducted, imprisoned, punished and otherwise tormented or humiliated by an older, authoritative man. The young prince/hero bears all of this and through his submissiveness and acceptance eventually melts the older man's heart so that, in the end, a relationship of tenderness (not a sexual relationship) is achieved between them.

In AF's version of the third phase of the girl's fantasy, there is a happy ending. The girl succeeds. In the stories she becomes a boy, but AF's case presentation does not, unlike her father's, close off the possibility that she might still accede to femininity and heterosexuality; she is not definitively placed outside of sexuality. We might read this paper as suggesting that the submissiveness and passivity of the 'boy hero' and his/her focus on an authoritative male as object could serve as the ground for a later 'feminine', heterosexual object choice.

What was AF saying to her father in this paper in 1922, approaching the end of her first period of analysis with him? Ostensibly she had entered analysis because of lassitude, anxiety, depression, eating disorders and indecisiveness about her future and career, obsessional behaviours, demands for attention and affirmation. Freud attests this in various correspondence (with Lou Andreas-Salome). From other evidence, AF's letters to Salome and both Freud's and AF's papers on beating fantasies, there was more to it. The girls in the papers by the two Freuds overcame the beating fantasies and compulsive masturbation in childhood or around puberty – an outcome necessary to project them into the Oedipus. AF did not. These fantasies and masturbation were still with her in her twenties and into her thirties. In 1922 she was telling her father that, through analysis, she was now 'well' and had overcome it all; she had decided on being an analyst rather than a teacher and was showing him that she was worthy and able to do that. Going further, one might say that she was declaring that she was dedicating herself to him and his brainchild, her twin, psychoanalysis.

Freud had introduced AF to Lou Andreas-Salome.[8] In January 1924 AF wrote to Salome that her 'nice stories' and masturbatory activities had come back, and that these were shameful, especially when she did 'it' between seeing patients (quoted in Young-Breuhl 2008: 121). In May 1924 she announced to Salome that she was returning to analysis with her father because of the daydreams 'combined with an increasing intolerance – sometimes physical as well as mental – of the beating fantasies and of their consequences which I could not do without' (ibid.: 122). She also told Salome that her daydreams had been: 'pulled apart, analysed, published and in every way mishandled and mistreated' (ibid.: 121), presumably by her father and herself. The tone of this remark is jocular, but it is intriguing. In AF's analysis with her father there was obviously a dialogue between them, and her paper also represents a continued dialogue with him and his essay of 1919. If, as I have suggested, in 1922 she was telling him what he wanted to hear and what she wanted him to hear, that does not mean that what they said was untrue. However, the sequel, AF's return to analysis, indicates that there were things that were not said, not resolved, one might suspect both in the analysis and in the written traces. What we cannot know is what these absences and ellipses actually were.

The lesbian question

Was AF a lesbian? This question haunts considerations of her life (Burlingham 1989; Young-Bruehl [1988] 2008, 1998), and if we read her father's writing from 1919 onwards psychoanalytically, it hovers there too. It is bound to arise for us, knowing that she and Burlingham were together for approaching 50 years. Does it mean – do we want to know – whether their relationship was sexual in the sense that it involved genital acts? Is that what we take a sexual relationship to mean? Is it asking whether AF had a sexual identity exclusively focussed on a female sexual object? Is that what we take 'lesbian' to mean?

As far as we know, Freud never asked his daughter this question directly – there is no evidence. In his writing, references to female homosexuality, as he called it, are sparse; the two key cases where he came up against it – the 'Dora' case ([1905]

1985) and 'Psychogenisis of a Case of Homosexuality in a Woman' ([1920] 1981) were incomplete, broken-off failures. In his later works, attempting to deal with femininity and female sexuality, the possibility of female homosexual object choice is raised, but is not examined in any detail. It is hard to credit that Freud, seeing his daughter's attachments to Loe Kahn, Eva Rosenfeld and above all Dorothy Burlingham, would not have asked himself this question. I shall return to this. But first, I want to turn to MM.

It is perhaps unexpected that a spectre of female-to-female desire flits in and out of accounts of Monroe. Reading about her and AF in tandem, it is interesting how the lesbian question is broached and, for the most part, then recedes, or is taken into a wider narrative. Regarding both MM and AF, it also takes us back into Freudian formulations of femininity and sexuality.

Marilyn: Venus

As Churchwell points out, speculations on what she terms MM's bisexuality focus on the drama coach Natasha Lytess and the putatively spurned acting rival Joan Crawford. Churchwell shows that the accounts largely see this as a further symptom of MM's rampant (object-indifferent and primarily narcissistic) sexual appetite, her manipulation of her desirability to further her career, and/or her need for mothering (2004: 205–210). Such explanations were ready-to-hand in the 1950s and 1960s and have not disappeared in popular culture since. As a woman, MM could be seen simultaneously as sexually rapacious (insatiable) and indifferent (frigid); as manipulative (femme fatale) and manipulated (victim); dissembling, cunning, vindictive; sweet, trusting; extrovert, exhibitionist; shy, unconfident; vain, artificial; natural, instinctual; clever and articulate; or just a dumb blonde. According to the accounts that Churchwell surveys, MM longs for a father in her relationships with men, for a 'good' mother in her relationships with women, and for a child, which will make her a 'real' woman. All of these interpretations are not very far from, and are actually very close to, Freud's conceptions of femininity. In their repetition, these contradictions appear to make sense; they become believable.

Supposing we see representations of MM in terms of a long-lasting cultural form – the mythological Venus. Venus is an image of desire, an image that excites the desire *of* others but does not necessarily represent her desire *for* others; she represents desirability rather than desirousness. In Freud's terms, she is woman and femininity, wanting to be wanted and to fit herself to another's desire, passive in that she does not actively desire the other but wants the other to desire her. However, Venus is also a temptation and, through her seductiveness, a threat. The stories of Monroe conjure up Venus, Helen of Troy and other women real or imagined – tales that are familiar and frequently have dire consequences.

Churchwell considers that 'bisexuality' in tales of MM 'seems to operate as a contemporary form of nymphomania' (ibid.: 209) and adds that biographers do not take it seriously because 'episodic bisexuality is cute, even titillating' (which itself suggests that bisexuality as an enduring identity is more problematical for those who conceive themselves as heterosexual). Bisexuality, in the Freudian schema, is a difficult term to tie down. Churchwell uses this term rather than lesbian, which itself implies that 'lesbian' might designate a long-term or even permanent same-sex object choice and also an identity; 'bisexuality' might also indicate a long-term or permanent capacity to be attracted to people of either sex and therefore an identity, but also, as here, designates a temporary oscillation in object-choice within a primarily heterosexual life. The lesbian question is not of major import to Churchwell – she sees it more as a narrative trope in the accounts, functioning to emphasize the notion of excessive sexuality. Appignanesi and Rose do not mention it at all. Only Lois Banner (2014) accords this question significance. Her reading of this is in no way queer, in the sense of opening up a space for consideration of femininity and female sexuality beyond the parameters of heteronormative conceptions of desire.

At the beginning of her book, Banner states that: 'Significant among my discoveries about Marilyn are her lesbian inclinations' (2012: 4) and that, despite three marriages and numerous reported affairs with men she 'desired women, had affairs with them, and worried that she might be lesbian by nature' (ibid.). By the end of the book, Banner makes a leap, not merely asserting that MM had 'inclinations', but saying: 'she was the world's heterosexual icon who *preferred* women as sexual partners' (ibid.: 422, my emphasis). The evidence cited for this and other claims is not only previous biographies (although she does acknowledge her extensive use of them, in particular Anthony Summer's book *Goddess* (1985) and the collection of interview notes and other documents he made available to her). Alone of all the feminist writers considered here (including those concerned with AF), Banner brings MM and the psychoanalysts AF and Greenson together in such a way that their diagnoses are brought forward as evidence of MM's 'lesbian inclinations' and the part these purported inclinations may have played in her death.

Reading Banner's book along with a host of other writings, it is clear that MM is repetitively presented as an enigma, even though the terms in which it/she is represented are very recognizable and familiar. The idea of enigma is central to conceptions of femininity, before Freud, for Freud, and subsequently. In both Summers' and Banner's biographies MM appears as a figure constantly peeled away to reveal what lies underneath. The treatment of her resembles, to an uncanny degree, that of the Anatomical Venus (see Ebenstein 2016). These life-sized wax figures were produced from the seventeenth century into the nineteenth, modelled on dissected female corpses for the instruction of men of science. On the outside they present a body that is both beautiful and apparently ecstatic, as if post-coitally asleep and dreaming. The body can be taken apart layer-by-layer to reveal all the organs and viscera. In the most famous one, the last section reveals a foetus in the womb. The eroticization of these Venuses is particularly uncanny to modern eyes, even though the connotations of these figures can be easily read, because we already know them. With their smiling, half-open mouths, they seem to invite investigation, penetration beneath their surface beauty to lay open an unlovely truth underneath. From the first, any such figure was seen as a *momento mori*. This has both a moral and scientific dimension.

For science, the figures enabled a delving into the body of woman to demystify processes such as childbirth – male doctors gained knowledge. Morally, the eroticization of the figures associates female sensuality, seductiveness and sexuality with death – their own, and the threat of death to their (male) viewers.

Banner presents a catalogue of diseases and disorders, physical and psychic, in her portrayal of MM. The 'lesbian inclinations' become associated with all sorts of other afflictions and sufferings, some of them self-inflicted, but rooted in MM's disrupted childhood, her lack of a father, her mother's mental illness and the sexual abuse she experienced as a foster child. According to Banner and the analysts she references, MM was plagued by her same-sex desire. Of course, Banner does not claim that lesbian desire is itself pathological, only that it was for MM. Banner states that in 1956, in one of her analytic sessions with AF, the two played a game with marbles. MM launched these one-by-one toward AF, who concluded that MM wanted to have sex with her and that she was afraid of men. As Banner says: 'the analysis seems overblown, but we don't know what else happened in their interactions' (2012: 261).

Banner states in the prologue to her book (2012) that she had found AF's notes on this analysis, but does not say where. On page 261 a footnote refers the reader for information about AF's analysis of MM to a book by Berthelsen (1987) based on interviews he conducted with the Freuds' elderly housekeeper Paula Fischl. Young-Bruehl ([1988] 2008: x) considered this book and Fischl's testimony unreliable and refused to use it. In 2006, a book by Michel Schneider came out in France, translated into English as *Marilyn's Last Sessions: A Novel* ([2006] 2011). In it, Schneider relates the AF analysis in very similar terms to Banner and also references Berthelsen. Schneider tells readers that he relied entirely on published sources for the background to his novel and also that he made things up, quoted documents that have not been found and might not exist ([2006] 2011: 1–2).

Banner carried out 'deep readings' of Greenson's psychoanalytic writings (2012: 8) including those that may have been based on MM. At Churchwell's talk in 2013 Banner stated that she had located and read Greenson's notes on his analysis of MM, apparently not in the official archive at UCLA (where much material is still embargoed). The material she discusses also draws on Greenson's correspondence with Marianne Kris and AF. She therefore uses the opinions of the analysts as evidence of MM's 'inclinations' and their significance. An opinion attributed to Greenson was that MM could not bear even the hint of anything homosexual and yet she fell into situations that had 'homosexual coloring [*sic*]'. She recognized her own tendency, but then projected it on to the other person involved, who then 'became her enemy' (Banner, 2012: 385, quoting Greenson).

Much of this relates to Greenson's attempts to deal with MM's alleged paranoia and her possible 'borderline' status; after her death, it involved attempts to counter rumours of his involvement (accidentally or otherwise) in that death and in a much disputed cover-up involving the Kennedy brothers, the Mafia, the Teamster's union, the FBI, the CIA, you name it (see Spoto 1994). Banner says that Greenson told his family and wrote to Kris (letter of 20 August 1962) that MM had killed herself 'because she couldn't handle her lesbian urges' (2012: 422). Banner's verdict on Greenson's view is:

> There may be some truth to this assertion. The European tabloids were soon to run Natasha Lytess's lurid story of their affair, which would be a considerable humiliation to Marilyn as well as a public exposure of her deepest secret. *(Ibid.)*

MM had dealt with revelations before – about posing for a nude calendar when she was young and needed money; about saying, early in her career, that her mother was dead when she was in fact in a mental institution. Even rumours about affairs with women had been published earlier on and she had not seemed perturbed. To claim that this was her 'deepest' secret, or even that it was a secret, seems far-fetched, and rests on Greenson's interpretations. These interpretations are classically Freudian, following quite precisely Freud's line of argument in his 1922 paper 'Some Neurotic Mechanisms in Jealousy, Paranoia and Homosexuality'. Here Freud bases theoretical pronouncements on just two cases, one of jealousy and the other of persecutory paranoia, both of them, incidentally, male. He claims that both projected feelings that they did not want to recognize in themselves on to the other person, the most-loved person of their own sex ([1922] 2001: 226). Freud says this projection comes about because of an ambivalence of feeling, exacerbated by a refusal by the other of the patient's claims for love. In both cases the persecutory paranoia and the jealousy served 'as a defence against homosexuality' (ibid.: 227), which enabled the two patients' homosexual desires to remain unconscious.

For Greenson and Banner, MM was aware of her homosexual desires and these were so toxic to her that she killed herself. This diagnosis also seems far-fetched, and falls back upon a view of homosexuality, in men and in women, that is rooted in a binary notion of masculinity and femininity, whereby an excess of masculinity in a female and of femininity in a male may lead to homosexual object-choice.[9] Banner, following Greenson and despite some caveats, ups the ante on the lesbian question, which she foregrounds. However, neither she nor Greenson have anything to say about female-to-female desire per se – there is no analysis of it, merely an association of lesbian or bisexual desire with shame, fear, possibly disavowal. For Greenson it is associated with destructive and self-destructive behaviours, and for Banner it is not much different, since MM's 'inclinations' figure as a possible explanation for her suicide. Conversely, when the lesbian question arises concerning AF, commentators play it down.

Anna: vestal virgin

Princess Marie Bonaparte, Freud's friend, an analyst who trained with him and the patron who secured the Freud family's flight to England in 1938, is credited with describing AF as a vestal dedicated to preserving the flame of her father's work and reputation (Young-Bruehl [1988] 2008: 137). Such a designation re-inscribes AF's sublimation of sexuality to another cause, which is the general consensus in accounts of her, and might be true, for all we know. Young-Bruehl certainly concurs with Marie Bonaparte, and with Freud's view in 'A Child is Being Beaten'.

In 1998 Young-Bruehl wrote about the circumstances through which she ended up writing the biography. She was asked to do it by AF's literary executrix and spoke to the woman's husband, an analyst who had known AF and Burlingham. She told him she did not want to write the biography, asked if the two women's relationship had been sexual and said: 'Would it be the biographer's task to brave the homophobia of psychoanalysis with a lesbian life story?' He replied: 'Sweetheart, these two ladies lived together *harmoniously*, really *harmoniously* for *fifty years* – now I ask *you* could that be a sexual relationship?' (Young-Bruehl 1998: 9, original emphasis). What was he saying? That it must have been a sexual relationship, or that it could not have been? Young-Bruehl reported this conversation to her own analyst, as she ran through all the reasons why she could not write the biography. Her analyst laughed and at the end of the session told her he thought she had changed her mind. She wrote the biography, and her answer to the lesbian question was 'no'.

She tells us that what she wanted to write was the story of an AF who managed to create a family life with another woman who had children, without being their father or her husband, without being 'the mother or the wife' but being 'everything'. As Young-Bruehl puts it, this relationship would be 'conventionally unclassifiable'. But then admits that this was not the biography that she wrote (ibid.: 4). Young-Bruehl is circumspect, an analyst who says something yet does not quite spell it out.

The biographer also tells us that she had to overcome some antipathy towards AF. She could not identify with her 'very restricted sexuality' nor with 'the severest parts of her superego' (ibid.: 21). She came across a business letter in which AF recommended refusing a homosexual applicant for training. One sentence brought her 'to a screeching halt' and she hated it. The sentence said that it was no good for a course or any institution 'to permit people with sexual abnormalities' (ibid.). Subsequently, she read AF's unpublished clinical reflections on male homosexuality, which, she said, made her understand what the sentence in the letter meant to AF 'how it protected her, how it represented her' (ibid.), but she does not elaborate. If AF were fending off the possibility of reputational damage to the institution and practice of psychoanalysis, it might be understandable, but it does not sound like that. I take the licence to read this as saying that AF was protecting herself from people prying into her private life, from rumours, from any implications that she and her steering of the Freudian movement might not be fitted to the task. The 'protection' amounts to saying, in my view: 'I am not that'.

In AF's correspondence with fellow analyst Max Eitingon in 1926 she told him something about herself in relation to Burlingham and the Burlingham children, two of whom, Robert (Bob) and Mary (Mabbie), she had taken into analysis.

AF wrote: 'I think sometimes that I want only to make them healthy but also, at the same time, to have them, or at least something of them, for myself' (quoted in Young-Bruehl [1988] 2008: 133). She added: 'Towards the mother of the children it is not very different with me'. In the same letter she described this as an '*Etwas-Haben-Wollen*', wanting to have something for herself. Whatever this was, and she described it as a dependency (ibid.), might not have been sexual (in relation to the mother) but was not undesirous. She told Eitingon that she was ashamed of this, especially in front of her father, and therefore did not tell him about it. She recalled that she had tried to discuss it with Lou Salome, who was 'enormously distanced from it', to the extent that they had 'complete inability to understand each other' (ibid.). AF had previously told Lou Salome that she was ashamed of an 'it' – the recurrence of beating fantasies and masturbation, and in this instance she was again ashamed, and Salome did not understand this 'it' at all. What was this 'it' – the same as previously or different?

Michael John Burlingham, in a biography who wrote of his grandmother, asked the lesbian question (Burlingham 1989). He says that AF was afraid that Bob (his father) had homosexual tendencies and that she set out to reorientate him to heterosexuality: 'By laborious work with his superego, it was her intent to reawaken Bob's original oedipal rivalry with his father for Dorothy, and thereby set Bob back

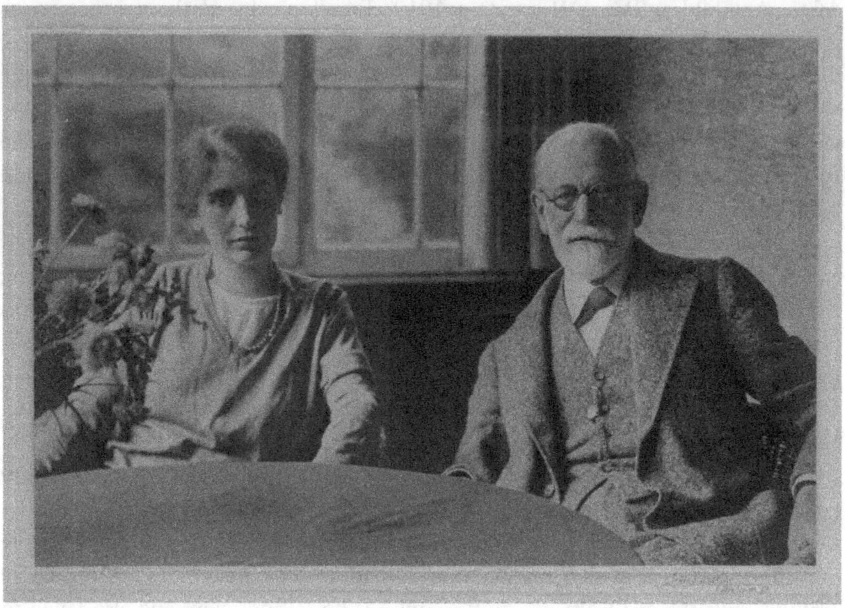

FIGURE 10.2 After: Anna Freud and her father in 1929, after her analyses with him had finished, after she had formed a bond with Dorothy Burlingham and when she no longer told her father everything.

Source: Used with permission, copyright Freud Museum, London.

on the heterosexual track' (ibid.: 173). AF's analysis of Bob follows Freud's precepts ([1922] 2001: 223–232), both in ascribing male homosexuality to an unbroken identification with the mother and in equating 'normal' masculinity with activity. AF's position as analyst and also as surrogate mother to the children is complicated, particularly since she takes on the role of the authoritative Oedipal father in her attempt to break Bob's identification with his mother. Michael Burlingham says the relationship was not lesbian 'in the sexual sense of that word', and adds that it would have taken a hypocrite to discourage homosexuality in Bob while 'revelling' in it herself and 'Anna Freud was not hypocritical' (1989: 291–292).

Young-Bruehl and Michael Burlingham judge that the AF–Burlingham relationship was not lesbian, was not sexual, because AF particularly was ascetic. Banner concludes that MM did have sex with women. Churchwell does not make a judgement, except to say that bisexuality can be titillating and in accounts of MM functions primarily as an indicator that she was oversexed. None of these accounts really has anything to say about woman-to-woman desire, how it might feel, come about, operate. It is just a matter of deciding 'Was she or wasn't she?' 'Were they or weren't they?' – this 'it' either just is, or just isn't. The same spectal presence/ absence occurs in the Freudian sources.

The Freuds and femininity

After 'A Child is Being Beaten' in 1919, Freud produced three papers concerned with femininity and female sexuality – 'Some Psychical Consequences of the Anatomical Distinction Between the Sexes' [1925] 1981: 323–343); 'Female Sexuality' ([1931] 1981: 367–392) and 'Femininity' ([1933] 1973: 145–169). He wrote many other things within this period and it may be coincidental that 'The Psychogenesis of a Case of Homosexuality in a Woman' came out in 1920 and 'Some Neurotic Mechanisms in Jealousy, Paranoia and Homosexuality' in 1922.

In the three femininity papers, Freud does little to revise basic premises set out earlier in *Three Essays on the Theory of Sexuality* ([1905] 1981) and 'A Child is Being Beaten' ([1919] 1997), but is more concerned than before to account for the girl's turn away from the mother and toward the father. In 1925, Freud continues to see female development as centred on the penis as both revered and desired for herself. The girl sees a penis and immediately recognizes that it is superior to her own genitals; she does not have one and is therefore inferior, castrated. Consequently she falls 'a victim to penis envy' ([1925] 1981: 335). She develops a 'masculinity complex', either recognizing her state of castration but hoping to get a penis by some means, one day, or by refusing to accept castration and continuing to believe she does have one, which may compel her to act as a man (ibid.: 337). These attitudes split the girl from her mother, who is herself deficient and also failed to supply her daughter with the proper genital equipment. According to Freud, dissatisfaction with the clitoris may turn the girl against masturbation – but not all girls; as we have seen, not AF. Girls who succeed in attaining 'normal' femininity substitute their wish for a penis with a wish for a child, initially taking their father as love object for the purposes of this wish. These girls/women abandon the clitoris in favour of the vagina as the organ of sexual pleasure. Hence, 'normal' femininity consists in a change of love object and organ of stimulation. However, he says, sometimes the girl's attachment to her father may go wrong, so that she identifies herself with him and 'may return to her masculinity complex and perhaps remain fixated in it' (ibid.: 340). She does not modify her penis envy into a wish for a 'penis-child', nor switch from clitoris to vagina, nor from father-object to another man; in short she does not attain 'normal' femininity, i.e. heterosexuality.

In 'Female Sexuality' ([1931] 1981) Freud builds on the 1925 essay to set out three pathways or lines of female development. On all three paths, girls rebel against their castration, but in different ways: they all want a penis of their very own. On the first path, the girl's dissatisfaction with her clitoris makes her give up her 'phallic activity' (masturbation) and with it 'her sexuality in general as well as a good part of her masculinity in other fields' ([1931] 1981: 376). On the second path, the girl clings to her masculinity and hope of getting a penis and becoming a man. This 'masculinity complex', Freud says, 'can result in a manifest homosexual choice of object' (ibid.: 376). Only the third path, which is 'very circuitous' (ibid.) results in 'normal' femininity. The girl turns away from her clitoris and her mother, turns her wish for a penis into a penis-child, turns to her father as object in order to get this and then transfers this wish to another man.

When we consider these pathways, they are all a little bleak. On the first pathway, then, the girl/woman is likely to have no sexual desire at all and to lose any ambition she might otherwise have had, for instance to pursue a profession. She is a woman, she looks like one and acts like one, particularly in her passivity. In fact, it is quite easy to see that women of this type conform to what we might identify as a nineteenth-century notion of acceptable (middle-class) womanhood: the dutiful daughter or wife whose loyalty and fidelity are guaranteed because she does not herself desire anything. It is also a convenient explanation for female frigidity (which Freud touches on in his 1933 lecture). On the second pathway, the girl/woman believes herself to be a man, or at least a man-in-waiting, and behaves as such, with active desire and also possibly with social or professional ambition; she might even be a feminist. She might also become a lesbian, but need not necessarily. It is not difficult to recognize, in this depiction, the type of the mannish lesbian, a stereotype well known in early twentieth-century European culture. They are masculine 'underneath', but still female, and therefore, by inference, play at being men. They are hence delusional and ultimately deficient. Those on the third path manage to negotiate their way to femininity and female sexuality: but what does this amount to? They want to be feminine and want to be desired as such, but their own desire is not for another person, not for sex as pleasure, only as a means to get the child that they want as a penis substitute.

Where did AF sit on these three pathways? Clearly not on pathway three, even though she did acquire children and made them the centre of her practice. Burlingham and the professional leadership of the psychoanalytic movement were also central to her life. It is evident that pathway one relates back to the girl who becomes an observer of beating fantasies and takes herself out of sexuality: in 1919 this was her father's view of AF. The trope of vicarious enjoyment that Freud put forward in 1919 chimes with two mechanisms of ego defence that AF set out much later ([1936] 1993) 'altruistic surrender' and 'identification with the aggressor'. Interestingly, AF based the discussion of 'altruistic surrender' on a case of a governess, who might well (again) have been AF herself (Young-Bruehl [1988] 2008: 210). Her father had discussed a defence in similar terms, calling it 'retiring in favour of another' in his 'Psychogenisis of a Case of Homosexuality in a Woman' ([1920] 1981) and in 'Some Neurotic Mechanisms in Jealousy, Paranoia and Homosexuality' ([1922] 2001). AF consistently presented herself, and has been represented, as reluctant to take on leadership of the psychoanalytic movement, and as only doing so on behalf of her father and the importance of his ideas; in other words, out of ambition for him rather than herself. But this hardly rings true. She pursued a different branch of psychoanalysis – child analysis – and different methods and aims from those of her father: observation and experiment instead of free association; education to strengthen the ego and superego for adaptation to social norms (for more on this see Stewart-Steinberg 2011). The battle for supremacy in the field of child analysis she undertook with Melanie Klein, despite being couched as a defence of her father's key concepts, tends rather to suggest that she was ambitious on her own behalf.

AF did not abandon ambition. In her father's terms, she would seem to be an amalgam of paths one and two. Indeed, both she and her father assented to AF's 'masculinity complex' and her identification with her father is impossible to ignore. For Freud, such an identification was a condition for fixating the masculinity complex. This would have put AF on path two in the 1931 formulation, where lesbian object-choice is posed, but not seen as inevitable. It seems – certainly to me – that for both Freud and his daughter it was preferable that she should be ascetic, outside of sexuality, undesiring, a consummate sublimator, rather than an active, desiring lesbian. Of course, it might be true that she was that. The 'it' that her letters refer to may have been masturbation. It might equally have been female-to-female desire. It appears that, whatever 'it' was, she controlled it and refused it to the end of her life.

'Femininity', Freud's last words on the subject, was a response to the work of female analysts[10] who were at the time exploring pre-Oedipal mother–child relationships; reading the paper, it is clearly also a riposte to unnamed feminists who had taken exception to his views on women and femininity. Here he reiterates the centrality of penis envy for femininity and of the Oedipus Complex for everyone, along with the propensity to bisexuality in women – if not in object-choice, at least in their tendency to switch between feminine attitudes (with passive aims) and masculine ones (with active aims). The necessity of the girl/woman being split away from the mother is emphasized, not only for the attainment of 'normal' femininity but for women on all three pathways. He says that even female homosexuals must take their father as object and enter the Oedipus for a time and it is only disappointment with the father that causes her to 'regress' into the masculinity complex. The bisexuality of women is the ground for these statements, backed up by remarks, said to be derived from clinical observation, on the 'practices of homosexuals', who 'play the parts of mother and baby with each other as clearly as husband and wife' (Freud [1933] 1973: 164). He attributes to Helene Deutsch a finding that 'the erotic actions of homosexual women reproduce the relations between mother and baby' (ibid.: 165).

Whatever else one might think about these statements, it is clear that Freud in 1933 conceives of female homosexuality in terms of his conception of heterosexual relations. It appears that for him there always has to be a masculine/father player and a feminine/mother player and also playing at being the baby for the other. Across this cluster of writings about femininity and homosexuality from 1919 onwards, it is also evident that Freud regards identification with the father as an essential component in lesbianism, as identification with the mother is in male homosexuality. The supposed inherent bisexual tendency in women is necessary to his formulation of lesbian relations, because it allows partners to switch between different positions and roles. We might consider that, for Freud, male homosexuals, in identification with the mother, in a sense fall into femininity and are thereby 'bisexualized', become what we might term 'shifters' in similar ways. I have to ask you, queer reader, if you are out there, is this what bisexuality means to you? Is it what homosexuality – male or female – means? Could this be a sexual relationship?

What about femininity itself? Not only is the path to 'normal' femininity 'circuitous', the state itself is said to be precarious, unstable. According to Freud, mature women can so readily lose their sexual appetite, can become indifferent and frigid, can focus all their emotional energy on their child or children, if they have them. Freud says that a mother only gets 'unlimited satisfaction' through her relationship to a son, which is 'the most free from ambivalence of all human relationships' (ibid.: 168) and that a marriage is only secure when the wife makes her husband her child and mothers him (ibid.). The propensity in women, all women, to 'switch' and to 'regress' to masculinity, in Freud's formulation, surely carries within it the possibility of any woman at any time forming a passionate relationship with another woman? He does not acknowledge this.

The notion of penis envy is the bedrock of Freud's conceptions of femininity and female sexuality. Yet it is precisely this concept that falls out of favour, through the twentieth and into the twenty-first centuries after Freud's death, even though the whole circus cannot revolve without it. And yet, so many aspects of the Freudian schema of femininity still persist in popular conceptions of women, and in representations of women even today.

The fluid and the fixed

Freud was a man of his time, his complex background, and his views on femininity and sexuality were inevitably coloured by these, despite his self-analysis. There is something particularly curious and queer in Freud's works on femininity. In 1933, he turned his attention on one hand to mother–daughter relations in childhood and, on the other, to sexuality as phenomenon in mature women. There he stated that those who had managed to attain 'normal' femininity could fall back into masculinity, frigidity, disappointment. Femininity, but actually it was 'normal' femininity – heterosexual womanhood – that was unstable for Freud, always susceptible to regression. The daydreaming, masturbating girl who takes herself out of sexuality in the 1919 essay remains fixed outside of it. The girl who regresses to her masculinity complex early on similarly remains fixed and either becomes asexual while retaining social or professional ambition, or becomes sexually active through homosexual object-choice; the latter, for Freud, operating along the same lines as a man might, through the chivalrous scenario he imposes on the 'psychogenisis' case and that he sees as masculine desire. A paradoxical note of fixity and fluidity sounds through the 1933 essay.

The 'normal' woman can fall into illness, and strikingly Freud proclaims that she, at around the age of 30, 'frightens us by her psychical rigidity and unchangeability' ([1933] 1973: 169) because her libido has become fixed and she is incapable of development. All that analysis can do, faced with this intractability, is to alleviate her symptoms (and these of course, go back to his earlier works on hysteria). He proposes that all the changes that the 'normal' woman has had to make to attain this femininity have worn her out. Clearly, then, the 'normal' woman, in her inherently unstable and yet paradoxically fixed state is highly prone to becoming neurotic. If all analysis can then do is to relieve symptoms by 'doing away with her neurotic conflict' (ibid.) one wonders what else Freud wanted to do? What was it that he had been hoping to cure? Perhaps her unhappiness in being placed as she was in the culture of his time, in the familial structures that he cast in mythological and therefore ancient and unchanging terms; rather, it seems as if he wanted to cure her of femininity itself, as he conceived it to be.

Freud, unlike his daughter, did not believe that diverting or re-orientating homosexual desire was possible. What is striking in his examination of female sexuality is that female homosexuality is the only pathway on which a woman can maintain a desire that is actually sexual and object-oriented, and that might even be satisfying. This is, of course, because he sees lesbian desire as masculine, but he does not really consider how this might work outside of a heteronormative framework. What he has to say about mature female heterosexuality suggests that it does not work very well.

Hence, I claim that the spectral presence of female-to-female desire is crucial, essential to Freud's conceptions of femininity; that it remains marginal, relatively unexplored, denied or with caveats and get-out clauses, not only in relation to AF but to femininity as a concept, is equally essential.

Anna/Marilyn: queer tales and a final twist

The corpus of writing about MM demonstrates that Freud's conceptualizations linger on, not only in the 1950s and 1960s, when MM was alive and under analysis, but even today, in popular culture and in more scholarly examinations, as accounts such as Lois Banner's show. Banner, like many others, paints MM in terms of illness and damage, physical and mental. This characterization makes MM's aspirations and achievements brave and heroic, but doomed nevertheless. Churchwell and Rose are attracted by and celebrate the bravery of MM's attempts to be herself despite all the projections thrust upon her. For Rose, MM was a kind of scapegoat, burdened with the insecurities and fantasies of US society (around troubled masculinity) in particular after World War Two. For Churchwell too, MM as icon of uber-femininity has carried all the baggage of fantasy, fear and contempt that femininity evokes and to an extreme, and therefore revealing, extent. The trouble is, that MM does seem to have accepted and internalized conceptions of femininity that circulated in her lifetime, including psychoanalytic ones. What is evident is that the myriad characterizations of her femininity, thus femininity itself in this extreme or absolute form, is cast as the seat of pathology. Female homosexuality is just one more facet, one more confirmation that 'abnormality' infects or at least constantly threatens femininity through and through, shading through utter abrogation of desire, active masculinity as denial of femininity and also as a stubborn insistence on desire (which may include female-to-female desire), and the rocky road of 'normal' femininity that can always fall back into (and actually begins with) a desire that is not primarily sexual and can easily be lost.

What about AF? Her father, probably with her consent, placed her as ascetic, asexual, with her masculinity complex fixed and fixated on him as father. This is what her father made of her and it was possibly what she made of herself; perhaps it was true. Certainly, it enabled her to remain the daughter that Freud called his Anna-Antigone, helpmeet to his Oedipus in old age. This insistence on AF as amalgam enabled her to avoid neurosis, to retain social and professional ambition, to pursue it, to become her father's heir. We might even say that it enabled AF to have it all – a lifelong emotional, affective relationship, children (at a remove), a successful career, acclaim, respect; everything except a sexual relationship? It might also have afforded her a representation, a protection and one might add a disguise for her own ambition couched as ambition for others through 'altruistic surrender' and also for the profound differences between her own and her father's psychoanalytic methods and practice. Who is to say that AF did not also disguise from others her sexual desire for women, perhaps for one woman in particular? If she felt it and refused it, controlled and sublimated it, that does not mean that it was not there. Reports of MM's 'lesbian inclinations', on the other hand, cannot be taken as proof that she experienced lesbian desire, or that she acted upon it. What is significant is that woman-to-woman desire haunts the accounts of these two women, and, as I have argued, haunts conceptualizations of femininity since Freud, as a 'third term', an occluded but pivotal point in constructions of female desire.

In a final twist, in the early 1940s, AF made notes on a series of dreams that eventually became the basis for her paper 'About Losing and Being Lost', which she drafted in 1948, gave as a lecture in 1953 but did not publish until 1967. Young-Bruehl quotes extracts from these notes, translated from German ([1988] 2008: 276–314). There is a recurrent dream in which the dead Freud is lost and wandering about and calls her to walk with him. He shows her tenderness, which makes her cry and that she says he hardly ever showed her in life. She thinks he should not have called her; that this undoes some progress in her mourning (ibid.: 286). Reading this recalls the 'tenderness' that was the outcome and goal of the younger AF's 'nice stories', but the dream is different. In associations to it, AF considers that her wish to leave the house at Maresfield Gardens, to acquire a retreat or an escape at Walberswick in East Anglia with Dorothy Burlingham, might have been a stimulus for this recurrent dream (ibid.: 287).

AF's resultant paper is a response and dialogue with her father's 'Mourning and Melancholia' ([1915] 1917), through the lens of her own mourning for him. In the associations to this recurrent dream, AF identifies Freud as Odysseus, not Oedipus, and reproaches him for being unfaithful to her. She casts herself as Penelope, the faithful wife who weaves a shroud by day and unpicks it at night so as to avoid finishing it and having to marry someone else (ibid.: 287). Behind this AF identifies a self-reproach, that she is being unfaithful to him, which, in AF's paper is expressed as a stage of mourning where the contradictory urges to remain loyal to the dead are opposed by urges to 'turn toward new ties with the living' (ibid.: 291). AF did turn toward the living, to Dorothy and their work. She ostensibly remained faithful to his memory and ideas, but pursued her own way, which was markedly different from his. AF and Dorothy did get their country cottage and yet made the house in Maresfield Gardens their home, despite its ghosts. They wove a life together, in whatever way, and who can say what that life was; what was a cover and a disguise?

In the end, I find that the sexuality of MM and of AF, whatever each might have been, no longer matters to me, or only in this respect: concepts of femininity, psychoanalytic and conventional, shaped them and the lives written about them and that shaping still persists. The Freudian legacy, despite its revisions and critical interventions, still makes me a spectre, not like MM, not like AF, yet not entirely unlike. I know I am not a spectre; I am not that but am, like them, a woman whose desire remains inadequately represented and theorized in psychoanalysis with its Freudian legacy.

Notes

1 The terms 'co-incidence' and 'coincidence' occur here in an attempt to distinguish between the several meanings of one word. 'Co-incidence' privileges the spatial and temporal senses: i.e. that an object, entity, idea, occurrence, occupies the same space or place as another, or that an occurrence or experience is taking place at the same time as another occurrence/experience. 'Coincidence' refers primarily to a meaning that the Shorter Oxford English Dictionary (5th edition, 2002: 445) defines as 'a notable concurrence of events or circumstances *without apparent causal connection*, (emphasis added). This is the popular sense that is applied to events (including thoughts) that are seen as only apparently linked, which come about by happenstance, which merely appear similar but are actually accidental juxtapositions. This meaning is pervasive; so that a coincidence is frequently understood as not meaningful. In psychoanalysis, such apparently random conjunctions, particularly when repeated, are not seen as accidental and

are never without cause. 'Coincidence' also carries another sense, that of correspondence, '*exact agreement*' whether in substance, nature, character or value, between one entity and another (ibid.). This latter sense – that one thing is in some aspect the same as another thing – is not employed or intended her in relation to Anna Freud, Marilyn Monroe and accounts of them; they were not the same and accounts of them do not exactly correspond. However, despite this contrivance, the several meanings of co-incidence/coincidence cannot really be contained: they all sound whenever the word appears. The spatial and temporal senses might make us think of the linguistic operations of metaphor (substitution) and metonymy (contiguity – side-by-side-ness); from there it is no great step to the psychic and psychoanalytic conceptions of displacement and condensation as keys or clues to decipherment of hidden or obscured meanings. Indeed, the various meanings of this word 'coincidence' might well make us think about the unconscious and its operations. Always present, and in the continuous-present tense, the unconscious or its operations is yet abstracted, not normally accessible, disguised, forgotten, but making its presence felt in signs that need to be interpreted, hazarded. Nothing, no symptom or slippage, no affect that takes place and is repeated is unmotivated for psychoanalysis.

2 This is a nod towards Lacan's *point de capiton* or 'quilting point', although not used or elaborated in his developed, technical sense (for a simple definition, see Evans 1996: 149). It is intended here to suggest that there are points where accounts of the two women, and interpretations of them touch on each other or are brought into relationship, not by similarity but their relationship to something else that is familiar and recognizable through repetition and consequently becomes meaningful and takes on a truth-value. I aim to show that familiar conceptions of femininity, in their repetition, act in this way to make accounts of women – not just Anna Freud or Marilyn Monroe – seem fixed, believable and even true.

The reference also introduces an extended metaphor and also a metonymy that will play out throughout this piece. Lacan's reference is to upholstery; mine is to the craft practices, generally seen as particularly female or feminine, of knitting and more particularly weaving. This takes us to the notion of a clue, or clew – a thread that in the myth of Theseus the woman gives him to get out of the labryrinth, and that in detective stories and psychoanalysis is sought and followed, as narrative, interpretation and possibly solution.

3 As we shall see, her father said this in so many words. Despite his caveats, masculinity and femininity are binaries and central to his thought, masculinity linked to active aims and femininity to passive ones. His contention (in several works) that females are particularly inclined to bisexuality revolves around notions that some women never achieve true or normal femininity, and even those who do are prone to regressing into masculinity. Bisexuality, then, becomes an ambiguous term, which may but does not necessarily relate to object choices or to sexuality as such, but rather to oscillations of identification across the binary and actually between a tripartite familial structure of father/mother/child.

4 Unfortunately, there is not space to examine Stewart-Steinberg's sophisticated and fascinating arguments here.

5 I use the terms 'normal' and 'abnormal' as Sigmund and Anna Freud used them. I do not concur with those designations, but take them as a talisman, like the term 'queer', against a heteronormative presumption that shapes desire in its own faulty image.

6 As another coincidence, in the late stages of redrafting this chapter I read Jennie Greengrass' novel *Sight* (2018), where she also meditates on AF's living with her father's ghost and also, weirdly, considers the wax figures of the Anatomical Venus (see below).

7 In this lecture Freud quoted Heinrich Heine's poem 'Nordsee', which does not ask a question about femininity but rather asks 'what signifies man'.

8 Freud introduced Lou Andreas-Salome to AF in a move that we might consider analogous to his advice regarding the unnamed young women in 'Pathogenisis of a Case of Homosexuality in a Woman'. There he broke off the analysis and advised that the young woman, or her parents, seek out a female analyst. Freud provided an analytically trained, very feminine woman for his daughter. In early 1922 AF went to stay with Andreas-Salome and started to write her paper, with Lou's help.

9 There is a great deal more to be said about this, but no space to elaborate it here beyond what is said below, in the section on the Freuds and femininity in particular.
10 He names Ruth Mack Brunswick, Jeanne Lampl-de Groot, Helene Deutsch and perhaps significantly does not mention Melanie Klein and others.

Bibliography

Appignanesi, L. (2008) *Mad, Bad and Sad: Women and the Mind Doctors*. New York: W. W. Norton.

Appignanesi, L. and Forrester, J. (1993) *Freud's Women*. London: Virago.

Banner, L. (2012) *Marilyn: The Passion and the Paradox*. New York: Bloomsbury.

Berthelsen, D. (1987) *La Famille Freud au jour le jour: Souvenirs de Paula Fichtl*. Paris: Presses Universitaires de France.

Blass, R. E. (1993) Insights into the Struggle for Creativity: A Reading of Anna Freud's 'Beating Fantasies and Daydreams'. *Psychoanalytic Study of the Child*, 48, 67–97.

Buchthal, S. and Comment, B. (eds) (2010) *Fragments: Poems, Intimate Notes, Letters by Marilyn Monroe*. London: Harper Collins.

Burlingham, M. J. (1989) *The Last Tiffany: A Biography of Dorothy Tiffany Burlingham*. New York: Atheneum, Macmillan.

Churchwell, S. (2004) *The Many Lives of Marilyn Monroe*, New York: Picador.

Churchwell, S. (2013) *The Many Minds of Marilyn Monroe*. Freud Museum event, 21 November.

Cohler, B. and Galatzer-Levy, R. (2008) Freud, Anna and the Problem of Female Sexuality. *Psychoanalytic Inquiry*, 28, 3–26.

De Lauretis, T. (1991) *The Practice of Love: Lesbian Sexuality and Perverse Desire*. Bloomington, IN: Indiana University Press.

Derrida, J. [1995] (1998) *Archive Fever: A Freudian Impression*. Trans Eric Prenowitz. Chicago, IL and London: University of Chicago Press.

Ebenstein, Joanna (2016) *The Anatomical Venus*, London: Thames & Hudson.

Evans, D. (1996) *An Introductory Dictionary of Lacanian Psychoanalysis*. London and New York: Routledge.

Freud, A. [1922] (1974) Beating Fantasies and Daydreams. In *The Writings of Anna Freud Vol. 1 1922–1935*. Madison, WI: International Universities Press.

Freud, A. [1936] (1993) *The Ego and the Mechanisms of Defence*. Trans Cecil Baines. London: Karnac.

Freud, A. [1953] (1967) About Losing and Being Lost. In *The Writings of Anna Freud Vol. IV*. New York: International Universities Press.

Freud Museum (2013) 'Mad, Bad and Sad': Women and the Mind Doctors. Exhibition leaflet.

Freud, S. [1905] (1981) Three Essays on the Theory of Sexuality. In *Pelican Freud Library Vol.* 7. Harmondsworth: Penguin.

Freud, S. [1905] (1985) Fragment of an Analysis of a Case of Hysteria. In *Pelican Freud Library Vol. 8*. Harmondsworth: Penguin.

Freud, S. [1915] (1917) Mourning and Melancholia. In J. Strachey (ed.) *Standard Edition of the Complete Works of Sigmund Freud, Vol XIV*, London: Hogarth Press.

Freud, S. [1919] (1997) A Child Is Being Beaten. In E. S. Person (ed.) *On Freud's 'A Child is Being Beaten'*. New Haven, CT and London: Yale University Press.

Freud, S. [1920] (1981) 'The Psychogenisis of a Case of Homosexuality in a Woman. In *Pelican Freud Library Vol. 9: Case Histories II*. Harmondsworth: Penguin.

Freud, S. [1922] (2001) Some Neurotic Mechanisms in Jealousy, Paranoia and Homosexuality. In J. Strachey (ed.) *The Standard Edition of the Complete Psychological Works of Sigmund Freud, Vol. XVIII.* London: Hogarth Press.

Freud, S. [1925] (1981) Female Sexuality. In *On Sexuality, Pelican Freud Library Vol. 7.* Harmondsworth: Penguin.

Freud, S. [1933] (1973) Femininity. In *New Introductory Lectures on Psychoanalysis, Pelican Freud Library Vol. 2.* Harmondsworth: Penguin.

Greengrass, J. (2018) *Sight*. London: John Murray.

Hecht, B. [1974] (2007) *My Story*. Lanham, MD: First Taylor Trade Publishing.

Mailer, N. [1973] (2012) *Marilyn*. London: Virgin Books.

Midgley, N. (2013) *Reading Anna Freud*. London and New York: Routledge.

Oates, J. C. (2000) *Blonde*. London: Fourth Estate.

Person, E. S. (ed.) (1997) *On Freud's 'A Child is Being Beaten'*. New Haven, CT and London: Yale University Press.

Phillips, A. (2014) *Becoming Freud: The Making of a Psychoanalyst*. New Haven, CT and London: Yale University Press.

Rose, J. (2014) *Women in Dark Times*. London: Bloomsbury.

Schneider, M. [2006] (2011) *Marilyn's Last Sessions. A Novel.* Trans: W. Hobson. Edinburgh: Canongate.

Smith, M. (2003) *Victim: The Secret Tapes of Marilyn Monroe*. London: Century.

Spoto, D. (1994) *Marilyn Monroe. A Biography*. London: Arrow.

Stewart-Steinberg, S. (2011) *Impious Fidelity: Anna Freud, Psychoanalysis, Politics*. Ithaca, NY and London: Cornell University Press.

Summer, A. (1985) *Goddess: The Secret Lives of Marilyn Monroe*. London: Victor Gollancz.

Young-Breuhl, E. [1988] (2008) *Anna Freud: A Biography*. New Haven, CT and London: Harvard University Press.

Young-Breuhl, E. (1998) *Subject to Biography: Psychoanalysis, Feminism and Writing Women's Lives*. Cambridge, MA: Harvard University Press.

11

TIRESIAS

Bracha L. Ettinger and the transgression with-in-to the Feminine

Sheila L. Cavanagh

This chapter is about Tiresias, the blind Theban prophet in the Oedipal trilogy and how he[1] animates what Israeli feminist psychoanalyst Bracha L. Ettinger calls an Other sexual difference. This Other sexual difference must be distinguished from Oedipal (or phallic) sexual difference theorized by Freud in terms of psychosexual development and later by Jacques Lacan under the auspices of sexuation whereby there are two possible sexual positions – man and the Woman – demarcated by the phallic signifier. Tiresias appears in Greek mythology and plays an important role in Sophocles' *Antigone* and in *Oedipus the King* as seer. Tiresias also appears in Homer's *Odyssey*, in Ovid's *Metamorphosis*, and in T. S. Eliot's *The Waste Land*, among other literary and dramatic works. In this chapter, I consider the significance of Tiresias to Ettinger's formulation of the Other (feminine) sexual difference. The Other sexual difference is an unconscious time-space of emergence, fading and transformation. It involves an unconscious process whereby we are borderlinked to Others (who Ettinger calls our non-I's)[2] in a matrixial web. The borderlinking is an encounter-event in the Real at the basis of what Ettinger calls feminine sexual difference. As Griselda Pollock explains, the Other sexual difference "generates a specific proto-ethical dimension in all human subjectivity irrespective of later gender identifications as masculine or feminine subjects under the sign of the Phallus" (2013: 167).

Although Tiresias is an ancient Greek shape-shifter and not transgender by contemporary definitions, his centrality to Ettinger's writing on the transgression with-in-to the Feminine (Ettinger 2000) is relevant to transgender cultural studies (Stryker and Whittle 2006; Stryker and Aizura 2013). Transgender cultural studies is based, in part, on a study of somatechnical (Murray 2016) transformations, transsexual transitions, desire and diverse embodiments – some of which resonate with Tiresian mythology. As such, there is an important convergence between Ettinger's feminist psychoanalytic theory and transgender studies that can be narrativized through the character Tiresias. Ettinger is, to the best of my knowledge, the first post-Lacanian feminist scholar to address the central importance of Tiresias in the Oedipal-trilogy. Certainly, Judith Butler names Tiresias in her discussion of the Oedipal-trilogy in *Antigone's Claim* (2000) and Hélène Cixous and Annette Kuhn (1981) mention the Theban prophet in their work on castration and decapitation. But there is curious neglect of the character in the now substantive body of feminist psychoanalytic scholarship. Perhaps this is due to unacknowledged transphobia and the consequent neglect of trans-like characters in psychoanalytic studies of mythology. It may also be due to a reluctance to consider the interrelationship between feminist psychoanalytic theory and transgender studies.

My supposition is that Ettinger's theory of the matrixial-feminine has something to offer transgender studies, if only because the character Tiresias, who changes sex, is central to what Ettinger refers to as the transgression with-in-to the Feminine. I have argued elsewhere that there is a discourse and an aesthetic particular to trangender that is not only submerged in psychoanalysis but rendered pathological or psychotic (Cavanagh 2017). Although Ettinger is not a transgender studies scholar and, to the best of my knowledge, has not worked analytically with transgender clients, her conception of the transgression with-in to the Feminine gives us a template to think about Tiresian-like transitions. A Tiresian-like transition is not the same as a transsexual transition (but the later may involve the former). It is, in Ettingerian terms, an entry into the matrixial whereby we co-emerge, transmutate and change with Others in unconscious and asymmetrical ways.

Tiresias indexes an Other sexual difference in Ettinger's formulation of the matrixial and this is, consequently, relevant to transgender studies. But the transgression of interest to Ettinger is matrixial. As such, it involves the "possibility of transgressing between male and female with-in a matrixial feminine dimension where Other and Outside are fatally engaged with I and inside" (Ettinger 2000: 198). The transgression with-in to the Feminine is not about becoming a woman in an identitarian sense but, rather, about entering into a feminine dimension of experience that refuses binaries between outside and inside, self and Other, male and female and so on. Referring specifically to Tiresias, Ettinger writes that the

> transgression between male and female is not a passage to the radical Other nor transcending to the ultimately exterior, but a metramorphosing with-in-out of selves with-in-to the Feminine that passes along the threads that turn, like a Mobius strip, the inside into the outside and the outside into the inside.
>
> *(Ibid.)*

As I will explain in what follows, the Tiresian origin-story involves an encounter-event with copulating snakes and Goddess Hera, in Peleponnese, which enable a metramorphic change. For Ettinger, a metramorphosis is a borderlinking and co-affecting relation in the matrixial web whereby partial-subjects are changed in/by the encounter-event with an Other. As she explains, metramorphosis "draws a nonpsychotic yet *beyond-the-phallus* connection between the feminine and creation" (Ettinger 2006: 64). Metramorphosis is a co-affective borderlinking, which enables change akin to the Deleuzian notion of "becoming". The metramorphic transgression enables the subject to access a "surplus beyond" the phallic axis. This surplus is about the transformation of what Ettinger calls phallic limits into thresholds.

In the myth, Tiresias turns into a Woman and enters into what Ettinger calls an Other axis of difference. While I focus on an Other sexual difference theorized by Ettinger in this chapter, let us remember that there are other dimensions of difference yet to be narrativized in psychoanalysis. It is an established fact that transpeople are subject to erasure, discrimination and are denied access to public space: the transphobic bathroom laws in the United States are but one contemporary example. But I am here concerned about the space of the clinic, the state of psychoanalytic theorizing and the Feminine (as an axis of difference) more generally. We have yet to account for the multiple harms engendered by the negation and expulsion of transpeople in psychoanalysis at the level of the International Psychoanalytic Association, its constituent organizations, the clinic and its training curriculum. The collateral damage done by the omission and pathologization of transpeople under the auspices of Oedipal psycho-sexual development is increasingly well established.[3] We can no longer ignore or sideline the contributions made by transgender scholars, artists, clinicians and analysands to the psychoanalytic scene.

Bracha Ettinger

Ettinger began to publish her writings on the Feminine and the matrixial borderspace inspired by her art and her psychoanalytic work with patients in the 1990s. The corpus of her theory is inspired by the writings of Wilfred Bion, Sigmund Freud, Jacques Lacan, Emmanuel Levinas, Maurice Merleau-Ponty, Gilles Deleuze and Félix Guattari and Donald Winnicot, among others. Her theories of the matrixial, along with her painting and art notebooks, have been written about by Griselda Pollock, Catherine de Zegher, Jean-François Lyotard, Christine Buci-Glucksmann and Brian Massumi. She is now a professor at the European Graduate School in Switzerland, a practising artist and analyst. Her oeuvre is offered as a supplement to and extension of Lacan's writing on feminine sexuality and subjectivity. Like other feminist psychoanalytic theorists including, but not limited to, Julia Kristeva, Luce Irigaray and Hélène Cixous, Ettinger contends that there is a discourse and aesthetic particular to the Feminine that is submerged in Lacanian psychoanalysis and in modernity more generally.[4] Ettinger's (2006) writing on the matrixial borderspace is designed to give theoretical form to a missing discourse and aesthetic of the Feminine.

For Ettinger, the Feminine operates through affective and aesthetic fields. Building upon Levinas, Ettinger explains that the Feminine is the "irreducible difference inside subjectivity: precisely what makes it human" (2006: 190). The matrixial borderspace is a feminine sub-stratum that coexists alongside what she refers to as the phallic (Symbolic) stratum theorized by Lacan.[5] The Other axis of sexual difference is foreclosed by the phallic signifier, but signifiable in an expanded sub-symbolic where (and when) we are attuned to Others and non-I's in the matrixial web (Ettinger 2006). The Other sexual difference in the matrixial is not about the One (and its binary oppositions between object and subject), but about "thinking transmissivity and co-affectivity" (ibid.: 183). It is about the unthought time-space of borderlinking in the matrixial that is trans-subjective (as distinct from transgender to be discussed below). This dimension of difference is, for Ettinger, primordial, occurring before, alongside, and after Oedipal sex difference but irreducible to it. The Feminine axis of difference is not based on phallic cuts, splits and severance but, rather, severality. The Ettingerian Feminine is thus not reducible to male or female, masculinity or femininity in a sociological sense. The Other sexual difference is based on trans-connectivity and trace connections to Others known and unknown in familial and extra-familial matrixes. In the Feminine dimension, the subject is more than one and bound to others in asymmetrical difference. This is why she refers to partial-subjects, as opposed to individual subjects. Ettinger does not theorize individual subjects who can be said to relate in the terms offered-up by object relations theory. Her focus is on partial-subjects who exist in relation to Others and non-I's in a non-conscious matrixial borderspace.[6]

Although Ettinger uses the metaphor of the mother-to-be and the subject-to-be in the pre-birth encounter as a model to think about the matrixial borderspace, the matrix should not be used as a synonym for maternity. Indeed, the matrixial is an axis of difference that transcends conception, gestation and birth. The female bodily specificity that Ettinger refers to in her writing on the matrixial involves corporeality but is not reducible to it. The matrixial is

> the site, physically, imaginatively, and symbolically, where a feminine difference emerges, and through which a "woman" is interlaced as a figure that is not confined to one-body, but is rather a hybrid "webbing" of links between several subjectivities, who by virtue of that webbing become partial.
>
> *(Ibid.: 141)*

As Griselda Pollock notes, the matrix is a signifier of "transformative transferential potentialities in a shareable resonance sphere" (Ettinger, as quoted by Pollock 2006: 21). We are always with Others in "reciprocity without symmetry, creating joint compassionate and eroticized aerials, to be further shaped by following traces of their further affective irradiation" (Ettinger 2000: 199). What Ettinger calls erotic aerials intercept aesthetic traces relevant to a shared matrixial web. In other words, a transgression with-in-to the Feminine is aesthetic and leaves trace-like imprints linking several partial-subjects in a shared web. It is the transformative capacities of the matrixial that the character Tiresias helps us to understand. By focusing on Tiresias and Ettinger's feminist psychoanalytic theory of the matrixial, I am not suggesting that those who are transgender, by contemporary standards, are ultimately "women" or "feminine" (although some are). Those who are transgender, like those of us who are not transgender, are all differently gendered in what Ettinger calls the phallic landscape. As Ettinger explains, access to the Feminine dimension of experience is open to everyone regardless of gender or sexual positioning in the phallic stratum of difference theorized by Lacan.

Tiresias animates, and helps us to understand, the trans-subjective elements of human experience explicated by Ettinger. While the linguistic similarity between "transgender" (or "transsexuality") and "trans-subjectivity" in Ettinger's theorization is significant, they are, in fact, different concepts. Transgender usually refers to those who dis-identify with their sex assignment at birth and/or to those who are gender variant. Transsexuality often refers to those who undergo social and/or medically assisted transitions that may involve gender confirming surgeries, hormone therapies, hormone blockers, etc. In Ettinger's formulation, "trans-subjectivity" does not have anything to do with gender. Nor does it refer to transpeople. Rather, trans-subjectivity refers to our status as partial-subjects in the matrixial web. In essence, the trans-subjective is used by Ettinger to account for the matrixial elements of the partial-subject in the Feminine sub-stratum (defined below). Trans-subjectivity should also not be confused with intersubjectivity because intersubjectivity depends upon singular subjects (in the phallic landscape) who can relate to one another in conscious ways. We are not singular subjects in matrixial terms but, as stated above, partial-subjects. Ettinger defines the partial-subject as several (more than One) and also refers to "subjectivity-as-encounter" in the matrixial order of things. In the transubjective weave, partial-subjects are co-affected by Others in non-symmetrical ways and thus partners in difference. Trans-subjectivity also involves "co-emergence" and "co-fading" in/through/ by metramorphosis (defined below). It thus contains transformative potentiality, which is relevant to transgender studies.

Tiresias and the Oedipal legacy

Before I advance my argument, let me offer a brief biographical sketch of Tiresias, the ancient Greek mystic. The original story told by Ovid (1986) in *Metamorphoses* begins as follows: Tiresias comes across two snakes copulating on Mount Kyllene in Peloponnese. Somehow upset by the inter-coiled snakes, Tiresias kills the female snake with his staff. Hera, the Goddess of women, marriage and fertility is furious. As a Goddess well known for acting upon impulse, she turns Tiresias into a woman in body and mind as punishment. But the curse may have been a blessing in disguise. By all accounts, Tiresias adjusts well to life as a woman. Tiresias marries, has three daughters, becomes a renowned prostitute and priestess. Seven years later Tiresias again encounters two mating snakes. Having learned Hera's lesson, Tiresias leaves them be and his masculinity is magically restored. We are to assume that by respecting not only the female snake but the act of copulation itself – a feminine dimension – Tiresias frees himself from Hera's spell.

But all was not well for long. Hera and her husband Zeus were fighting over who – man or woman – experiences more sexual pleasure in lovemaking.

Zeus insists it is the woman while Hera insists it is the man. Being unable to reach consensus they consult Tiresias who is said, in the myth, to have experiential knowledge of both masculine and feminine sexual pleasures. Tiresias answers to the Olympian court: "Of ten parts a man enjoys one only, but a woman enjoys the full ten parts in her heart" (Hard 1997: 171). Hera was incensed by the Tiresian-testimony and again moved to fury. She strikes Tiresias blind. Zeus takes pity on Tiresias but cannot undo his wife's spell. Instead, the masculine god gives Tiresias the gift of prophesy, second sight and long life. Over the course of his long life, Tiresias faithfully serves the Greek god Apollo. The blind-seer relays Apollo's words to the Lacanian letter. From a Lacanian perspective, we may infer that Tiresias, like a good analyst, attends to the particularity of the word and to the speaker's discourse.

In fact, Tiresian wisdom is known and respected throughout the Theban kingdom. His counsel is sought by king Oedipus and king Creon but both refuse Tiresian-guidance and suffer for it. Tiresias is, as a result, troubled by the impossibility of his job as prognosticator. Tiresias knows that hostility, denial, ignorance and projective identification on the part of the kings incite war. After telling Creon that in order to save his kingdom he must sacrifice his own son, Tiresias laments:

> Anyone who practices the art of prophesy is a fool. If he reveals offensive things
> he will reap resentment from all who hear his omens;
> but if, out of pity for those who come to him, he lies,
> he wrongs the gods. Only Phoebus should
> tell the gods' will to men, for he has no one to fear.
>
> *(Euripides 1994: 111)*

Exasperated by the plight of Oedipus and his refusal to see in *Oedipus the King*, Tiresias says, "How terrible – to see the truth when the truth is only plain to him who sees!" (Sophocles 1984). Tiresias discourages Oedipus from pursuing the truth – that he is the enemy he seeks (the one who killed his royal predecessor) – because he is cognizant of the tragedy awaiting King Oedipus who learns too late in life that he is not who he thought he was. Oedipus is not son of King Polybus and Queen Merope, but son of King Laius (who he has killed) and Queen Jocasta (who he marries). Tiresias knows that knowledge of patricide and incest will be too much for Oedipus and Jocasta to bear. But Oedipus, like a petulant child, insists upon knowing a truth he cannot handle. Upon hearing the truth he gouges his eyes out with his mother's brooch.

For the psychoanalytic record, Tiresias is also never wrong. Let us consider his oracular resume and demonstrated capacity to handle male protagonists in crisis: in Homer's *Odyssey*, Tiresias tells Odysseus how he may navigate treacherous waters on route home from the battle of Troy. In Euripides' *Phoenician Woman* Tiresias foretells that Oedipus' sons will ultimately kill each other in their warring anger and greed. In *Antigone*, Creon the King is less than thrilled to hear from Tiresias that he must withdraw his indictment against Antigone to save his family.

Like Oedipus before him, the King cannot accept Tiresian wisdom until it is too late; as a result his loved ones die and the Kingdom falls.

The Feminine in Lacan and Ettinger

At a conference on feminine sexuality at the University of Amsterdam in 1960, and later published in *Ecrits* (2006), Lacan said that we should not be fooled by the myth of Tiresias. In Ettinger's assessment, Lacan intimates that the Theban character cannot know anything more about feminine sexuality than we do, which is nothing. Ettinger's concern with Lacan is that he depicts feminine sexuality as unknowable. For her, Lacan is mistaken in assuming that the structure of language and thus, the unconscious, prohibits us from knowing anything about feminine sexuality. This, she insists, is only true in the phallic (Symbolic) stratum. While Lacan acknowledges limits to what can be known about the Woman due to what he calls a Real problem of language and logic, Ettinger's scholarship attempts to turn those limits into thresholds whereby something can be known about the Feminine – albeit in an expanded Symbolic that she calls the sub-symbolic (or sub-stratum). The Feminine sub-stratum does not generate signifiers (word-images) in Lacanian terms: it is Real. But from a matrixial perspective the Feminine can be apprehended.

Ettinger is critical of the way Lacan defines Woman as not-all, as object and as symptom of man. She reasons that he can only apprehend the Woman from the phallic angle. It is vital, she believes, to re-write the Woman in terms that can address her as several in a matrixial sense. The post-Lacanian Ettingerian formulation of Woman views her as a co-affecting and co-emergent borderlinking to Others (as partial subjects) in a matrixial borderspace. The Ettingerian Woman is best characterized as an assemblage, a co-affecting encounter-event between partial-subjects in a given matrixial web. Moreover, as Pollock writes, Ettinger's conception of Woman can be understood as "different conditions of subjective co-emergence[s]" (2006: 31). In the matrixial substratum Woman "digs an-other area of difference with its specific apparatus, processes, and functions" (Ettinger 1997: 367) that resonate in aesthetic fields through erotic aerials and aesthetic traces in a shared web. The Woman is, for Ettinger, not out of Symbolic bounds but can be apprehended in a matrixial sub-symbolic. In Pollock's reading, "Woman means different conditions: not just object or subject but the structure of transitivity" (2004: 46).

In her article "Transgressing with-in-to the Feminine" (2000), Ettinger revisits the myth of Tiresias to counter Lacan's claim at the Amsterdam conference that we can know nothing of the Feminine dimension. She explains that Lacanian psychoanalysis is bound to a phallic axis of difference while there is, in her formulation, an Other sexual difference that is matrixial (feminine) and applicable to everyone. There is, for Ettinger, a Woman in the matrixial feminine dimension that can be symbolized. A Woman is not a self-subject but a non-regressive transitive relation. In the matrix Woman is a "border-Other, a becoming in-ter-with the Other, never a radical alterity" (Ettinger 2001: 129). Ettinger also explains that the

Woman is the "co-emerging partial self and Other, or a different kind of relations to the Other" (2006: 72). As she reminds us, a father and son can be a Woman. Feminine cognizance of a non-I (or Other) in-relation to the I (as partial-subject) is, for Ettinger, based on a matrixial trans-sensitivity open to everyone. It is, for her, a feature of that which makes us human (and thus grounds for ethics). There is no one isolated subject in a matrixial web, only a Woman, defined as a condition of co-emergent relations between at least two partial-subjects. The matrixial Woman apprehends Others (as non-I's) as partners in difference.

While Lacan contends that a man (who experiences only phallic jouissance) cannot become a Woman (who experiences phallic jouissance along with an Other jouissance), Ettinger asks how Tiresias (or any partial-subject for that matter) cannot know something of/about the Other feminine jouissance. Ettinger's point is not that Tiresias can become a woman in a sociological sense (although he can) but, rather, that the story of Tiresias can tell us something about the transgression with-in-to the Feminine. Tiresias transgresses the difference between masculine and feminine sexual positions in the phallic axis theorized by Lacan. This places him in the matrixial-feminine dimension. Ettinger explains:

> Under the matrixial light, the transgression in the figure of Tiresias between man and woman is not a transgression of a frontier between known maleness and unknown femaleness. Rather, since the matrixial *I* carries traces of experiences of the matrixial *non-I*, inasmuch as *I know in the other* and my other *knows in me*, non-knowledge of the feminine, in the matrixial borderspace, is impossible, by virtue of the transgression itself.
>
> *(2000: 189, original emphasis)*

Ettinger reasons that the Tiresian transgression with-in-to the Feminine involves a metramorphic engagement with an Other (as non-I). The Other sexual difference is, as explained above, transitive. A man can thus become a Woman. But more than this, from Ettinger's standpoint it is impossible for anyone to not know something about the Woman (as co-affecting assemblage) in the Feminine dimension.

Sex difference in the matrixial is not about the One (and its binary oppositions between object and subject), but about "thinking transmissivity and co-affectivity" (Ettinger 2006: 183). It isn't about *having* (man) or *being* (Woman) the phallus, for example, but about the unthought time-space of borderlinking in the Real. Ettinger explains that the sexual coefficient in the matrixial is not between individuated subjects and their Others (intersubjectivity), but between the Other in the subject and the subject in the Other (trans-subjectivity). Tiresias is, for Ettinger, a matrixial figure because he transgresses sexual positioning in Lacanian terms. She writes, "what I would like to emphasize is that this kind of transgression between the sexes is a transgression with-in-to the feminine in a matrixial borderspace—whatever its direction [transition] is" (Ettinger 2000: 206).

Tiresias also reveals something of the Feminine dimension pertinent to desire and jouissance. Although Ettinger does not focus on Tiresian desire, she does write about matrixial desire. Matrixial desire is to borderlink and to differentiate within a "transgressive encounter-event and for the entirety of movements which create and fulfill such encounter-events, which, in passing by transformation would leave imprints for upcoming later transgressive encounter-events" (Ettinger 2007: 119). For Ettinger, borderlinking in the Feminine sub-stratum is ongoing and never, finally complete. In the matrixial, no one undergoes a transgression alone. Significantly, Tiresias does not instigate his own transition, it is caused by Hera (as partner-in-difference). He enters into a transgressive space whereby there is an event-encounter with Goddess-Hera and, of course, the snakes. There is also a borderlinking with the God Apollo to whom Tiresias is faithful. It must be remembered that Tiresias is a prophet, a seer and possesses knowledge outside the bounds of his own mortal and personal experience. Tiresian knowledge of, for example, incest and patricide in the House of Oedipus is not born of his own experience. In fact, it is, miraculous. Tiresian wisdom exceeds what can be known by any other character in the Sophocles trilogy.

As T. S. Eliot wrote in a footnote to *The Waste Land*, "all the women are one woman, and the two sexes meet in Tiresias. What Tiresias sees is, in fact, is the substance of the poem" (2001: 23). It is not surprising that Ettinger chooses Tiresias as a character who can transgress with-in-to the Feminine dimension but who can, also, tap into another axis of knowledge. Ettinger explains that, "Matrixial desire is an aspiration and an inspiration from a feminine *jouissance* toward the edges of a wider Symbolic" (2006: 113). In other words, there is for Ettinger a "feeling knowledge" that exceeds the phallic Symbolic. Lacan and Ettinger agree that feminine jouissance is characterized by a unique orientation to knowledge and logic. Ettinger reasons that matrixial desire is attuned to the trans-subjective field and is, ultimately, knowledge of transgression and borderlinking. It is, in other words, knowledge of the Feminine dimension. My supposition is that Tiresias is also a matrixial figure in Ettinger's formulation because he can see what Oedipus cannot. Not only does the Tiresian truth – that Oedipus killed his father and married his mother – lead to dramatic climax in the play, but it gestures to the boundaries of what can be known, at least without tragedy, in the phallic stratum represented in the play by the Kingdom of Oedipus.

Tiresias is also a matrixial figure because he is bound to Others who he does not repudiate. Unlike Oedipus, Tiresias avows his connections to Others (like, for example, Apollo), even as the God causes him pain. There is, in Ettingerian terms, a non-Oedipal sublimation and investment in Others that is feminine. Tiresias embodies this non-Oedipal sublimation. Ettinger explains that the Other sexual difference "produces for men and women a different, non-Oedipal sublimation where, in the search for *non-I*(s), the *jouissance* is of the borderlinking itself" (2001: 110). This feminine difference is symbolized by Tiresias, his transgression with-in-to the Feminine and his divine knowledge of an Other (Godlike) order of difference. Indeed, Tiresias turns the House of Oedipus on its head. Pollock writes that feminine desire might "signify something of profound importance for discussions of human subjectivity and indeed sociality"

(2006: 22). Likewise, Tiresias and transgender studies might signify something of profound importance to psychoanalysis.

Oedipus

Ettinger's writing on Tiresias and the matrixial gives us a new perspective on the Oedipal-life-tragedy that is germane to much psychoanalytic theorizing. As evidenced in *Oedipus the King*, Oedipus cannot tolerate or recognize Others in his familial web – at least not very well. He abandons his adopted parents on the road to Thebes, misrecognizes his birth parents, begets offspring by his mother, who are also his siblings, and in his old age at Colonus, treats Antigone, his daughter-sister, like a nurse maid. I think we can agree that Oedipus has more than his fair share of family troubles. It is an unacknowledged fact that he does not set a good therapeutic example. Apart from the fact that he kills his father and marries his mother, he disowns his sons who are at war with each other for what was originally their father's throne. Refusing Antigone's advice to yield to his sons and relent upon his anger, to the older Polynices, Oedipus says: "Die by your own blood brother's hand – die!" (Sophocles 1984: 365). Antigone is left to contend with her father-brother's traumatic legacy and tragically, takes her own life to give her brother, Polynices, a proper burial. Oedipus eventually dies in exile at Colonus. As Tiresias told the Theban king years before his actual death: "No man will ever be rooted from the earth as brutally as you [Oedipus]" (ibid.: 183). The Tiresian truth comes to pass and Oedipus dies a painful death in Colonus.

What Ettinger's oeuvre adds to psychoanalysis is a way for us to see how the plight of Oedipus is structured not only by a disavowal of his traumatic life-legacy (involving patricide and incest), but of the Feminine dimension. Oedipus lusts for his mother and over-identifies with his father, as indicated by his literal usurpation of his father's marital-bed and position as king. While Freud thought *Oedipus the King* had an impressive following because it reveals universal incestuous and patricidal desire – hence the Oedipal complex – the play is, in my Ettingerian reading, a classic because it reveals the tragic outcome associated with the negation of an Other sexual difference. Oedipus is primarily suffering from an un-symbolized loss: a feminine loss involving others in the matrixial web. What does his very public transgression of the incest taboo reveal if not a yearning for a way to borderlink with others from whom he has been separated? Oedipus could not apprehend his kin who stand-in for Others (non-I's) in the Feminine dimension. Tiresias could see this lack of apprehension and knew it would lead to tragedy. Let us be clear about the fact that the tragedy in each of the three Sopholean plays is born of exile, excommunication and war between cities: incest and patricide come after the fact. In other words, Oedipus is primarily affected by the traumatic rupture to his familial web and exile from his city-home. His position as king and patriarch prevent him from recognizing Others in his family and country to whom, from a matrixial perspective, he is ultimately bound.

Conclusion

I appreciate the role Oedipus has played in the choreography of psychoanalysis, but it is high time to make room on the psychoanalytic stage for other characters, like Tiresias, who tap into Other axes of difference. The mythology of Tiresias gives life and form to a configuration of feminine difference that supplements the Lacanian formulation of sexuation. Whether we accept Ettinger's critique of Lacanian writing on feminine sexuality or, alternatively, choose to theorize a feminine dimension of experience within Lacanian (phallic) parameters, it is important to embrace non-Oedipal characters, myths and stories in psychoanalytic theory. The Tiresian transgression with-in-to the Feminine is, in my Ettingerian reading, beyond the Lacanian limit mediated by the phallic structure. The transgression is, more precisely, into the matrixial order of things where no One is alone.

The story of Tiresias prompts us to consider an Other sexual difference relevant to a trans-psychoanalytic (Cavanagh 2017) turn in the clinic. Tiresias is ideally positioned to tell us something in retrospect about what Ettinger calls the matrixial order of difference that is, like the phallic order of difference, sexual. In other words, we are not lone actors on the stage of life but several and co-affecting in Ettingerian terms. By evoking Tiresias as emblematic of the Other sexual difference, we should not assume that transgender is a Rosetta Stone or unencumbered road to matrixial ethics or to an otherness beyond the phallus. As explained above, the matrixial is available to everyone regardless of gender, transgender status and sexual orientation. Transgender life experience may, however, prompt us to consider another axis of feminine difference because there can be an acute awareness of the Other sex in the One. As Ettinger explains, there are multiple ways to write the Woman in the matrixial. Transgender subjectivity may be one such way – at least for those identifying as trans-feminine or with the Tiresian-transgression with-in-to the Feminine.

Acknowledgements

I thank Bracha L. Ettinger for encouraging words on the development of this chapter at the Psychoanalysis in Our Time: Psychoanalysts and Femininity conference in Gdansk Poland (8–10 April 2016), organized by Agnieszka Piotrowska and Ben Tyrer. I am also indebted to Caitlin Janzen for her critical commentary on the Feminine and for her editorial assistance. I acknowledge the generous financial support of the Social Sciences and Humanities Council of Canada under research grant number 890-2014-0026.

Notes

1 I am using the masculine pronoun to reference Tiresias because the prophet lives most of his life as a man.

2 Ettinger refers to the non-I in the metramorphic encounter-event as a site of transmission to be distinguished from an Other as subject.

3 See, for example, the recent special issue of *Transgender Studies Quarterly* (2017) on "Transgender and Psychoanalysis".

4 Ettinger (2006) offers her theorization of the Other sexual difference as an alternative to the formulation of the semiotic and the Chora (which means womb and uterus) developed by Julia Kristeva. Although both the Chora and the Matrix are anchored to maternal encounters, Ettinger contends that the Chora cannot be symbolized in Kristeva's theory. The Chora is, for Kristeva, a precondition for the semiotic and ultimately a basis for language but is, for Ettinger, confined to psychotic discourse or to poetic discourse.

5 Ettinger refers to the Other (Feminine) axis of difference as a sub-stratum that coexists alongside what she calls the phallic axis of difference. The phallic axis of difference is the stratum whereby identity, intersubjectivity and sexual positioning (as man or as Woman) make sense. In the Feminine sub-stratum we are all trans-subjective because we are moored by Others and non-I's, partners in difference particular to a given matrixial web.

6 The I and the non-I are names for the partial-subject and its Other. "The I is a pulsating pole of co-poiesis. The I and non-I are pulsating poles of co-poiesis along a shared psychic string" (Ettinger 2006: 193). Together, these fields with their multiple I's and non-I's form matrixial webs.

Bibliography

Adams, P. (1996). *The emptiness of the image: psychoanalysis and sexual differences*. New York: Routledge.

Bertelsen, L. (2004). Matrixial refrains. *Theory, Culture & Society*, 21(1), 121–147.

Butler, J. (2000). *Antigone's claim: kinship between life and death*. New York: Columbia University Press.

Caldwell, C. and Keshavan, M. S. (1991). Schizophrenia with secondary transsexualism. *Canadian Journal of Psychiatry/La Revue Canadienne de psychiatrie*, 36(4), 300–301.

Cavanagh, S. L. (2017). Introduction. *Transgender Studies Quarterly*, 4(4).

Carlson, S. T. (2010). Transgender subjectivity and the logic of sexual difference. *differences*, 21(2), 46–72.

Chiland, C. (2000). Some thoughts on transsexualism, transvestitism, transgender and identification. In G. Ambrosio (ed.) *Transvestitism, transsexualism in the psychoanalytic dimension*. London: Karnac.

Cixous, H. and Kuhn, A. (1981). Castration or decapitation? *Signs*, 7(1), 41–55.

Elliot, P. (2001). A psychoanalytic reading of transsexual embodiment. *Studies in Gender and Sexuality*, 2(4), 295–325.

Eliot, T. S. (2001). *The waste land*. New York and London: W. W. Norton.

Ettinger, B. L. (1997). The feminine/prenatal weaving in matrixial subjectivity-as-encounter. *Psychoanalytic Dialogues*, 7(3), 367–405.

Ettinger, B. L. (2000). Transgressing with-in-to the Feminine. In P. Florence and N. Foster (eds.) *Differential aesthetics*. London: Ashgate.

Ettinger, B. L. (2001). Matrixial gaze and screen: other than phallic and beyond the late Lacan. In L. Doyle (ed.) *Bodies of resistance: new phenomenologies of politics, agency, and culture*. Evanston: Northwestern University Press.

Ettinger, B. L. (2006). *The matrixial borderspace*. Minneapolis: University of Minnesota Press.

Ettinger, B. L. (2007). Diotima and the matrixial transference: psychoanalytical encounter-event as pregnancy in beauty. In H. Viljoen and C. N. Van der Merwe (eds.) *Beyond the threshold: explorations of liminality in literature*. New York: Peter Lang.

Euripides (1994). The phoenician woman. *The Classics Pages*. Available at: www.users.globalnet.co.uk/~loxias/phoenissae.htm.

Glocer Fiorini, L. and Gimenez de Vainer, Á. (2003). The sexed body and the real: its meaning in transsexualism. In A. M. Alizade (ed.) *Masculine scenarios*. London: Karnac.

Freud, S. (1917). Mourning and melancholia. In J. Strachey (ed.) *The standard edition of the complete psychological works of Sigmund Freud, Vol. XIV*. London: Hogarth Press.

Gherovici, P. (2010). *Please select your gender: from the invention of hysteria to the democratizing of transgenderism*. New York: Routledge.

Goldner, V. (2011). Trans: gender in free fall. *Psychoanalytic Dialogues*, 21(2), 159–171.

Guattari, F. (1996). Ritornellos and existential affects. In G. Genosko (ed.) *The Guattari reader*. Oxford: Blackwell.

Hard, R. (1997). *Apollodorus: the library of Greek mythology*. Oxford: Oxford University Press.

Lacan, J. (2006). *Écrits: the first complete edition in English*. New York: W. W. Norton.

Laufer, M. E. (1991). Body image, sexuality and the psychotic core. *International Journal of Psychoanalysis*, 72(1), 63–71.

Millot, C. (1990). *Horsexe: essays on transsexuality*. New York: Autonomedia.

Morel, G. (2011). *Sexual ambiguities: sexuation and psychosis*. London: Karnac Books.

Murray, S. (2016). *Somatechnics: queering the technologisation of bodies*. London: Routledge.

Ovid (1986). *Metamorphoses: A New Translation by A. D. Melville*. Oxford: Oxford University Press.

Pollock, G. (2004). Thinking the feminine aesthetic practice as introduction to Bracha Ettinger and the concepts of matrix and metramorphosis. *Theory, Culture & Society*, 21(1), 5–65.

Pollock, G. (2006). Introduction. Femininity: aporia or sexual difference? In B. L. Ettinger, *The matrixial borderspace*. Minneapolis: University of Minnesota Press.

Pollock, G. (2013). From horrorness to compassion: re-facing Medusan Otherness in dialogue with Adriana Caverero and Bracha Ettinger. In *Visual politics of psychoanalysis: Art and the image in post-traumatic cultures*. London: I. B. Tauris.

Prosser, J. (1998). *Second skins: the body narratives of transsexuality*. New York: Columbia University Press.

Salamon, G. (2010). *Assuming a body: transgender and rhetorics of materiality*. New York: Columbia University Press.

Shepardson, C. (2000). *Vital signs*. New York: Routledge.

Siomopoulos, V. (1974). Transsexualism: disorder of gender identity, thought disorder, or both? *Journal of the American Academy of Psychoanalysis*, 2(3), 201–213.

Sophocles (1984). *The three Theban plays: "Antigone", "Oedipus the King", "Oedipus at Colonus"*. New York: Penguin Classics.

Stryker, S. and Whittle, S., eds. (2006). *The transgender studies reader*. New York and London: Routledge.

Stryker, S. and Aizura, A. Z., eds. (2013). *The transgender studies reader 2*. New York and London: Routledge.

12

A SPECIMEN OF A COMMENTARY ON LACAN'S *'L'ÉTOURDIT'*

A. R. Price

The commentary that follows, specimened from more extensive discussion, bears on a segment from the section of 'L'étourdit' *that falls on pages 19–23 of* Scilicet *4 1973.*

* * *

C'est de fait le scandale du discours psychanalytique. Following the now well-established pattern, beyond the reference strophe-sentences heading the new section the construction loosens into a freer scheme that compels a parsing of larger word groupings.

An outrage is asserted, pertaining not to an analytic community or history but to the very discourse itself, indexed above in its newly formalised combinatory, and so the scandal must be intrinsic to psychoanalysis, not the result of local incident. This reading can be quickly confirmed in reference to the Seminar material, where as early as the fourth in the series Lacan could be heard to assert that 'analysis partakes of a sort of scandalous notion of man's affective relations'; above and beyond the role accorded to sexuality, this scandal in analysis 'introduced the notion of a paradox, of an essential difficulty, that is inherent, so to speak, in the approach to the sexual object' (Lesson of 12 December [1956–1957]). While this passage predates by over a decade the sloganizing of 'no such thing as sexual relation', the alertness to absence of harmony between human subject and sexual object as isolated discursively in analysis is here lent unequivocal formulation, and indeed ascribed to the fundamental Freudian articulation. Specifically, to pursue Lacan's indication, in the *Drei Abhandlungen zur Sexualtheorie* the first sexual object, the mother, carries the qualification *unverwendbar*, that is to say, 'unutilisable' (cf. James Strachey's corrected translation in Freud [1905] 1987: 94, 119), and the object is preserved so in memory throughout the latency period, conditioning its 're-finding' as an insuperably discordant partner.

This scandalous aspect of acknowledged sexual discordance finds enhancement in '*L'instance de la lettre*', delivered then redacted in May 1957 and so concurrent with the fourth seminar: 'The intolerable scandal at the time when Freudian sexuality was yet to be sanctified, was that it was so "intellectual"' (Lacan 1966: 523). It may be inferred, then, that this is about the unwelcome prompt to a seizing of absence by the intellect.

The present paragraph, like the two preceding, has been construed by some commentators as somehow pointing exophorically to an epistemic failing on the part of the analytic community adequately to address feminine 'otherness' (cf. Fierens 2002: 135; Soler 2006: 9–10, 190), but the same thereby rehearse the very confounding of the feminine and the absolute Other that already in the 1958 '*Propos directifs pour un Congrès sur la sexualité féminine*' was declared to arise from the 'phallocentric dialectic' (Lacan 1966: 732). However potentially scandalous such a tendency may be, here the focus is pitched otherwise: the matter is what has been actualised 'in deed', in such fashion as thereby to have openly and effectively scandalised, which is precisely what this substantivised 'scandal' implies. And so the opening *C'est* is indubitably endophoric, picking up the forcing of ab-sense from the previous sentence.

, et c'est assez dire où les choses en sont dans la Société. The International Psychoanalytic Association was an altogether different institution in 1972 from the one that Freud left behind in the 1930s, and even from the one that would have been familiar to Lacan in the 1950s and early 1960s. Any attempts such as there were to mimic the secret committee of the 1920s with an eye to orienting and doctrinally unifying the widely spread societies of the post-war period were ineffective, while Freud's carefully pressed recommendations on lay analysis were not heeded in the United States until the law suits of 1985, and only then with great reluctance and a peculiar disengagement from the considerable ethical stakes (see the long-drawn-out and thoroughly noncommittal account by then president Robert S. Wallerstein [1998]). Perhaps in using the denomination *Société* rather than *Association*, the local French seat of the IPA is here being fingered. As one of the members of the *Société psychanalytique de Paris* observed in a commemorative report, having ostracised Lacan in 1964, the contributors to the SPP Congress of 1965 ensured that he would be 'nevertheless quite present, by his very absence': in their new-found confidence, a number of papers gave loose rein to geneticist and ego-psychological perspectives hitherto contained during the years of his influence (see de Mijolla 1991: 34).

qui le supporte. Again both verb and pronoun operate bivocally, tendering an undiscerning reader the bait of a psychoanalytic society that 'supports' discussion, but on more careful inspection rebuking this seat of officialdom for merely 'putting up with' the scandal inherent to the analytic discourse.

, que ce scandale ne se traduise que d'être étouffé. The copulative and existential senses of *être* are once more exploited, this time to isolate a 'hushed-up scandal' that

simultaneously localises a 'stifled being', the latter designating a state both pre- and post-translation, to drive at spatial and temporal conveyance rather than linguistic rendering. By further implication, the *Société* in question cannot be the native ground of the psychoanalytic discourse and its inherent scandal, only that of its reluctantly tolerated implantation. In the terminology of . . . *ou pire*, this stifling is 'the institutionalised silence of psychoanalysis on this matter of there being no such thing as sexual relation' (Lesson of 8 December [1971–1972b]).

, si l'on peut dire. A common locution is again lent fresh tenor as one of the key signifiers of '*L'étourdit*' now makes its second appearance in this same sentence: there would be *dire* enough would that such muzzling might allow for so saying, in deed.

In the oral teaching of 1972, Lacan twice alludes to the gagging action of the IPA: in his own regard, citing the 'sitting officials' who 'dealt me one of those blows that diminishes your voice' (Lesson of 8 March [1971–1972b]); and with respect to Ignacio Matte Blanco, whose work on bi-logic had been subjected to a 'stymie', to be lifted only in 1975 with the publication in English of *The Unconscious as Infinite Sets* (*entretien* of 1 June [1971–1972a]; the belated publication may have been part-indebted to Lacan's attentions, though Matte Blanco's 'Acknowledgements' contain no such mention).

, au jour. The reader is put to the task of making the concluding remark cohere either with the scandal of a smothering in broad daylight, acknowledging a likely pun on '*étaler au jour*' ('to divulge' or 'to bring to light'), perhaps even at its very moment of coming to light of day, or with a potential fact of saying 'in this day and age'.

* * * *

Au point que. The sentence opens as a subordinate clause to the previous sentence, straining to a degree the otherwise conspicuous paragraph break which is thus to be read as ordering the first in an itemisation of corollaries ensuing from the *scandale* and its smothering.

c'est un monde. Initially a hyperbolic locution used to remark on unexpectedly grand scale of architectural space or human congregation (cf. the letter of 29 September 1680 from the Marquise de Sévigné to her daughter, the Comtesse de Grignan: '*C'est une république, c'est un monde que votre Château; je n'y ai jamais vu cette foule*' [1775: 363]), the more general use of '*c'est un monde!*' for exaggerated expression of disbelief first gained ground in the nineteenth century.

By 1972, the discussions on female sexuality of 40 years hence could fairly be described as 'a world away'. Few were able to claim a direct connection with the events of the 1920s and 1930s, one among scarce exceptions being Helene Deutsch who was to outlive Lacan himself (12 years her junior), passing away in 1982. The locution here connotes also the microcosm of the pre-war psychoanalytic community, presently to be fractured both geographically by the events in Europe and factionally by the tangential loyalties that set the following generation at loggerheads.

à soulever. The pun works tautologically: a world of extreme effort to raise a world dead and gone, here raised as comment-worthy issue. The connotation of 'raising the dead' is subtly lifted from *être étouffé* in preparation of a sustained metaphor of expiry.

que. The grammatical hinge of this single-sentence paragraph appears to function not as a conjunction but adverbially, further to heighten the exclamatory tone (cf. the examples in Claude Buffier's 1709 *Grammaire française sur un plan nouveau*, translated into English as *A French Grammar on a New Plan*: '*c'est une passion dangereuse que l'amour*'; or '*ce seront toujours des tourmens que les désirs*' [1734: 214]).

ce débat défunt. Where in 1958 the pre-war debate on female sexuality was being qualified as *délaissé* (Lacan 1966: 687), like an item dropped or given up in the flight from *Mitteleuropa*, here it is more despairingly reckoned to lie beyond retrieval and reanimation. As noted, the *défunt* is thematically redolent of the asphyxiated being of the previous sentence.

des années 30. What is here denoted in relaxed mode as a debate from the 1930s refers to what had been more specifically, though divergently, designated in two of the written texts from 1958. While '*La signification du phallus*', delivered in Munich on 9 May and printed without modification in the *Écrits*, cites a 'discussion on the phallic phase' echoed and pursued in various writings published *between 1928 and 1932* (1966: 687), in '*Propos directifs pour un Congrès sur la sexualité féminine*', penned in 1958 but not published until 1962, reference is made to a question that raged *between 1927 and 1935* (ibid.: 777).

These dates coordinate usefully, both in their convergence and slight divergence. First, they together exclude the early writings on the topic of female sexuality that predate Freud's 1925 paper on '*Einige psychische Folgen des anatomischen Geschlechtsunterschieds*' (. . .) Second, they omit some of the first responses to Freud's 1925 paper (. . .) Third, they set down an end-date that debars the pre-war pursuance of the debate in Horney's lecture to the German Psycho-Analytic Society on 23 December 1936, printed as 'The Neurotic Need for Love' in the posthumous collection *Feminine Psychology*, (1967), itself a foretaste of her sociological position developed soon thereafter in *The Neurotic Personality of Our Time* (1937).

(. . .)

The divergence between the two sets of dates is perhaps more telling. By bringing forward by one year the opening of the debate, the '*Propos directifs*' effectively include the contributions from the 1927 Congress in Innsbruck (. . .) Conversely, by pushing back the closing date by three years, there is a pronounced embracing of: Freud's piece on 'Femininity' in the *New Introductory Lectures* of 1933; Horney's paper on 'The Denial of the Vagina: A Contribution to the Problem of the Genital Anxieties Specific to Women' (1933) and her 1933 lecture in Washington DC on 'The Problem of Feminine Masochism'; together with Jones' paper on 'The Phallic Phase', and most especially his taking stock of the whole debate in the famous address to the Vienna Psycho-Analytical Society on 24 April 1935 (. . .) These later papers are almost certainly an influence on this more vague reference in '*L'étourdit*' to a debate 'from the 1930s', though still the 1958 description of Jones' 'Early Female Sexuality' as having 'scorched the earth for any contribution since' (Lacan 1966: 728) maintains its currency.

non certes pas qu'à la pensée du Maître. Just as previously the bivocal masculine pronoun was exploited to enable conflation between Freud and the *pourtout*, here the *Maître* is both Freud in his role of mentor and mastermind of psychoanalysis, and the master-signifier as instanced from its command position in thought structuring.

ne s'affrontent pas Karen Horney, Hélène Deutsch. The debate on female sexuality and the phallic phase was brought to a pitch of intensity by three contributions each from Helene Deutsch and Karen Horney, the 'most eminent' women to participate in the debate according to the terms of '*La signification du phallus*' (Lacan 1966: 687).

Deutsch read 'The Significance of Masochism in the Mental Life of Women' at the Oxford Congress of 1929. Published first in English in the *International Journal* of 1930, then in German in 1930 in the *Internationale Zeitschrift für Psychoanalyse* and in 1931 in the *Almanach der Psychoanalyse*, it was followed in 1932 by '*Über die weibliche Homosexualität*', initially intended for the 1931 Congress which in the event did not take place (published in English in 1933 as 'Homosexuality in Women'; it is noted that the paper is being printed in response to Freud's recently published 'Female Sexuality'). Then came 'Motherhood and Sexuality', one of five papers delivered to the Vienna Psychoanalytic Society in the summer of 1932, published the following year in *The Psychoanalytic Quarterly*.

As for 'affronting' the *Maître*, if the latter is to be understood as the master 'himself', in these contributions Deutsch takes issue just once, and gently, with a Freudian tenet. 'Homosexuality in Women' reasserts the girl's 'swing towards passivity' first posited in her 1925 book, but now couples it with an early 'swing towards activity' that lays down the 'foundationstone' for feminine homosexuality ([1931] 1933: 55), thus openly challenging Freud's focus on the later pubescent period in 'Psychogenesis of a Case of Homosexuality in a Woman'.

Karen Horney's defiance is far more pronounced. In 1932, she published her paper '*Die Angst vor der Frau Über einen spezifischen Unterschied in der männlichen und weiblichen Angst vor dem anderen Geschlecht*'; also printed that same year in English as 'Observations on a Specific Difference in the Dread Felt by Men and by Women Respectively for the Opposite Sex' (1932: 348–360). The argumentation pursues the same line as Horney's articles of the late 1920s, yet with renewed vigour following Freud's public admission that her notion of a secondary *penisneid* 'does not tally' with his impressions ('Female Sexuality'). Here, Freud is criticised for failing to give due consideration to, and thus adequately to account for, the factor of anxiety in the fetishist's abhorrence of the vagina (ibid.: 352). In similarly confrontational tone, Horney proceeds to revise Freud's note on the boy's 'impulsion to inquire into things', amplifying instead the 'desire to penetrate' first posited in Müller-Braunschweig's paper on 'The Genesis of the Feminine Super-Ego' (ibid.: 354); considerations that play a role in the concluding revision where 'once we realize that masculine castration-anxiety is very largely the ego's response to the *wish to be a woman*, we shall not altogether share Freud's conviction that bisexuality manifests itself more clearly in the female than in the male' (ibid.: 359).

As noted above, Horney's paper of 1932 was closely followed by the papers on 'The Denial of the Vagina' and 'The Problem of Feminine Masochism'. In the former, a selection of Freud's key theoretical assertions are again cast in doubtful light: 'It seems to me that analytic experience alone does not sufficiently enable us to judge the soundness of some of the fundamental ideas which Freud has made the basis of his theory' (1933: 59); in particular, Freud's statement that male and female character are sharply differentiated only from puberty onwards is singled out for attack, Horney adding that she struggles to reconcile the young girl's spontaneous coquetry or 'maternal solicitude' with 'Freud's view of the initial masculine trend of the little girl's sexuality' (ibid.: 60). Drawing again on Josine Müller's 1925 text (published posthumously in 1932), 'A Contribution to the Problem of Libidinal Development of the Genital Phase in Girls' ([1925] 1932: 361–368), and her own earlier paper 'On the Genesis of the Castration Complex in Women', but now further bolstered by recent remarks from gynaecologist Wilhelm Liepmann and analyst Felix Boehm, Horney challenges anew Freud's assessment that the vagina remains 'undiscovered' by the young girl, and proffers the evidence of phantasies that 'do not in fact stop short at quite indefinite ideas of an act of violence, through which one gets a child' in support of an 'instinctive knowledge of the existence of the vagina as the organ of reception' (1933: 63–64). 'I have never been wholly convinced', opines Horney, 'by Freud's explanation why girls suppress direct genital masturbation more easily and frequently than boys', proffering the 'dread of vaginal injury' as an alternative to Freud's 'narcissistic mortification' (ibid.: 65).

Meanwhile, in 'The Problem of Female Masochism', Horney makes bold to say of *penisneid* that, 'it must be realized, however, that this hypothesis is an hypothesis, not a fact; and that it is not even indisputably useful as an hypothesis' ([1933] 1935: 243), later asserting in a footnote that to deduce women's jealousy from *penisneid* 'is not convincing' (ibid.: 255n8). Tellingly, however, in this same note, *penisneid* is qualified as a 'more purely individual anatomical-physiological' source, which itself provides a foreshadowing of the evacuation of subjectivity that would become central to Horney's later culturalist position, and concomitantly, of how her 'affront to the master' was above all a resistance to the status of the phallus as master-signifier.

, voire Ernest Jones. Here the sense of *voire* is 'even' rather than 'indeed', given Jones' hitherto unstinting declarations of loyalty to Freud. The details of this dissension are addressed further on in this section.

, d'autres encore. The equivoque is this time potentially multifarious: probably 'yet others' from the 1930s; but conceivably 'others still' (in the late 1960s and early 1970s), such as Kate Millett for her *Sexual Politics* (1969), Germaine Greer for *The Female Eunuch* (1971) or Eva Figes for *Patriarchal Attitudes* (1971); while again *encore* carries the already pronounced 'en corps', acknowledging that the attempted riposte to the Freudian account of the phallic phase was couched predominantly in reference to bodily phenomena.

* * * * *

Mais le couvercle mis dessus depuis, depuis la mort de Freud. With this second corollary of the stifled scandal, likewise introduced in subordinate clause, the funereal thematic as here sustained in allusion to a coffin lid sealed shut insinuates an unceremonious wake, the 'dead and gone' debate silently committed to its casket only once its instigator could no longer be counted on to revive it. Keeping a lid on the debate falls to the same culprits who perpetrated its smothering, who will see to its anonymous potter-field burial.

(. . .)

, à suffire. The tightly sealed lid is deemed sufficient for the action for which it was destined, a judgement implicating in turn the *Suffisance* of the psychoanalytic hierarchy which '*n'a à suffire à rien, puisqu'elle se suffit*' ['need not suffice for anything, since it suffices unto itself'] ('*Situation de la psychanalyse et formation du psychanalyste en 1956*' [Lacan 1966: 475]). In Lacan's 1956 text, *Suffisance* apparently renders the Greek *αὐτάρκεια*, a state of independent self-sufficiency, also a contentedness with one's lot, there employed to denounce the cooptative trend in the IPA as further enabled by Balint's model of the end of analysis as identification with the analyst. The antique *πόλις* in which *δημοκρατία* is made by and for the masters alone, prefigures the institutionalised analytic community that coheres into a self-sufficient class radically incompatible with any mode of insufficiency, to the extent that in matters of sufficiency there are no degrees (ibid.: 476). The paradoxical effect of this *Suffisance* is that within the community, whose rightful task ought to be the maintaining of the analytic discourse, '*le silence règne en maître, et (. . .) son temple repose sur deux colonnes tactiturnes*' ['silence reigns supreme, and its temple sits on two taciturn columns'], that of the '*Suffisances*' themselves and that of the '*Petits Souliers*', the 'Eggshell-walkers' who form the recruiting ground of trainees cautiously expectant of preferment (ibid.: 477). Lacan would return briefly to this theme in remarks during the *entretien* of 1 June [1971–1972a] on the trend of '*ça se préfère soi*' among psychoanalysts, and then again in his address, coeval with redaction of the second portion of '*L'étourdit*', to the Belgian School of Psychoanalysis on 14 October ([1972] 1981: 6–7).

à ce que n'en filtre plus la moindre fumée. Special care will have to be taken to ensure that no whiff of what was once such lively and vivid debate should seep from its pall. The fumes still rising suggest hasty or premature burial, perhaps even the consequence of a vivisepulture.

, en dit long sur. The silence is thus purported to be eloquent, in yet further demonstration that no human deportment falls out of range of the unconscious and its logic. As dissected in '*Temps logique et l'assertion de certitude anticipée*', hesitation, interruption and lagging behind instantiate as 'suspended motions' (Lacan 1966: 202–204) that carry signifying value and participate in symbolic process as a dropped beat (ibid.: 206). Even institutional taciturnity, therefore, can assume the status of a protracted *dit.*

la contention. While the French word *contention* loans to the cognate 'contention' in English, its full range of signification does not since the French encompasses an eighteenth-century addition of the sense of 'tension' to refer to a medical splint or immobilisation, and similarly to a restraint device in psychiatric contexts.

à quoi Freud s'en est, dans son pessimisme, délibérément remis. Lacan's text of 1956 on the then situation of psychoanalysis and training was as much a response to the recently published second volume of Jones' biography of Freud and its disclosures on the situation of the 1910s and 1920s. Jones reveals that the first impulse to form a secret steering committee had been his own, in 1912, following the defections of Adler and Stekel and the increasingly strained relations with Jung. Lacan's text quotes directly from the biography: first a portion of Freud's letter to Jones, 'This committee would have to be *strictly secret* in its existence and actions' (1955: 153); then from a letter to Eitingon, 'The secret of this Committee is that it has taken from me my most burdensome care for the future, so that I can calmly follow my path to the end' (ibid.: 154). The first quotation is offered in evidence of the 'free play' ('*blanc-seing*') accorded to the Committee, in independence from Freud himself; the second, in evidence of the security he drew from it. Together they figure the two faces of the Committee's *contention* function: secretly to contain and contend dissenters; and to contain Freud's anxious foreboding. And so the founder of the IPA fell back on the project, deliberately and willingly, in the wake of his 'past disappointments with men' (ibid.) and avowed habit of preferring 'to repudiate in silence and go my own way' (ibid.: 149).

pour perdre, à vouloir le sauver, son discours. In the 1956 text, Lacan denounces the secret Committee as having instilled a Cominternism in the IPA, regulating the far-flung societies from a central hub in the same manner as the Third International was controlled by a junta-inclined Comintern that took full advantage of its Soviet prestige. The text proceeds to expose the sectarian drift endemic to a community organised around an ideal; a configuration diagnosed by Freud himself, but not until 1921 in his *Massenpsychologie* when the Committee was already on the cusp of its second decade of exercise.

Freud's discourse, which is strictly the psychoanalytic discourse, is thus miscarried in entrustment to the discourse of the master, hence the appeal at the end of Lacan's 1956 text to Poe's short story, 'The Facts in the Case of M. Valdemar': likening the IPA to a mesmerised cadaver sustained only by Freud's ventriloquising, the Word that could awaken from hypnosis is the very same that would constitute a final commendation. For the phrasing of these last words, Lacan turns to the first book of Augustine's *City of God* (I.12), '*conditio sepulturae*', or more specifically to a rendering thereof by François Martin Thiébault in his Explanation of the Second Epistle to the Thessalonians, '*les soins d'une sépulture décente*' ('Instruction III, Consolation de la mort, ou amis chrétiens après la mort les uns des autres', 1858: 1282). Here, *conditio* is the genitive of *conditiōnis*, thus 'making' or 'creating'; this as respected in Joseph Bingham's rendering, 'the building of a sepulchre' (Bingham 1840: 442), and also in that of Marcus Dods: 'the equipment of the tomb' (Augustine 1888: 20). More recently, R. W. Dyson has given 'the place of interment' (Augustine 1998: 21), while Henry Scowcrofy Bettenson's paraphrastic translation is closer to Thiébault's rendering: 'a decent funeral and a proper burial' (Augustine 1972: 21). Whether or not the specific wording of the fuller Augustinian source was known to Lacan, the concealed citation adds special nuance to his conclusion, intimating perhaps that this is no petition for an honourable mausoleum for a great man but on the contrary a plea to heed Augustine's *détournement* of the Lucan dictum (disdained by Thiébault): *caelo tegitur qui non habet urnam* ['He who lacks an urn has the sky to cover him'].

In founding the IPA, Freud 'wanted to establish the safeguarding of a kernel of truth'; instead, the upshot was a body of members who seek 'to draw consideration thereof to themselves, even if they declare this kernel to be modest' (Lesson of 10 May [1971–1972b]). The lesson for the learning, therefore, is that vital preservation of the analytic discourse invariably comes at the cost of deigning to forego certain respectable rites and insignia.

Compare the account here of Freud's 'losing' with Lacan's account of his own witting participation in a match lost in advance, in the *entretien* of 1 June [1971–1972a].

*** ***

Indiquons seulement que les femmes ici nommées. Here the bivocation falls on the definite article: *the* women here named are of course Helene Deutsch and Karen Horney, but women *as such* are here mentioned nominally, or indeed 'nominated', for the first time in this section, a surprising deferment given that in its entirety it pertains ostensibly to passage from male to female sexuation. This second reading serves as a reminder that one does not pass from one side to the other as one passes between contrary positions defined by logical negation, conjunction, disjunction or implication (*entretien* of 3 March [1971–1972a]); nor is woman predetermined as such in her Being; rather, here is anticipated the development below on the subject who '*se propose d'être dit femme*', thus being nominated to womanhood.

, *y firent appel.* To what, or against what, did these women lodge their appeal? If the paragraph is to be taken as a further subordinate clause, running to a third the list of sequential corollaries to the stifling of the psychoanalytic scandal of sexual non-relation, the *y* may denote this institutional reticence as the target of their entreaty. Alternatively, the somewhat obtrusive comma may be designed to force *ici nommées* into an aside, interrupting the sentence in such fashion as to imply that the women – a wider group delimited only by such contextual markers as may legitimately attach to the past simple verb – drew upon or appealed to whatever is designated by *y*: perhaps the Cominternist *contention* of the previous sentence, which would accommodate an allusion to the rise to power of the likes of Anna Freud and Melanie Klein in England, Marie Bonaparte in France, Jeanne Lampl-de Groot in Holland and Phyllis Greenacre in the United States. Here the silent ending of the third-person plural facilitates a plausible homophony with '*firent rappel*', their appeal doubling as a call to order.

– c'est leur penchant dans ce discours – . The 'leaning' or 'weakness' designated by the French *penchant* can carry negative connotation absent from its English cognate. Such signification of 'decline' is attested, for example, in the adjectival use in *L'Ombre des jours* by Anna Elisabeth de Brancovan, Comtesse de Noailles, '*un soir si penchant et si triste*' (1902: 146), or in the second tome of Anatole France's *Vie de Jeanne d'Arc*, '*leur cause penchante*' (1908: 343).

This parenthetical remark anticipates the fuller assertion eight years later in the single-session Seminar of 15 January 1980, transcribed and printed 11 days thereafter in *Le Monde*, that women are '*les meilleures psychanalystes – les pires à l'occasion*' ['are the best psychoanalysts – occasionally the worst']; a text which offers useful clarification in its stipulation:

> *C'est à la condition de ne point s'étourdir d'une nature antiphallique, dont il n'y a pas trace dans l'inconscient, qu'elles peuvent entendre ce qui de cet inconscient ne tient pas à se dire, mais atteint à ce qui s'en élabore, comme leur procurant la jouissance proprement phallique.*
>
> *(Lacan 1980)*
>
> [It is on the condition of on no account getting worked up over some antiphallic nature, of which there is no trace in the unconscious, that they [these women] may hear what of this unconscious is not intent on saying what it is, but attains to what is elaborated thereof, as bringing them the jouissance that is properly phallic.]

Retrojecting the extract to read the present turn in '*L'étourdit*', here it is the woman in the analytic discourse who runs the risk of incarnating the *étourdie* by inflecting her penchant for importunity with anti-phallic claims, yet in this same leaning, opening fresh prospect of audition of the ab-sense of the unconscious.

de l'inconscient à la. The construction is designed to suggest a movement running 'from . . . to', though the *à la* form may equally denote 'in the style or manner of'. The question arises therefore as to whether the unconscious is by this reckoning the provenance of the appeal or rather, or also, its content, as an unconscious determined in the body and its voicings.

voix du corps. The unconscious as manifested through the *voie du corps*, the way of the body, might adequately describe the conversion symptom, the phenomenon that came to constitute the native ground of psychoanalysis, but here it is the *voix du corps* that is at issue, the voice of the body as though it were the defining condition of the unconscious, effectively upending Rousseau's adage: *La conscience est la voix de l'âme, les passions sont la voix du corps* (*Émile ou de l'éducation*, 1762). While the body, and the female body especially, is a constant presence in the work of Horney and Deutsch, not least in the debate on vaginal sensation in young girls, the allusion here seems as much to encompass Melanie Klein's notions of symbol formation through transfer of emotions and anxieties on to parts of the subject's own body or those of his mother (implicit throughout her writings but most succinctly expressed in the posthumously published 'Some Reflections on *The Oresteia*' [1963]), or her view that the body interior is the representative of the superego and the unconscious ('Contribution to the Theory of Intellectual Inhibition' [1931]). This more widely cast reading is largely supported by Lacan's remarks to the Belgian School of Psychoanalysis in October 1972, where it is noted that women 'have incontestably always been more interested in what truly constitutes the reference of analytic experience, the body as such' ([1972] 1981: 20), but with the danger that language might be allowed to give more *corps langagier* to this body than it actually possesses (ibid.: 21), whereupon Klein is invoked for her efforts in child analysis to do 'all she can for something of this corporeal activity to be deposited' (ibid.).

Klein, it may be added, was also receptive to the hypothesis of an 'unconscious realization of the existence of the vagina' in young girls, as endorsed by Deutsch and Horney (see the chapter on 'The Effects of Early Anxiety-Situations on the Sexual Development of the Girl' in Klein 1932).

, comme si justement ce n'était pas de l'inconscient que le corps prenait voix. In rectifying the mishmash, Lacan reinstates the primacy of the unconscious as the condition for the bodily yield of the object voice, and in so doing echoes Freud's own reprimand addressed by letter to Müller-Braunschweig on 21 July 1935:

> Your work fits into that of authors such as Horney, Jones, Rado, etc. who do not come to grips with the bisexuality of women and who, in particular, object to the phallic stage. The frequency seems in itself proof that something is missing, undiscovered or unsaid at this point (. . .) I object to all of you to the extent that you do not distinguish more clearly and cleanly between what is psychic and what is biological, that you try to establish a

> neat parallelism between the two and that you, motivated by such intent, unthinkingly construe psychic facts which are unprovable and that you, in the process of so doing, must declare reactive or regressive much that without doubt is primary. Of course, these reproaches must remain obscure. In addition, I would only like to emphasize that we must keep psychoanalysis separate from biology just as we have kept it separate from anatomy and physiology; at the present, sexual biology seems to lead us to two substances which attract each other.
>
> *(Freud 1971: 328–329, published in August 1971 after being made available by Dr Edith Weigert and translated by Dr Helm Stierlin)*

The phrasing of Lacan's countermand also reinforces the *à la* form mooted above, in that to assert in confutation the prevalence of the unconscious over the body implies as its target a notion of an unconscious *equated with* the body, not a movement from the unconscious to the body, which is here in the refutation asserted.

Il est curieux de constater, intacte dans le discours analytique. The final sentence of this sixth paragraph reasserts the context of the analytic discourse laid out at the start of the third as the setting to be maintained throughout this sequence of corollaries to its stifling. Here, what may indeed be most 'curious' is that the scarcely credible impetus behind the effect of authority pulled up in the closing words is located within the discursive mechanics of psychoanalysis, and not merely in an historical contingency of the psychoanalytic movement.

, la démesure qu'il y a entre l'autorité dont les femmes font effet. If an invitation is indeed being extended to read this absence of measure between effect and purported or apparent cause in reference to the discourse of the analyst, might it then be situated specifically on the lower level of the formalised scheme, where the analyst's knowledge (S_2) is held in check and radically partitioned from the master signifier (S_1) that is the discursive product? This reading offers an unexpectedly dynamic approach to the ascendency of feminine authority in analytic circles, even coalescing with the above remark from 1980 that the analytic discourse brings women the 'jouissance that is properly phallic' on consenting to devote their attentions to what is elaborated in the unconscious, in relinquishment of spurious antiphallic drift. In this tentatively offered extrapolation, the S_1 that stands all alone as the product of the discourse is the source of authority attaching to the person of the female analyst, and which she acquiesces to incarnate.

et le léger des solutions dont cet effet se produit. It is difficult to escape the sense of a gently pressed insinuation in this passage directed at the various psychoanalytic 'matriarchs' – Marie Bonaparte, Anna Freud, Melanie Klein – much rather than at the comparatively limited, yet by no means negligible, institutional roles and influence of Horney and Deutsch after their respective relocations to the United States.

Melanie Klein in particular was often derided, even by her allies, for the disparity between the sway she commanded and her intellectual rigour, John Bowlby for one claiming her to be 'inspirational, the antithesis of what I aim to be' (Interview of 23 November 1981, quoted by Phyllis Grosskurth, 1985: 404n); Grosskurth reports numerous further comments of like tenor (see especially ibid.: 406).

The *léger* that here predicates *solutions* cannot help but implicate its antonym 'depth' which was so insistently and intrusively bandied in qualification of their interpretations by the circle around Klein in the 1940s that Edward Glover issued a series of pleas for more scrupulous vocabulary-use, culminating in his charge that the Kleinians had sought to

> pre-empt the use of the word 'deep' implying thereby that other types of interpretation were both superficial and therapeutically ineffective. Clearly the arrogation of propriety rights, however effective as a political policy, offends every canon of objectivity. It may intimidate an opponent but it does not dispose of his point of view.
>
> *(Glover 1955: 280–281)*

Meanwhile, the noun *solutions* itself strikes as mildly incongruous when restricted to designating of analytic interventions and so is doubtless to be read as operating widely to tender a chemical metaphor of 'light solutions', thereby alluding to the watering down of Freudian doctrine into more palatable doses, dissolving it beyond recognition.

*** * ***

Les fleurs me touchent. Clearly this remark is pitched as a preliminary to facilitate allusion to 'flowers of rhetoric', yet in so doing the gardenist thematic from the start of the second part of '*L'étourdit*' is hereby extended beyond the specifically Freudian reference. The author positions himself passively with respect to this sensual receptivity, taking a courteous and conceivably gallant line of approach to his object as though respecting the implicit 'touch-me-not' injunction of an *Impatiens noli-tangere*. Perhaps also this is a repayment in kind of the 'metaphors' to which the *représentantes du sexe* confined themselves (Lacan 1966: 728). A vulvic allusion can hardly be doubted here, chiming too with Freud's sweeping dream symbolism, still being asserted in 1916 to seduce the Viennese audience of the *Introductory Lectures*: '*Blossoms* and *flowers* indicate women's genitals, or, in particular, virginity. Do not forget that blossoms are actually the genitals of plants' (Lecture X, 'Symbolism in Dreams', in [1916–1917] 1987: 192). Compare also Lacan's passing remark in Seminar XVII that woman plunges her roots, 'like the flower, in jouissance itself' (Lesson of 11 February 1970 [1969–1970]).

, d'autant plus qu'elles sont de rhétorique. The *Flores Rhetorici*, also known, in three of the four extant manuscripts, as the *Dictaminum radii*, is a treatise traditionally

attributed to Alberic of the Benedictine abbey of Monte Cassino and dated to 1087 (an Englishing by Joseph M. Miller may be consulted [1973: 131–161]), though this attribution has been more recently contested (by Florian Hartmann [2014: 74]). Its lengthy discussion on the 'Properties of a proemium' is followed by a consideration of the *colores*, under which are listed figures and tropes, followed in turn by examples of 'vices of diction'.

In the late fifteenth century there appeared the anthology of courtly poetry, *Le Jardin de plaisance et fleur de rethoricque*, compiled by an anonymous collator known only as '*l'infortuné*', made available in *editio princeps* by Antoine Vérard in 1502. The thematic pairing of horticulture and ornamental rhetoric would become a staple of Renaissance scholarship, as instanced in English most prominently by Henry Peacham's 1577 *Garden of Eloquence, Conteyning the Figures of Grammer and Rhetorick*. Compare also Sidney in the first book of *The Countesse of Pembrokes Arcadia*, where a crudely officious public speech is denounced as 'such a kinde of Rhetorike, as weeded out all flowers of Rhetorike' (1593 composite edition, I.6; sig. B5v; 95). The term was still being employed, seemingly with un-ironic intent, in the nineteenth century, notably in the title of Ralph Sharp's 1819 glossary, *The Flowers of Rhetoric: The Graces of Eloquence and the Charms of Oratory; Depicted by Men Celebrated for Their Taste, Genius, Diction, and Erudition.*

Lacan would almost certainly have been familiar with Jean Paulhan's, *Les fleurs de Tarbes ou la Terreur dans les Lettres*, published in 1941 but collecting articles from 1936. The eponymous flowers are derived from the second chapter, rueing the decline of rhetorical ornament in recent prose:

> A sign at the entrance to the Tarbes public park reads as follows:
>
> IT IS FORBIDDEN TO ENTER THE PARK CARRYING FLOWERS
>
> The same sign can be found these days at the entrance to literature. How nice it would be, though, to see the young girls of Tarbes (and young writers) carrying a rose, a poppy, a bouquet of poppies.
>
> *([1941] 2006: 9)*

'*L'étourdit*' here self-references its richly ornate style in direct contravention of the prohibition lamented by Paulhan, while forewarning the reader of imminent recourse to 'rhetorical' arguments in the material ahead.

dont Karen, Hélène. It is unlikely that Lacan was on first-name terms with either Horney or Deutsch, and so these given names are to be taken as a rhetorical shift of register into a more intimate societal setting. A further allusion to the floral thematic may draw tentative support from the long attested borrowing of women's names from botanical nomenclature (Daisy, Erica, Hyacinth, Iris, etc.), though neither Helen, Karen, nor their associated forms, carry any association in this respect.

– laquelle n'importe, j'oublie maintenant. The offhand tone of this parenthesis stands in curt contrast to the chivalrous register established in the opening words, descending even into a simulated attitude of caddish indifference. In this, the already highly worked-up bivocation in the sketching of the theoretical positions finds expression in a burst of emotive charge.

, car je n'aime pas de rouvrir mes séminaires –. In opening the lesson of 28 November 1956 from the fourth Seminar, Lacan informs his audience that he has been reading a host of first- and second-generation analytic texts on female sexuality, and from the second term onwards these can be seen informing his approach to *frustration* and *privation* (supra in '*L'étourdit*') through the analysis of Freud's texts '*Über die Psychogenese eines Falles von weiblicher Homosexualität*' and '*Ein Kind wird geschlagen*'. Horney is mentioned by name in the lesson of 27 February 1957 (the mentions in the Seuil edition of Horney on page 31 and pages 97–98, and of Deutsch on page 31, are editor's interpolations), and Lacan returns to consider the theme at greater length the following year with mentions of both Horney and Deutsch in the lessons of 12 and 19 March 1958.

dont donc Horney ou la Deutsch. The feigned testiness of the parenthesis now holds sway over this resumption of the main clause, marked by the *sprezzatura* repetition of *dont*. The given names are dispensed with, seemingly in favour of surnames, but why the definite article before Deutsch? Willy van Langendonck makes the following general remark on articles before personal names:

> [I]n many article languages the definite article adopts an emotive function, at least with personal names. Usually this function is of an augmentative nature. In Dutch (Flemish) dialects the article *de* 'the' is used before men's names and sometimes before women's names to express familiarity with respect to the name bearer, e.g. *de Jan* 'the John', *de Marie* 'the Mary'. In German, the article has almost lost its expressivity with first names because of its frequency in discourse (e.g. *der Johann*).
>
> (*§ 3.2.1 in 2007: 158*)

This use is met also in Romance tongues, including French, but here the surname is at issue, not the given name. The effect is more akin to an epithet, with a possible Germanic characterisation, but Helene Deutsch was of Polish nationality and spent more time in Austria than Germany (medical studies in Munich and a year in Berlin for analysis with Abraham). Could the text be playfully switching agnominations, with '*la Deutsch*' designating the German-born Karen Horney, while 'Horney' functions as a macaronic pun on the English 'horny' to designate the 'masochistic' jouissance of Helene Deutsch? This interchange of names would thus be in keeping with the carelessly brisk tone of one who is keen to move on from past conquests.

meublent le charmant doigtier. The earliest attested use of *doitier* (without *g*) is from the *Registre criminel du Châtelet*, where it denotes a cylinder on which rings were slid as a means of storage. By the late fifteenth century it was being used to describe a piece of fabric or leather to envelop a finger (cf. Guillaume Tardif, *Lart de faulconnerie et deduyt des chiês de la chasse*, Vol. I, 1492), and by the nineteenth century as the brass thimble of a tailor or lace-maker, notably as employed in *passementerie*. In contemporary use, it refers to the medical finger '-stall', '-frock' or '-cot'. *Doigtier* is also one of the many common names in French for the flowering plant *Digitalis purpurea* (along with '*Gant-de-Notre-Dame*', '*Gant-de-bergère*', '*Gantelée*', '*Gantière*' and '*Gantillier*', which approximate the English nomenclature of 'foxglove' or 'lady's glove').

The verb *meubler* is here used in the more general sense of 'fill', mainly as for provision or enrichment (cf. Montaigne, *Essais*, Book I, Chap. XXIV, '*Du Pedantisme*': '*De vray le soing & la despence de nos peres, ne vise qu'à nous meubler la teste de science*', where *meubler* in the 1595 edition replaces *garnir* in the original 1588 edition).

French use of *charmant* aligns closely with its English cognate 'charming' to encompass the signification of 'likeable', 'affable' 'agreeable', 'admirable', etc. and also that of exerting a magical power that can fascinate or deceive. Ironic antiphrasis cannot be discounted here (cf. Flaubert's letter of 28–29 June 1853 to Louise Colet: '*Depuis la fin de février, j'ai écrit cinquante-trois pages! Quel charmant métier!*' [1899: 255]) in the somewhat crude genital analogy.

qui leur fait reserve d'eau. The *doigtier* is made to serve as a waterskin-type receptacle, forcing yet further the vaginal metaphor with allusion to lubrication during arousal, and possibly also extending the tentatively identified paronomasia on 'horny'.

au corsage. This use of *corsage* seems closer to the English adoption of the word, which abbreviates the French '*bouquet de corsage*' where *bouquet* denotes the spray of flowers and *corsage* the bosom of the blouse or corset to which it is appended. Derived from *corps*, the term was formerly used to refer to the bust or the central trunk of the body, especially a woman's, or, with greater rarity, to the 'body' of a fabric, in the sense of a full, consistent quality. The figuration here suggests a posy inserted in a receptacle supplied with water for hydration.

tel qu'il s'apporte au dating. Modern tradition has it that a woman's gentleman 'date' should present her parents with a bouquet of flowers from which a nosegay is then selected and pinned to her dress front. The extended metaphor is thus consummated by this phallic corsage 'brought along' by the gentleman squire, the near homophony with '*tel qu'il se porte* . . . ' hinting at the subsequent transition from bestowal to adornment: the item the man comes bearing is reinvested to become the woman's bearing as such, thus effecting a re-arraying from his *having* to her *being* the phallus, just as *corsage* itself finds once more its original bodily signification. Yet the ambiguous phallic status of *corsage* is not without reproducing the strained phallicisation of female genitalia that Lacan mocks in the '*Question préliminaire*': the egalitarian principle of 'to each their own' whereby the boys have their *phalle* and the girls have their c . . . (1966: 554; *phalle* is mentioned on page 214 of Pierre Le Loyer's 1605 *Discovrs, et histoires des spectres, visions et apparitions des esprits, anges, démons, et âmes, se monstrans viſibles aux hommes*, as '*Et de Phalats indubitablement viennent les Phalles, membres virils des hommes, que les Payens portoiét en leur pompes, Proceſſions & feſtes ſolennelles*'; and again on page 239 of the third tome of the 1752 *Dictionnaire de Trévoux*, under the lemma PHALLE: '*Selon Héſychius, c'eſt ligneum virile*'; Queneau fetched the term back into use in *Les Enfants du limon* [1939: 36]: '*ce qui lui évitait de détailler les phalles de messieurs et les mottes de dames, que ni d'Adam ni d'Ève elle ne connaissait*', where the naturist vogue of the interwar period is implicitly likened to the antique *Phallogogia* feasts).

On the oscillation between concealment and display with regard to the vagina, consult Horney in 'On the Genesis of the Castration Complex in Women':

> I further conjecture that the difference in the dress of men and women, at least in our civilized races, may be traced to this very circumstance – that the girl cannot exhibit her genital organs and that therefore in respect of her exhibitionist tendencies she regresses to a stage at which this desire to display herself still applied to her whole body. This puts us on the track of the reason why a woman wears a low neck, while a man wears a dress coat.
>
> *(1924: 53)*

, soit ce dont il semble qu'un rapport s'en attende. This attention to modern dating ritual is reminiscent of Lacan's contemporaneous appreciation of the singing jousts between troupes of young men and young women described in Marcel Granet's *Danses et légendes de la Chine ancienne* (1926), or the rites and ceremonies surveyed in *Sexual Life in Ancient China* by Robert Hans van Gulik (1961). Human courtship seems wrought not to facilitate sexual relation as do mating rituals in the animal realm, but to contrive its expectation. When Lacan refers to Granet's descriptions of 'herd behaviour' in terms of 'ethology', the appellation is puckish: there is no biological programme; it is a matter of 'materialising the universal' by means of a mirage (*entretien* of 3 March [1971–1972a]).

, ne serait-ce que de son dit. The concluding bivocity is operated by the preposition: since the *en* has already duplicated the *dont* – perhaps to effect a distribution between the preliminaries to the date (the hopeful presentation of the corsage) and the date itself – this *de* can bind *son dit* to *rapport* either as what is said *thereof* or as what is said *therein* and *thereby*. The single-sentence paragraph thus returns to its opening assertion: the corsage is a flower of rhetoric, sexual by dint of carrying over to speech, not by essence.

*** ** ***

Pour Jones, le biais de cervice. The importation of the Latin *cervīce* to condense 'service' and 'cervix' from the close of the previous section is now enlisted to describe Jones' serviceable angle of approach to Freud.

(cf. dernière ligne avant le dernier intervalle). As an intratextual prompt, this reminder is somewhat extraneous given how '*L'étourdit*' has already postulated consistently an engaged and assiduous reader not given to memory lapse, and may therefore operate dually as a punning allusion to the anatomical position of the cervix, the last line of passage before the ultimate cavity that is the uterus.

qu'il prend à qualifier la femme de la deutérophallicité, *sic*. Jones first coined the term 'deutero-phallic' in the afore-mentioned paper on 'The Phallic Phase' to label what he hypothesises as a second phallic phase, noting that, 'Freud would, I know, apply the same term, "phallic phase", to both, and so has not explicitly subdivided them'. Nor did Freud do so implicitly. Jones lays out his hypothesis as follows:

> The first of the two – let us call it the *proto-phallic* phase – would be marked by innocence or ignorance – at least in consciousness – where there is no conflict over the matter in question, it being confidently assumed by the child that the rest of the world is built like itself and has a satisfactory male organ – penis or clitoris, as the case may be. In the second or *deutero-phallic* phase there is a dawning suspicion that the world is divided into two classes: not male and female in the proper sense, but penis-possessing and castrated (though actually the two classifications overlap pretty closely). The deutero-phallic phase would appear to be more neurotic than the proto-phallic – at least in this particular context. For it is associated with anxiety, conflict, striving against what is felt to be reality – *i.e.*, castration – and over-compensatory emphasis on the narcissistic value of the penis on the boy's side with a mingled hope and despair on the girl's.
>
> *([1932] 1933/1948: 453–454)*

In a footnote, Jones goes further in explaining how his hypothesis is a partial integration of Freud's position and that of Horney:

> In agreement with Freud is the fundamental view that the passage from the proto- to the deutero-phallic phase is due to fear of castration at the hands of the father, and that this essentially arises in the Œdipus situation. Freud would, I think, also hold that the feminine wishes behind so much of the castration fear are generated as a means of dealing with the loved and dreaded father: he would possibly lay more stress on the idea of libidinally placating him, whereas I have directed more attention to the hostile and destructive impulses behind the feminine attitude. On the other hand I cannot subscribe to the view of sex ignorance on which Freud repeatedly insists (. . .) and I regard the idea of the castrated mother as essentially a mother whose man

> has been castrated. Nor do I consider the deutero-phallic phase as a natural stage in development.
>
> With Karen Horney there is agreement in her scepticism about sex ignorance, in her doubts about the normality of the (deutero-) phallic phase, and in her opinion that the boy's reaction to the Oedipus situation is greatly influenced by his previous relation to his mother. But I think she is mistaken in her account of the connection between these last two matters, and consider that the boy's fear of his feminine wishes (. . .) arise not in shame at his literal masculine inferiority in his relation to his mother, but in the dangers of his alimentary sadism when this operates in the Oedipus situation.
>
> *(Ibid.: 466–467)*

The comment that the deutero-phallic phase is not a natural stage in development is clarified in the conclusion to the paper:

> the typical (deutero-) phallic phase is a perversion subserving, as do all perversions, the function of salvaging some possibility of libidinal gratification until the time comes – if it ever comes – when fear of mutilation can be dealt with and the temporarily renounced hereto-erotic development be once more resumed. The inversion that acts as a defence against the fear depends on the sadism that gave rise to the fear.
>
> *(Ibid.: 484)*

Lacan's claim here in '*L'étourdit*' that Jones' term qualifies the woman's sexuality is thus an extrapolation that diverges to a degree from Jones' intention in 'The Phallic Phase'. A remark from Seminar X shows that this extrapolation was already present in Lacan's thinking in the 1960s:

> The fundamental dissatisfaction that's involved in the structure of desire is, if I may say so, pre-castrative. If it comes about that she takes an interest in castration as such, $(-\varphi)$, it's to the extent that she will venture into men's problems. It's secondary. It's deutero-phallic, as Jones quite rightly put it.
>
> *(Lesson of 27 March [1962–1963])*

This passage draws on Jones' subsequent intervention on the topic, the momentous 'Early Female Sexuality' delivered in Vienna, which Lacan uses as the basis of his remarks in the lesson of 12 March 1958 from Seminar V. In the Vienna intervention, Jones invokes his earlier paper, though with focus shifted almost entirely on to the girl:

> You may remember the distinction I drew in my Wiesbaden paper between the proto-phallic and the deutero-phallic phases, the separation between them being marked by the conscious discovery of the sex difference.

> This discovery often results in envy and imitation, which are the main characteristics of the deutero-phallic phase. One very important observation about which there is general agreement is that the passing of this phase – or rather the plainer evidence of femininity – is apt to be accompanied by unmistakeable hostility and resentment against the mother. Freud in his explanation has coupled these two events together not only chronologically but intrinsically.
>
> *([1935] 1948: 493)*

So, the shift in focus of the deutero-phallic phase on to feminine sexuality dates from 1935, but the unpicking and re-stitching of this purported 'coupling' dates from 1933.

Lacan's coining of a nounal *deutérophallicité* – which strictly speaking cannot be asserted as *sic erat scriptum* by Jones, who used exclusively the adjectival 'deuterophallic' – thereby integrates a pun on both the fallaciousness and the felicity of Jones' compromise position.

, soit à dire exactement le contraire de Freud, à savoir qu'elles n'ont rien à faire avec le phallus. In 'The Phallic Phase', Jones leads his reader down the following garden path:

> [W]hen I made the suggestion that the phallic phase in girls represents a secondary solution of conflict I was under the impression that by the phallic phase was meant what I now see to be only the second half of it, a misapprehension Professor Freud corrected in recent correspondence; incidentally, his condemnation of my suggestion was partly based on the same misunderstanding, since on his part he naturally thought I was referring to the whole phase.
>
> *([1932] 1933/1948: 467)*

Hence Lacan's remark in his tribute paper to Jones that he sets himself to '*le contre-pied des positions prises par Freud sur la phase phallique par la seule voie d'affirmations réitérées de s'y accorder entièrement*' ['the wrong-footing of the positions taken by Freud with respect to the phallic phase by the sole path of reiterated assertions of being wholly in agreement with them'] ('*À la mémoire d'Ernest Jones; Sur sa théorie du symbolisme*' in Lacan 1966: 703). Jones' argumentation prepares the ground for his claim two years later in Vienna:

> [W]e regard the deutero-phallic phase as essentially a defence against the *already existing* Œdipus complex. To us, therefore, the problem of why the defensive phallic phase comes to an end puts itself quite differently, being not altogether unlike the problem of why an infantile phobia ever disappears.
>
> *([1935] 1948: 494)*

Lacan seizes on this as the essence of the Jonesian position on female sexuality. By Jones' reckoning, 'the exit from the phallic phase has to be thought of as the recovery from a phobia' (Lesson of 12 March [1957–1958]). Thus, there is a reduction here whereby 'the phallus can only intervene as the means and the pretext for a kind of defence', and so the phallic phase becomes 'nothing but a pure detour in an essentially instinctual cycle' (ibid.). The remark here in '*L'étourdit*' to the effect that, according to Jones, women have nothing to do with the phallus, is to be understood in the sense that they will come to know it only through a detour taken in earnest, until they realise the error of their ways and conclude that such is not their business after all, freeing them to heed 'the promptings of an instinctual constitution' ([1935] 1948: 495).

, tout en ayant l'air de dire la même chose, à savoir qu'elles en passent par la castration. Since Jones has turned the phallus into a means of defence for the girl, he cannot read it as the signifier of castration, even though this is precisely what his argument 'anticipates' (Lacan 1966: 703). Indeed, the term 'castration' is strangely absent from the Vienna address of 1935, and one struggles to deduce any theory of the castration complex in women from Jones' writings. In 1927, he claims that the concept of 'castration' had 'in some respects hindered' any appreciation of the woman's fundamental conflicts, and proceeds to parry this, in his thinking, by the postulate of a threat of *aphanisis*, a 'blow of total extinction' striking at 'sexual capacity and enjoyment as a whole' ([1927] 1948: 439–440). But in respecting Freud's dictum that the concept of castration should bear on the penis alone, he is led by the close of the paper to divorce *aphanisis* completely from castration (ibid.: 450) ending up, as is his wont, with two distinct concepts applicable to two distinct genders. Therefore, the claim in '*L'étourdit*' that Jones sounds like he is saying the same thing as Freud rests above all on what Jones passes over in silence.

Bibliography

Alberic of Monte Cassino [1087] (1938) *Alberici Casinensis Flores rhetorici*, edited by D. M. Inguanez and H. M. Willard, Montecassino: Arti grafiche e fotomeccaniche Sansaini.

Alberic of Monte Cassino (1973) *Flowers of Rhetoric*, translated by J. M. Miller in *Readings in Medieval Rhetoric*, Bloomington: Indiana University Press, pp. 131–161.

Augustine (1888) *The City of God*, translated by M. Dods, Edinburgh: T. & T. Clark.

Augustine (1972) *Concerning the City of God Against the Pagans*, translated by H. S. Bettenson, London: Penguin.

Augustine (1998) *The City of God Against the Pagans*, translated by R. W. Dyson, Cambridge: Cambridge University Press.

Bingham, J. (1840) *Origines Ecclesiasticæ; or, The Antiquities of the Christian Church, and Other Words*, Vol. VII, Oxford: J. H. Parker.

Buffier, C. [1709] (1734) *Grammaire française sur un plan nouveau*, Paris: N. Le Clerc et al.; translated as *A French Grammar on a New Plan*, London: Hinchliffe.

de Brancovan, A. E. (1902) *L'Ombre des jours*, Paris: Calmann-Lévy.

de Mijolla, A. (1991) 'Le Congrès des Psychanalystes des pays romans: quelques éléments d'histoire', *Revue française de psychanalyse*, 55(1): 7–36.

Deutsch, H. ([1929] 1930) 'The Significance of Masochism in the Mental Life of Women', *IJP* 11: 48–60.

Deutsch, H. (1931) 'Der feminine Masochismus und seine Beziehung zur Frigidität', *Almanach der Psychoanalyse* 6: 147–162.

Deutsch, H. [1931] (1932) 'Über die weibliche Homosexualität', *Internationale Zeitschrift für Psychoanalyse*, 18(2): 219–241.

Deutsch, H. [1931] (1933) 'Homosexuality in Women', *IJP* 14: 34–56.

Deutsch, H. [1932] (1933) 'Motherhood and Sexuality', *Psychoanalytic Quarterly* 2: 476–488.

Dictionnaire universel françois et latin (*Dictionnaire de Trévoux*) (1752) Tome III, fifth edition.

Fierens, C. (2002) *Lecture de L'étourdit*, Paris: Harmattan.

Flaubert, G. (1899) *Correspondance*, second series, Paris: G. Charpentier.

France, A. (1908) *Vie de Jeanne d'Arc*, Tome 2, Paris: Calmann-Lévy.

Freud, S. [1905] (1987) *Three Essays on the Theory of Sexuality* translated by J. Strachey in *On Sexuality, Pelican Freud Library Vol. 7*, London: Pelican/Penguin.

Freud, S. [1916–1917] (1987) *Introductory Lectures on Psychoanalysis*, translated by J. Strachey in *Pelican Freud Library Vol. 1*, London: Pelican/Penguin

Freud, S. (1971) 'Letter of 21 July 1935 to Müller-Braunschweig', translated by H. Stierlin, *Psychiatry* 34: 328–329.

Glover, E. (1955) *The Technique of Psycho-Analysis*, London: Baillière, Tindall & Cox.

Granet, M. (1926) *Danses et légendes de la Chine ancienne*, Paris: PUF.

Grosskurth, P. (1985) *Melanie Klein, Her World and Her Work*, London: Maresfield Library.

Hartmann, F. (2014) 'Eloquence and Friendship: Letter-Writing Manuals and the Importance of Being Somebody's Friend', in Steckel, S., Gaul, N. and Grünbart (eds.) *Networks of Learning: Perspectives on Scholars in Byzantine East and Latin West, c.1000–1200*, Zurich: LIT Verlag.

Horney, K. (1924) 'On the Genesis of the Castration Complex in Women', *IJP* 5: 50–65.

Horney, K. (1932) 'Observations on a Specific Difference in the Dread Felt by Men and by Women Respectively for the Opposite Sex', *IJP* 13: 348–360.

Horney, K. (1933) 'The Denial of the Vagina: A Contribution to the Problem of the Genital Anxieties Specific to Women', *IJP* 14: 57–70.

Horney, K. [1933] (1935) 'The Problem of Feminine Masochism', *Psychoanalytic Review* 22(3): 241–257.

Horney, K. [1936] (1967) 'The Neurotic Need for Love', in *Feminine Psychology*, New York: Norton, pp. 245–258.

Horney, K. (1937) *The Neurotic Personality of Our Time*, New York: Norton.

Jones, E. [1927] (1948) 'The Early Development of Female Sexuality', *IJP* 8: 439–440; reprinted in *Papers on Psychoanalysis*, London: Baillière, Tindall and Cox, 1948, pp. 438–451.

Jones, E. [1932] (1933/1948) 'The Phallic Phase', *IJP* 14:1–33; reprinted in *Papers on Psychoanalysis*, London: Baillière, Tindall and Cox, 1948, pp. 452–484.

Jones, E. [1935] (1948) 'Early Female Sexuality', *IJP* 16: 263–273; reprinted in *Papers on Psychoanalysis*, London: Baillière, Tindall and Cox, 1948, pp. 485–495.

Jones, E. (1955) *The Life and Work of Sigmund Freud, Vol. II: Years of Maturity, 1909–1919*, New York: Basic Books.

Klein, M. (1931) 'Contribution to the Theory of Intellectual Inhibition', *IJP* 12: 206–218.

Klein, M. (1932) *The Psycho-Analysis of Children*, London: Hogarth.

Klein, M. (1963) 'Some Reflections on *The Oresteia*', in *The Writings of Melanie Klein Vol. III: Envy and Gratitude and Other Works 1946–1963*, London: Hogarth, pp. 275–299.

Lacan, J. (1956–1957) *Le séminaire IV, La relation d'objet*. Twenty-four lessons delivered at Sainte-Anne Hospital. [In the absence of audio recordings, cf. *Book IV, The Object Relation*, edited by J.-A. Miller and translated by A. R. Price, Cambridge: Polity, 2020.]

Lacan, J. (1957–1958) *Le séminaire V, Les formations de l'inconscient*. Twenty-eight lessons delivered at Sainte-Anne Hospital. [In the absence of audio recordings, cf. *Book V, The Formations of the Unconscious*, edited by J.-A. Miller and translated by R. Grigg, Cambridge: Polity, 2017.]

Lacan, J. (1962–1963) *Le séminaire X, L'angoisse*. Twenty-four lessons delivered at Sainte-Anne Hospital. Audio recordings (incomplete) available at archive.org/details/Angoisse.

Lacan, J. (1966) *Écrits*, Paris: Seuil.

Lacan, J. (1968–1969) *Le séminaire XVII, L'envers de la psychanalyse*. Thirteen lessons delivered in the Law Faculty of University Paris I–II. Audio recordings available at archive.org/details/Envers_20140516.

Lacan, J. (1971–1972a) *Le savoir du psychanalyste*. Seven *entretiens* delivered in the chapel at Sainte-Anne Hospital. Audio recordings available at archive.org/details/Savoir.

Lacan, J. (1971–1972b) *Le séminaire XIX . . . ou pire*. Twelve lessons delivered in the Law Faculty of University Paris I–II. Audio recordings available at archive.org/details/OuPire.

Lacan, J. [1972] (1981) 'Séance extraordinaire de l'École belge de psychanalyse, le 14 octobre 1972', transcript published in *Quarto* 5(1981): 4–22.

Lacan, J. (1980) *'Séminaire du 15 janvier 1980'*, printed in *Le Monde*, 26 January 1980.

Le Loyer, P. (1605) *Discovrs, et histoires des spectres, visions et apparitions des esprits, anges, démons, et âmes, se monstrans viſibles aux hommes*, Paris: Nicolas Buon.

Matte Blanco, I. (1975) *The Unconscious as Infinite Sets: An Essay in Bi-Logic*, London: Duckworth.

Montaigne (1595) *Essais*, fifth edition with 'C' additions, Paris: Langelier.

Müller, J. [1925] (1932), 'A Contribution to the Problem of Libidinal Development of the Genital Phase in Girls', *IJP* 13: 361–368.

Müller-Braunschweig, C. (1926) 'The Genesis of the Feminine Super-Ego', *IJP* 7: 39–49.

Paulhan J. [1941] (2006) *The Flowers of Tarbes, or Terror in Literature*, translated by M. Syrotinski, Urbana/Chicago: University of Illinois Press, 2006.

Peacham, H. (1577) *Garden of Eloquence, Conteyning the Figures of Grammer and Rhetorick*, London: H. Jackson.

Queneau, R. (1939) *Les Enfants du limon*, Paris: Gallimard.

Rousseau, J. J. (1762) *Émile ou de l'éducation*, Paris: N. Bonaventure Duchesne. [Disguised as 'Amsterdam: J. Néaulme', much reprinted and translated.]

Sévigné, Marquise Marie de Rabutin-Chantal de (1775) *Recueil des lettres de Madame la Marquise de Sévigné à Madame la Comtesse de Grignan, sa fille*, Tome 5, enlarged edition, Paris: Compagnie des Librairies.

Sharp, R. (1819) *The Flowers of Rhetoric: The Graces of Eloquence and the Charms of Oratory; Depicted by Men Celebrated for Their Taste, Genius, Diction, and Erudition*, London: William Fearman.

Sidney, P. (1593) *The Countesse of Pembrokes Arcadia*, composite edition.

Soler, C. (2006) *What Lacan Said About Women: A Psychoanalytic Study*, translated by J. Holland, New York: Other Press.

Tardif, G. (1492) *Lart de faulconnerie et deduyt des chiês de la chasse*, Vol. I, Paris: A. Vérard; edited with modern spelling by L'édition de Paris, 1882; reprinted by Geneva: Slatkine, 1980.

Thiébault, F. M. (1858) *Œuvres complètes*, Tome VII, Paris: J.-P. Migne.

van Gulik, R. H. (1961) *Sexual Life in Ancient China*, Leiden: E. J. Brill; revised edition, 2003.

van Langendonck, W. (2007) *Theory and Typology of Proper Names*, Berlin/New York: Mouton de Gruyter.

Vérard, A. [1502] (1925) *Le Jardin de plaisance et fleur de rethoricque* (*editio princeps*); facsimile print with introduction and notes by E. Droz and A. Piaget, Paris: Société des anciens textes français.

Wallerstein, R. S. (1998) *Lay Analysis: Life Inside the Controversy*, Hillsdale, NJ: The Analytic Press.

13

A #METOO MOMENT IN COMMUNIST POLAND

A short story

Agnieszka Piotrowska

When I look back at what has made me a woman, I remember so many episodes that did not seem particularly important or significant at the time but with hindsight (psychoanalytical 'deferred effect' Nachträglichkeit) they appear vital. Jacques Lacan reformulated Sigmund Freud's Nachträglichkeit as après coup, insisting that it is possible to change the meaning of a memory, through a shift of signifiers: the events remain but their traumatic significance can be altered. In part, for me, this story represents just such a shift in signifiers, as a schoolyard game incident becomes more than a trauma and retroactively emerges as the site of 'becoming woman' in both a biological and a political sense. The scene offers a vignette of teenagers working out what sexual difference might mean too, here against the background of the very powerful and masculine Big Other: the totalitarian regime.

My friend Joanna and I liked running around the schoolyard during the so-called 'running game'. The challenge was to outrun the boys. It seemed a healthy way to spend our lunch hour but in fact it was a little more complex than it appeared. Still, we were 12, about to turn 13 and the world was our oyster.

All schools in Poland in the 1970s were co-educational – for boys and girls. I went to one of these too of course. On the whole it was a rather good establishment. Our headmaster, Dr Jan Kowalski, was a communist of the old school: he believed in the doctrine, which heralded equality of opportunities for all. At that point we had only grimly realised that the version of communism offered to us involved a fair amount of corruption and Soviet control.

We entered the school at age 6 or 7 and stayed there until 14 or 15 before transferring to a school we were suitably gifted for – largely based on academic results. It was a good system and education was indeed one of the regime's indisputable successes. In due course, I was lucky to be allowed to go to a Lycée, a school based on the French curriculum and very good academically. But that is quite a different story and a different adventure. My primary school was an establishment with some academic and artistic aspirations and in healthy competition with another local school. I remember various incidents from these years but nothing that compares to the fiasco of the so-called 'running around' game that was popular among the middle schoolboys – the group between the ages of 11 and 12 or 13 at the most. After that both the boys and the girls usually found more exciting things to do. It was an unfortunate tradition. At lunch break boys would run around lifting girls' skirts to see their knickers. The girls usually would get away but not always. When I think about it today, some simple questions spring to mind, for example, why did we girls continue with the game if we disliked it? First, we did not dislike it to begin with. Second, we were all encouraged to be outside in the schoolyard during the spring and summer terms – part of the communist ideology was to persuade us of the importance of a healthy body, doing sports and exercise. It was important to be seen being physically active and not just sit around and read, for example during the lunch break. Education was important, yes, and easily available for 'the masses'. On the other hand, intellectual overstimulation was suspect, particularly when drawn from Western traditions, which usually smelled of bourgeois ideas that might encourage individualism and, God forbid, independence of thought. Healthy body and a well-educated mind were needed for the communist ideology to thrive, for the state of the working class to be able to develop and for the comrades to grow at the same pace, to share equally that which would be produced. That there was very little to be found in shops and that the only branch of activity truly thriving was indeed cultural and intellectual pursuits and individual achievements of artists who used satire to defy those in power were somehow uncomfortable truths hidden in their work, and often not completely clear to the regime. The events I am describing here took place in the late 1970s and perhaps could have taken place in the 1950s or the 1980s, during the time of martial law, but then soon after everything crumbled and changed and the new freedom with its own issues turned up. I often wonder if the nostalgia some people feel for the times of communism is the nostalgia for the knowledge that the profound lack of everything for everybody was a shared fate of sorts.

In any event, as we were told to hang out in the schoolyard weather permitting, the running game seemed as good a way to spend the lunch break as any. The game though with time turned pretty unpleasant and physical: the boys would not only lift our skirts but also touch – or attempt to touch – our private parts. This game went on for years without anybody giving it much thought. I guess we all felt it was just the way things were and we were very young. We never questioned the rules of the game, and we were encouraged on the whole not to question any rules. Nobody ever succeeded touching me up or my best friend Joanna – we could run fast and laughed at the boys. The game did not feel dangerous. By the time of this fateful afternoon I had grown quite tall and many boys in my year group were still a lot shorter and smaller, but the game continued. We did hear some girls complain at times but nobody paid any attention. It was just fun and good for you – the running that is.

And then all of a sudden things became different. One afternoon Joanna started her period, without quite knowing what it was. I knew. My mother had told me what was to come but it had not yet come for me. My mother was an educated person with some regrets in her life but she did believe in making 'the facts of life' clear early on. As soon as the class was over, Joanna pulled me into the school restroom and whispered, 'I think I might be dying: blood is pouring out of me'. She looked horrified so I didn't laugh. I explained basic things to her, trying to calm her down and then added: 'Don't worry, just go into the cubicle and get some toilet paper for now, there are only two lessons left and you will be home soon', and so she went to the toilet. When she got back she said she was worried about the game – we had a lunch break coming up straight after the maths lesson. 'What if the boys discover I am bleeding. Can you imagine?' I remember also being troubled at the prospect but thought we should be fine: we must run fast so they must not know her secret. 'We always outrun them,' I said nervously, 'so why not today? Nothing to worry about. Just run as usual. We will be fine.' I sounded confident. I lied. I was scared. 'What are we going to do if we don't outrun them today?'

It was the end of the summer term, so around June. The sun was shining. We wore school uniforms of sorts but as it was warm we had bare legs and knickers, no tights or other additional armour. 'Not good,' I thought.

The break began. The boys starting chasing us as usual. Joanna kept stopping, and whispering that she felt weak and looking at me in panic. 'I can't do it,' she said, 'I am in some pain.' 'Oh no,' I thought. 'Run!' I ordered her, and turned around, shouting to the boys, still running away. 'Hey guys, could you stop this?' I said, 'Joanna is not feeling well. OK?' But they laughed and they wouldn't stop – they wanted their usual thrill of chasing the girls and lifting our skirts and touching us, or imagining they were touching us. So we kept running. Any questions about why we stayed in the yard instead of going into the building and explaining the situation to the teachers, are useless here. The thought did not enter our minds until much later in the game. We were indeed unconsciously interpellated by the system and a small matter of the first period seemed too minor an inconvenience to bother with. We were stuck, or committed.

For now it all was going well, despite Joanna's paleness and her insistence on whispering to me, which I found near paralysing as she filled me with fear, without meaning to. 'Stop whispering as this is slowing us down,' I thought, but kept quiet. This time she raised her voice so I could hear her: 'I am scared that if I run about the usual way, the toilet paper will drop out or something. And then they will see and THEY WILL KNOW.' This worried me too. In my mind's eye I imagined the disgrace of it all, with a piece of rough cheap communist toilet paper suddenly falling out of my friend's knickers, the prospect of a bloody tissue right there in front of these boys made me feel nauseous. I tried to muster strength: 'Don't be silly,' I whispered back, panting and running on, 'you must just run as usual.' We got away from the boys temporarily. 'I am so tired,' Joanna said and started crying. Only then did I realise we were in big trouble, she could not run as fast as usual.

We had had it. I thought maybe we could run back to the school toilet. 'Ok, we will have to run for the school building,' I shouted to her and turned back sharply. We swerved to the nearest outbuilding but the school door was blocked by a group of older boys, who laughed at us menacingly. We knew this was no good. We kept running. The game continued, I felt short of breath, everybody kept at it, the boys chasing the girls, as they do, no doubt good naturedly, laughing and joking. We were petrified. I looked at my watch, a fancy present from my very important and very handsome grandfather who was also an influential Communist Party member. Time for once was going slowly, too slowly. Fifteen minutes to go. I myself had to slow down, feeling a sudden wave of tiredness, looking at pale Joanna, with sweat pouring down her forehead. 'Shit,' I thought. Fifteen minutes was too long. We slowed down.

Then it all exploded. One of our male classmates, Jasiu, caught up with us and pulled Joanna towards him in a gesture, which was unusually harsh and determined. She panicked and tore herself away, tripping over and falling to the ground. He still went after her and then did touch her knickers – her private parts, this time the panties hiding also the ugly bloody toilet tissue. Joanna yelled like I have never heard her yell before or since. The paper did not fall out, which she was grateful for and that I still worried about even at that moment. Jasiu yelled too but carried on trying to touch her at which point she became near hysterical and pushed him away, screaming her head off. 'Stop it!' I yelled at him and he turned to me, laughing, looking suddenly unfamiliar, sweaty and alien, not my old schoolfriend again, but suddenly a boy attacking me. He grabbed me. He lifted my dress, touching me too and then trying to touch me again, with the others boys being very near, ready to join him. I pulled away and tripped and fell on the ground too. Meanwhile Joanna was up on her feet again, screaming 'Nooo! Leave her in peace!' as I was lying there with another boy putting his hand right on my crotch. Everybody turned their attention to me now so Joanna tried to pull them away but they just pushed her away. We were in new territory, as this had never happened to us before. 'I am getting help!' Joanna yelled and ran off towards the school. I felt an overwhelming sense of fury coming over me, which was a novel experience too. 'This will not go on,' I thought as I gathered all my strength. This really was like in a movie. I said a quick prayer to my guardian angel just asking to be physically strong, no metaphors.

I was still on the ground but I kicked the boy who attacked me hard and jumped up. He fell back. It was then the original attacker, Jasiu, who pulled my skirt up again and I could feel his clammy hand right through my cotton knickers on the skin of my outer vagina.

It was not a moment of any great epiphany, but rather a primordial instinctual moment of self-defence and anger, and a rage that I can barely begin to describe even now, at his unspoken sense of entitlement that somehow it was OK that they did this to us, that we were expected to put up with this humiliation, that we had done so for years, and in one way or another would do for years to come. But I had grown bigger than these boys without anybody noticing and I was not going to let them touch me this way, my guardian angel's help notwithstanding. My rage propelled me forward.

I pulled his hair with one hand and hit his face with the other, hard. 'You will not forget this, my boy,' I hissed like a snake. 'And you will never touch me or any other girl in this schoolyard again this way and if you do, I will kill you.' I hit him again. He fell on the ground, yelling and at that moment exactly Joanna turned up with a teacher, Mrs Kolorowa. Jasiu, the boy I had just hit, was crying his eyes out – he was a good head shorter than me, but was standing up already and pointing at me accusingly. I could see the headmaster, Professor Kowalski, running towards us too. Mrs Kolorowa looked pale and started repeating rather nonsensically and waving her hands around, 'Please will you all calm down. Please calm down.' I cried. At this point exactly the headmaster caught up with us. I could see he was not happy.

'Pawlikowska,' he said to me 'What on earth are you doing here?' Jasiu was sobbing so badly he could hardly speak. I couldn't speak either. Joanna yelled: 'He attacked us. He touched our . . . things!' Jasiu kept crying and screaming. The headmaster was shaking his head. The school nurse turned up out of the blue too, putting a cold compress on Jasiu's forehead. He was sobbing. Joanna looked like she was going to faint. I still wondered whether she had time to run to the loo and change the make-do sanitary pad. At that point Jasiu and his friends pointed at me and yelled some more or rather, blurted out between the gasps for air: 'They are lying, they attacked us and she (pointing at me) kicked Marek and then hit Jasiu. Twice.' 'This is a complete lie!' Joanna yelled. The headmaster looked pale and furious. 'Will everybody now please stop yelling? And crying.' He did give Jasiu and his friends a cold look. Then he turned his attention to me. 'Did you do this indeed, Pawlikowska? Speak.'

I shook my head in defiance. Jasiu made a dreadful face and yelled again, 'She did!!! She kicked Marek, and she hit me. I am in great pain! I am allergic to any painkillers so this means I will be in this pain forever!' Mrs Kolorowa and the headmaster gasped. 'I am sure the pain will subside directly,' the headmaster said nervously. The nurse continued with the cold compress. I started crying now. 'Instead of these ridiculous tears, some kind of explanation would be appropriate,' said the headmaster, looking at me disapprovingly. I said nothing, and shook my head crying again, hot tears running down my flushed cheeks, and feeling confused and angry still. Joanna said nervously, 'This was self-defence. They attacked us!' The headmaster raised his hand.

> Silence! I am not interested any more in these stories. I see in front of me a boy in some distress who claims a girl assaulted two boys. This is a most irregular occurrence for a girl to behave this way. You should be ashamed of yourself, Pawlikowska. A very nasty conduct. Apologise immediately. Now.

Joanna tried to explain the situation again but he wouldn't listen and told her to go back to class – but she hovered, quietly. The headmaster was unfortunately into his pedagogical drive, using a deep tone of authority, which he had learnt from television broadcasts of the Party officials giving their speeches. A small crowd gathered around us. Jasiu was still sobbing but I stopped.

'Comrade Kolorowa,' the headmaster said grimly and Mrs Kolorowa shuddered. 'Is this girl one of your form pupils? Kolorowa nodded. 'This behaviour is utterly unacceptable. For anybody. But for a girl this is – well, monstrous. I have no words.' He looked at Kolorowa sternly. 'Well?' Kolorowa clearly had no words either as she just gasped again, looked at me and shook her head. 'This situation is unbearable,' he said again. Meanwhile, I blew my nose, wiped my tears and felt better. I did not feel bad about hitting Jasiu and I knew it was no big deal and that he was using the situation to evoke the greatest possible sympathy for himself and provoke the greatest possible punishment for me. I was quietly pleased with myself that I had made my point, and felt curiously elated, perhaps not quite appreciating the gravity of my situation. The headmaster looked at me with disgust, 'This situation is truly unbearable,' he repeated. I thought to myself, 'The headmaster really is given to a profound exaggeration – it is not that unbearable. What was unbearable was that these boys were running about touching our vaginas – for years. And nobody did anything about it.' I may not have quite thought it this way as I was 12, but the general feeling was there. I continued to stare at the boys and at our teachers. 'Comrade Kolorowa,' the headmaster repeated sternly, 'would you like to . . . well, discipline Pawlikowska? What will be your pastoral guidance here please?' Despite still feeling angry and scared, I almost burst out laughing: 'pastoral guidance my ass,' I thought. Kolorowa was a hopeless teacher, she did not know her subject, which was supposedly geography, and was said to have got the job only because her husband was some kind of minor Party apparatchik who knew Kowalski. She was continuing her studies with evening classes, and had a small child at home who her mother was helping her with. She appeared to hate her job, and us. Maybe she was just unhappy. She probably worked to supplement the family's meagre finances or perhaps because she would rather hang out at our school than at the small flat on one of these grey communist estates that were heralded as a great success at the time but now remain as a monument to a failed dream. This is where she lived, we knew it because a fellow pupil in our class walked with her, with a screaming kid and a mousy husband who somehow managed to be in a relatively good job, despite his utter lack of any discernible talent, except, that is, his moderate scheming ability which got him the Party job. We all knew she was exhausted with life and did not have a clue how to teach anybody anything, never mind give 'pastoral guidance'. She looked at me in exasperation and said: 'It is true that this is not very becoming behaviour for a young lady.' The crowd collapsed in laughter. The headmaster looked in desperation at Kolorowa and then at us. He cleared his throat nervously. 'Pawlikowska, you must not laugh here.' I wasn't. 'We are young socialists here, that is you are,' he cleared his throat again, 'so perhaps not so much a young lady but a young socialist! A young socialist girl! Yes. Are you a member of the scouts? I am sure you are. Did they not teach you respect for your fellow colleagues?' I nodded. Kowalski smiled triumphantly and looked at Kolorowa with a smirk on his face: he sometimes despaired over his teachers' lack of pedagogical talent. He praised himself on always being able to get through to a pupil. 'Sooner or later a breakthrough takes place. You must have the strength of conviction,' he would say to his team, 'and then the student will listen to you.' I re-gained my power to speak: 'But . . . Professor Kowalski . . . The boys were chasing us . . . and Jasiu touched my vagina . . . like really touched it . . . I had to do something. Young comrades are not meant to touch the girls this way I am pretty sure.'

Everybody giggled. Kowalski went paler still if it were possible. Kolorowa started coughing nervously and I knew things were not going well.

Joanna handed me a piece of toilet tissue, which she clearly must have kept on her because of her menstruation. Professor Kowalski looked at us with an expression of disbelief and horror.

'Pawlikowska, I am not interested in your shameful excuses. Your language speaks for itself, if I may say so. What on earth are you saying here? You must apologise to Jasiu and your other friends and colleagues immediately. Even if something untoward happened, which I do not believe for one second, then there are other channels for dealing with the matter.'

He coughed again. 'Did it not cross your mind for example to seek a teacher, to discuss the issue, to negotiate?' I went bright red again but a curious calm came over me. We looked at each other, the headmaster and I, this big man of about 50 and me, a month before my thirteenth birthday. I wiped my tears and thought to myself, 'Is this what it feels to become a grown up?' I took a deep breath and said calmly and quietly, looking right at him: 'Negotiate? I was lying on the ground, being assaulted. No time to negotiate. I kicked the attacker in self-defence.' Everybody laughed again, but this time it felt like they may have laughed at him, not me. Kowalski went grey. I saw small pearls of sweat on his forehead. He coughed. I could see I was in deep trouble.

'Enough. Pawlikowska, Enough. In your infantile desire to attract attention to yourself, you overstepped the mark. Now you need to apologise profusely and straight away – to Jasiu, to your colleagues, to Joanna, to me and comrade Kolorowa. Is that clear?'

He raised his voice. He yelled. The crowd around us stopped laughing. I felt frozen but knew already that I would not be apologising. Joanna looked at me in desperation. 'Apologise,' she whispered.

'I am listening,' the headmaster said, looking at me in disgust, with the boy Jasiu still crying and holding his red cheek, which I was sure was a totally unnecessary theatrical gesture on his part and somehow infuriated me further then and is still enraging me now as I remember it. 'Apologise immediately,' the headmaster repeated.

Everybody looked at me. I raised my head in a defiant gesture, looked him in the eye and shook it very slowly, which perhaps wasn't really necessary. I said nothing and met his eyes, and held his steely gaze well, despite now shaking all over. At last I said quietly but firmly: 'No.'

The silence became even deeper. The headmaster cleared his throat again and said in an ice cold voice, softly at first but then raising his voice yet again as he went: 'You will apologise. Mark my words. And if you don't – let me be absolutely clear – you will not be able to attend this school again – or perhaps any school. Not now, not ever. Do you understand???! I will make it my business. You will be expelled. You cannot behave this way and get away with it.'

He really yelled. 'Apologise! Now!' He got very close to me, too close, his large body overpowering. I could smell his sweat and it made me nauseous again. I took a small step back. Nobody was laughing any more. The silence was such that we could have heard a pin drop.

I did not apologise. I shook my head again. Joanna grabbed my hand. Kowalski looked at us all and took a deep breath, and looked at me. He then said firmly but quietly: 'Everybody goes back to class now. Except Antonia Pawlikowska. You go home. Your parents will be informed.'

And so I was suspended and sent home.

My mother was there, reading. She took one look at her watch and at me and said, 'So why are you home early?' And so I told her, 'I am not going back there. I will never apologise and the headmaster said that if I didn't I would never be allowed in the school again.' I sobbed. I liked my school – except for being scared that I might be touched up at lunch breaks. Other than that, it was a great school – or so we thought. My life clearly was in ruins.

My mother looked pale. Very unusually she put her book aside. 'OK then,' she said, 'tell me what happened exactly.' And so I did. About the game of running and touching, about my friend Joanna, about us not being able to outrun the boys this time because of her period, about getting flustered because she fell. Everything. I started crying. As I was telling these stories I realised the look on my mother's face changed. She looked angry too. 'Are you OK?' I said nervously. She seemed to have tears in her eyes. She tried to control herself. I could see that. She breathed more quickly though and I could see she wanted to gather her thoughts. 'Go to your room,' she said at last, 'and do your homework.' I sobbed louder. 'I don't know what the homework is because I was sent home early.' 'Read a book then,' she said, 'and stay in your room.' 'I am not apologising,' I said. She looked at me – it was such a strange look. 'Please go to your room and read and try to calm down.' She took a deep breath. She did not hug me and I stood looking at her, not a teenager yet, so small really and so stubborn. At last she stood up and embraced me, and hugged me hard. 'It will be Ok,' she said.

As I sat in my room trying to read, I could hear the phone ring and I knew it was the school. I couldn't make out what my mother was saying exactly but it was not a long conversation. Then I could hear her speak to my father on the phone too but again I could not hear what she was saying. The conversation was longer and she appeared more agitated. She then made another phone call and it was not clear who it might have been to, and what was being said as she whispered most of the time. Now I think she must have called her father, and my grandfather, a very powerful man, high up in the regional Party and the mayor of Gdynia. An hour later Joanna called me and said, 'Apologise to Jasiu. Say sorry to the headmaster and Kolorowa. What the hell. Come back to school. It was all my fault anyway. It is not worth it. Apologise and be done with it.' I whispered not wanting to create a further disturbance with my mother. 'I am not apologising to Jasiu or the headmaster. And if Jasiu does it again, or anybody, I will hit them all again. I have had enough. We are done with that game, you and I.' Joanna started singing to cheer me up – this was the kind of thing she would do, this is why we were so close, she was funny and creative but this time she was wrong. She still carried on, 'Yeah great, I get it. But what will happen if they don't let you come back to school? Didn't he say "any school"?' she whispered. I had no idea what would happen then but tried to sound defiant. 'I will study myself. At home.' I said, swallowing my tears. Joanna screamed at the other end of the phone. 'Oh no, no,' Joanna wailed, 'it is all my fault.' 'Don't be ridiculous,' I stopped her, 'We put up with this shit long enough. Now we are bigger than them and we don't have to run like this anymore. Obviously it is not good to hit people, it is also not good to let some cretinous boys touch you, right? This is stupid. We talk soon.'

I put the phone down. But the truth was I was truly petrified, and lost.

At supper nobody said anything and I couldn't eat much. After I went to bed, I could hear my parents having a heated discussion. I couldn't make out most of it – but I did hear my father say, 'Physical violence, even as a response, is never a way forward and you do know that. She should apologise.' I shuddered. I heard my mother answering quietly and then they switched on the telly, which was a gift from my grandfather, so I couldn't hear what they were saying – if anything. Then I heard my mother make another phone call. She talked at length this time.

I cried myself to sleep. I had nightmares featuring the 'running around' game, which I was losing and my friend Joanna's menstrual blood was flowing all over the schoolyard. I woke up. I then was lying for hours looking at the flickering light on the ceiling and wondering what jobs I could do in life without getting any education. I fell asleep about six o'clock but an hour later my mother woke me up and got me up as usual. 'Get up and have some breakfast and then we go. To school.' 'But I haven't apologised to the boy. And I can't. Don't make me don't make me.' I started sobbing again. My mother looked at me – a hard and determined look and a look full of love that I will remember all my life. She smiled her beautiful dazzling smile and said, 'Stop this nonsense now, go clean your face and put some clothes on. You are not apologising to the boy. No way are you apologising to any boys. In future, do not get involved in stupid games that you cannot possibly win, promise?'

I nodded quickly and said, 'I am so sorry.' And cried again a little. She wiped my face, and sent me to the bathroom. 'Let's go to school. You need to pull yourself together,' she said calmly, 'we must not be late.' And so we went.

The school was a ten-minute walk during which we said nothing to each other. I was fearful of the headmaster. I wonder what my mother was thinking about. Perhaps about her own life and how her father and my grandfather got her examined by a gynaecologist when she was 15 to see whether she was still a virgin or not. Or maybe she was thinking about her love affair with my father, 25 years her senior and a professor at the university she was studying at, who then did do the right thing and married her when she got pregnant. Or perhaps she was wondering how her political faith in communism was betrayed by Stalin, and then by Gomulka, and how she lost the inner strength to believe that anything could be truthful and that any meaningful transformation of this political system was ever possible. Maybe she was thinking about her unfulfilled promise of a successful academic career, as she dropped out of her studies after she got pregnant with me. Perhaps she was thinking about how my father had to leave his position at the university because he wouldn't join the Party. We said nothing.

When we arrived at the school, my mother sat me down in the hall and told me to wait while she went to talk to the headmaster. I do not know what happened during this meeting. Later I asked her what was said and at the time she said very little, but years later she said the headmaster laughed and told her to take me back home until I apologised to the boy. My mother apparently did not call my father, as perhaps she was not completely confident he would support her, but instead, she called my grandfather, the aforementioned patriarch of the family, who was also a despot controlling her every move as a child and a teenager. When I grew older, it became clear to me that it was a gesture of defiance against him, and love too, which got her into trouble with her professor and my father. At the time I knew nothing of any of it. Years later she did tell me it was my grandfather who demanded that I was reinstated at the school immediately. He was the mayor of our town and a high-ranking Party member and the headmaster just folded, he had no choice. I believe he might have been repaying a favour that they both knew he owed her – perhaps, in connection with the infamous gynaecological examination but also perhaps, more significantly, regarding the lack of support she had from her parents when she got pregnant. I did not know any of this as I sat on the hard bench in the hall, feeling sudden cramps in my lower stomach. 'Oh no not me now,' I thought, and ran to the bathroom, the very same bathroom that Joanna used only yesterday, when she got her first period. I used the rough cramped toiled paper she used too as a temporary sanitary towel, with blood pouring out of me.

I have no way of knowing what really happened during that meeting between the headmaster and my mother, but it seemed to have taken forever. I never learnt whether the running around game was discussed too during this conference but I do know that the game stopped completely for the remainder of my time at that school.

After the longest time, my mother and the headmaster emerged together and the headmaster just said to me, 'Go back to your class Pawlikowska and try not to beat the boys up in future please.' He looked somewhat embarrassed but not very – a man in his position in totalitarian Poland would have been very used to eating humble pie of many sorts. I smiled slightly, 'Professor Kowalski, thank you. I am sorry I didn't find a better way of negotiating this situation. I will try harder in future.' I said, and almost meant it. Kowalski just waved me on, shaking his head, and as I took my bag and marched on to the classroom, my mother smiled at me – the biggest sunniest smile you have ever seen. She winked at me too, and I knew that she was proud of me in a curious way. And not until years later, did I reflect that she still had to call upon a powerful man to save me – but I didn't care then, and I care even less now because the most important thing in the world was that my strong-mindedness or stubbornness was not broken at its inception right there and then, as a response to an incident that should never have happened. I know now how very close I was to losing any beginnings of any understanding of who I was or who I was trying to be. I made a choice but in truth it was not only my choice to make: I was but a kid after all, and I wanted to do well at school and I wanted for my parents to love me and be proud of me. A simple insistence on their part would have made me apologise, of that there is little doubt. That I did not have to do it, was a blessing indeed.

My mother was not a perfect parent. She was deeply unhappy, sometimes neglectful, at times too demanding, always preoccupied with her own despair. But the memory of that one moment wipes out everything else. She was there for me, fighting for my right to be stubborn and strong-minded against these boys, against the systems that somehow always worked better for the men, however much they were bad for everybody. That very moment defined her, and me and our relationship, or at least, after years in psychoanalysis this is what I choose to see it as.

14

VuLNeRaBILITies

Pia Hylén

Feeling disintegrating –
slowly dissolving into something
which lacks substance
and reference – other than of course that of overflowing
into nothingness
with no restrains
no borders no limits
no containing
no retaining
even the air gives way
more than usual
encouraging the abandonment
of that which
no longer has the power to keep its center

de-centrifying

sometimes
when you try to catch it
this de-centrification
it centrifies
and evaporates
sur le champs

My Vulnerabilities are
when I am not firm
when I let myself
be wrung through the wringer
and loose the tread
diffuse
an entropic endeavor?
if Lucien Freud thinks I'm clever
I can never
reach the firmament
of vulneraaaa . . . a . . . . a . . . . a
so ethereal
that the abilities
diffuses

You can keep paddling
but if you don't let go
you get ambushed
in the unforgiving cleverness
that
nevertheless
smothers
& never forgives
your fake ambition
at the detriment
of true
vulnerabilities

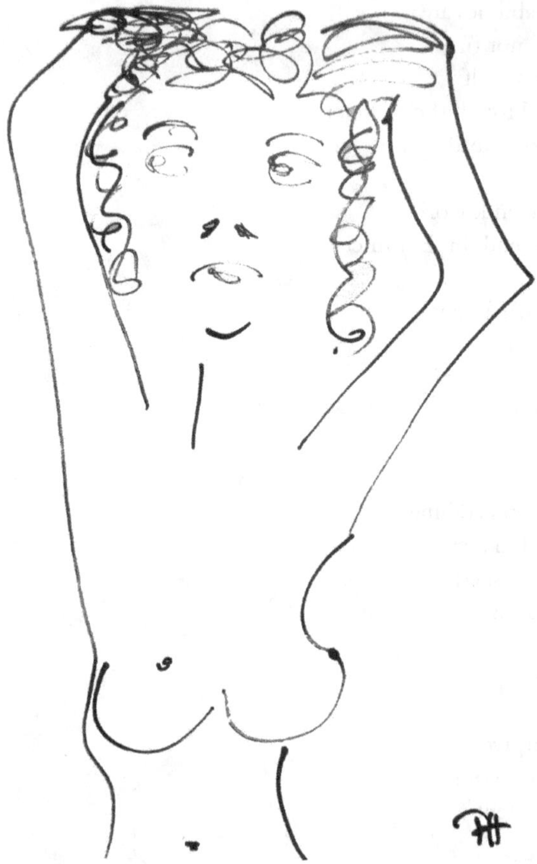

FIGURE 14.1 'Ravage' (2010). Drawing by the author. Encre de Chine on paper (30 × 40 cm).

Source: Courtesy of the artist.

INDEX